Design for Aging Post-Occupancy Evaluations

Design for Aging Post-Occupancy Evaluations

Lessons Learned from Senior Living Environments
Featured in the AIA's *Design for Aging Review*

EDITED BY

JEFFREY W. ANDERZHON, AIA

INGRID L. FRALEY, ASID

MITCH GREEN, AIA

The AIA Design for Aging Knowledge Community

FOREWORD BY Margaret Calkins, Ph.D.

THE AMERICAN INSTITUTE OF ARCHITECTS

John Wiley & Sons, Inc.

Published by John Wiley & Sons, Inc., Hoboken, New Jersey
Published simultaneously in Canada

Wiley Bicentennial Logo: Richard J. Pacifico

Limit of Liability/Disclaimer of Warranty: While the Publisher and the author have used their best efforts in preparing this book, they make no representations or warranties with respect to the accuracy or completeness of the contents of this book and specifically disclaim any implied warranties of merchantability or fitness for a particular purpose. No warranty may be created or extended by sales representatives or written sales materials. The advice and strategies contained herein may not be suitable for your situation. You should consult with a professional where appropriate. Neither the Publisher nor the author shall be liable for any loss of profit or any other commercial damages, including but not limited to special, incidental, consequential, or other damages.

For general information about our other products and services, please contact our Customer Care Department within the United States at (800) 762-2974, outside the United States at (317) 572-3993 or fax (317) 572-4002.

Wiley also publishes its books in a variety of electronic formats. Some content that appears in print may not be available in electronic books. For more information about Wiley products, visit our web site at www.wiley.com.

Library of Congress Cataloging-in-Publication Data:

The American Institute of Architects
  Design for aging post-occupancy evaluations / The American Institute of Architects ; foreword by Margaret Calkins.
       p. cm.
  Includes index.
  ISBN 978-0471-75714-6
  1. Long-term care facilities—Design and construction. 2. Long-term care facilities—Evaluation.
I. The American Institute of Architects. II. Title
  RA998.5.A53 2007
  725'.56—dc22
                                                          2007001272

Printed in the United States of America

10 9 8 7 6 5 4 3 2 1

Contents

Foreword By Margaret Calkins, Ph.D.   vii

Acknowledgments   ix

Introduction   xi

Part I

Independent Living Apartments   1

Chapter 1   Parkview at Asbury Methodist
            Village   3
Chapter 2   The Hallmark   13

Part II

Continuing Care Retirement Communities   24

Chapter 3   Avalon Square   25
Chapter 4   Bishop Gadsden Episcopal
            Retirement Community   37
Chapter 5   The Jefferson   49
Chapter 6   La Vida Real   61
Chapter 7   McKeen Towers   73

Part III

Assisted Living   85

Chapter 8   Dominican Center at Marywood   87
Chapter 9   Rosewood Estate of Roseville   99
Chapter 10   The Fran and Ray Stark Villa   111
Chapter 11   Sunrise of La Jolla   123

Part IV

Assisted Living for Those with Dementia   133

Chapter 12   Cuthbertson Village at
             Aldersgate   135

Chapter 13   Freedom House at Air Force
             Village   147
Chapter 14   The Forest at Duke   159
Chapter 15   The Village at Waveny Care
             Center   173
Chapter 16   Woodside Place of Oakmont   185

Part V

Nursing Care   197

Chapter 17   Abramson Center for Jewish Life   199
Chapter 18   The Green Houses™ at Traceway   213
Chapter 19   The Colorado State Veterans
             Home at Fitzsimons   223
Chapter 20   Foulkeways at Gwynedd   237

Part VI

Community-Based Services   247

Chapter 21   Cody Day Center   249

Part VII

Scandinavian Comparisons   259

Chapter 22   Tempe Health and Welfare Centre   261
Chapter 23   Swedish Elderly Homes   273

Conclusions and Next Steps   291

Appendix 1   Project Cost Update
             and Estimate   295

Appendix 2   Listing of Project Owners
             and Architects   297

Index   301

Foreword

By Margaret P. Calkins, Ph.D.

There is growing interest in evidence-based design, as there is in evidence-based medicine and evidence-based teaching. Even nonprofit organizations are increasingly expected to be able to evaluate the efficacy of their programs and services—especially if they want to continue to raise funds to support what they do. This increasing emphasis on systematic evaluation of the techniques and processes we use, regardless of the field, fundamentally reflects an interest in greater fiscal responsibility: making sure the dollars that are spent, be they for medical treatment, education, services, or construction, are well spent.

This is heartening progress for environment-behavior researchers, who have long labored to increase the knowledge base used for making design decisions. Nevertheless, relationship between research and design is complex. Ideally, design is based on research, but research on buildings is generally conducted on constructed buildings where the program, philosophy, operational aspects, and population served may not match those of the originally proposed building. Thus, designers interpolate the findings and develop hypotheses about how they think design elements will function within new parameters. Progress in this area is further complicated by the fact that many design professionals are not taught how to read and interpret environmental research, nor are most environmental researchers cognizant of the structure of information that designers find most useful. Thus, there are communication barriers between the designers and researchers that should be torn down.

In most design projects, there is limited documentation of the influence of research on the design or of the specific hypotheses used in designing the building. Even when there is an attempt to document retroactively once the building has been constructed and occupied, it is hard to pinpoint the hypotheses that should be tested. Andrew Seidel, in his publications on environment and behavior, distinguishes between *instrumental,* or direct, research use versus *conceptual,* or indirect, research use. Instrumental research use might include full documentation of specific design decisions that are based on behavioral research. In contrast, conceptual research use might include application or consideration of general notions, perhaps learned of through the popular press, to the design of buildings. General use of research-based concepts and ideas gleaned from site visits or from conference presentations would fall midway in the continuum between these types of research utilizations.

Post-Occupancy evaluation (*POE*) is a term used to describe a broad range of activities, from a quasi-research walk-through of a building by the designer to systematic research conducted longitudinally using validated assessment instruments. Many architects will tell you they routinely conduct POEs on their buildings, but these usually consist of meeting with the client a year or so after the building has been occupied, asking if there are any problems, doing a quick observational walk-through, and perhaps having a few casual conversations with users of the building. True, this is not very rigorous, but it provides at least some insights for both designer and client. Unfortunately, fear of being perceived as having made mistakes means that these POEs are seldom published; generally, they are used only for internal education by the design firm.

The evaluations in this book fall somewhere between these two levels of POEs. They were conducted by individuals from outside the design team—people who are less likely to be biased in their evaluation of the building. The teams were also interdisciplinary, involving architects and interior designers, providers and researchers; this breadth of experience encourages examination of the buildings from different perspectives. The POEs typically took place over two days, which, although still a relatively short time frame, gave the evaluation team a chance to spend some time in the buildings to see how they really functioned, not just hear about it from administrators and staff. These POEs included interviews with staff at all levels of the organization, not just administration. They also included tours of several rooms or apartments and usually conversations with the tenants of these spaces, though not necessarily conversations with a large number of residents.

The real strength of these POEs lies in what they tell us about reality versus what is published in the original

American Institute of Architects *Design for Aging Review* publications. The original descriptions were written by the designers and care providers, who wanted to show the best side of their work through professional photographs of strikingly clean (and often pre-occupancy) photographs. What we see in this book is much more honest: photographs that are not staged with professional lighting, showing the building as it is lived in; and evaluations developed through team observation, rather than carefully worded descriptive prose aimed as much at marketing as assessment.

I reviewed the 1992 AIA *Design for Aging Review* in preparation for writing this Foreword, just to see what the issues were then in comparison with the critical topics of today. In the nursing homes category, the 1992 jury was pleased to see that "privacy issues in semi-private rooms were responded to in some projects in unique ways. . . . Unfortunately several medical model units were also presented with traditional approaches to nursing patterns and room layouts. The jury rejected these as inappropriate responses to the needs of residents." This issue continues to be important today, as some providers are still building the traditional, hospital-layout, side-by-side bedroom that offers nothing but a piece of fabric for "privacy." A recently completed study that I conducted on the costs of private versus shared rooms shows that with a room rate differential as little as $5 per day—a rate that Medicaid will now pay—it takes less than nine years to recover any additional costs of constructing a private room, including debt service.

In the same 1992 *Design for Aging Review,* within the continuing care retirement community classification, the jury noted that "historical clichés such as 'Bell Towers' and 'Clock Towers' still abounded, as did 'Town Centers' and 'Pedestrian Malls' but more attention was being devoted to careful integration of parking, as well as dramatic grand scheme site plans." A perusal of the most recent *Design for Aging Review,* or of other similar publications, shows that clock towers and town centers are still appearing in new projects, and often still feel like clichés. It is not that creating meaningful public gathering space, where familiar social and supportive activities like shopping and banking can take place, is a bad idea. It is that the articulation of these spaces seldom feels real. It is not unlike being at Disney World—and living your life in Disney World is very different from an occasional visit to that theme park.

So, it appears that there is much that has not changed in the past two decades. We are still grappling with many of the same issues. One of the reasons we have not moved forward may be the lack of systematic evaluation of senior living environments, and the rigorous dissemination of the information gleaned from these evaluations. Perhaps, with an increased interest in evidence-based designs, there will be more focus on and more funding for research. We hope that some of this research will go beyond the information that can be gleaned from a two-day site visit. There is a critical need for research that specifically links design features and elements with the activities of individuals having specific needs, desires, and abilities. This book is a great step forward in that process. Unbiased evaluations of projects that were hailed, in their time, as being reflective of good design principles will be of tremendous value to both the design and care provision professions. Designers and providers alike should use the information contained herein to make explicit their hypotheses, which is the necessary first step in enabling more systematic or instrumental research to be conducted, so that in the future, projects truly reflect evidence-based design.

MARGARET P. CALKINS, PH.D. *is an internationally recognized leader in the field of environments for elderly, especially those with Alzheimer's and other dementias. She founded Kirtland, Ohio-based I.D.E.A.S., Inc. (Innovative Designs in Environments for an Aging Society) in 1991. The I.D.E.A.S. mission is to engage in research, education and consultation on the therapeutic potential of the environment—organizational and social as well as physical—particularly as it relates to frail and impaired older adults.*

Acknowledgments

"It takes about ten years to get used to how old you are."

UNKNOWN

As with any undertaking of this magnitude, there are many individuals who contributed much to its completion but whose names do not appear on the cover. These people fully understood the importance of taking a critical view of environments for aging so that those which follow can be better. These people, without exception, are focused in their belief that there is certainly a more compassionate way of celebrating the golden years of life. They contributed to the creation of this manuscript without any sort of compensation except the knowledge that this manuscript may benefit future environments for the aging. They are the unsung heroes and heroines, today's leading edge of forward thinkers on the relationship between the environment and the aging individual. They are collaborators, contributors, and colleagues, but most of all they are friends. We have shared a common experience that brings us all closer together and makes us more committed to the intent of this work. There can never be enough thanks to balance the debt we owe them all.

Kate Alvarez, simply on faith, joined the fray as a sounding board and language marshal and saved many a bad sentence from the dust bin of editing. She worked hard when she could have been playing elsewhere, and she cheerfully and diplomatically offered advice that was sage beyond the number of her years. Without her, this book would still be electronic files with odd notations in the margins.

Without the diligence of Cathy Nun, there would be no book. She has the talent of being able to extract schedules and dates from those unwilling and uncooperative and to do so with a sweetness that belies her determination. Her organizational skills rescued several evaluations that threatened to devolve into thin nothingness, and her encouragement rescued many "blue" moments.

By simply introducing us to Kate, Eleanor Alvarez deserves high praise. But she did far more than that. As an evaluator, she was superb in quickly getting to the kernel of operational issues; as a reader of many first drafts, she quickly applied the paring knife of concise writing. She was instrumental in the completion of a number of chapters in our deadline-driven race to the end. Most importantly, she was our very good friend, offering encouragement when we could see none and offering constructive suggestions when we thought we were at dead ends.

Without the able assistance of Melissa Strunk, there would be only an unfulfilled dream. She tirelessly located archived and forgotten documents and photos. She helped without as much as a frown when we were irritable and demanding—and she always offered an amazing smile when we most needed it.

Vanessa Williamson immediately shared our vision and quietly and skillfully shepherded it past many roadblocks. She found us necessary funds when we thought the well was dry. She never let us lose sight of the benefit of our mission when we were discouraged, and she nurtured us when we felt overwhelmed.

David Slack was able, as an evaluator, to ask the hard questions in a manner that was disarming but that solicited real answers. He showed us all how to be tough, gentle, intelligent, and unassuming all at once. He tirelessly double-checked data and entertained us all with his poignant and colorful experiences.

Eric McRoberts, Leslie Moldow, John Shoesmith, and Terri Zborowsky kept asking us if we needed help until we said yes. They then responded without hesitation and with great enthusiasm. They are undoubtedly the next standard-bearers. Special thanks go to Margaret Calkins and Mark Proffitt for their assistance. And to SAGE, which provided necessary assistance for two important evaluations.

Glen Tipton provided us all with direction and purpose. He unknowingly gave birth to an understanding that alone we could do good things, but together we could accomplish greatness. We owe Glen much more than can be expressed so briefly here.

Uno Claesson and Fredrik Zeybrandt worked hard to make the Swedish evaluations possible. Jason Reis made their inclusion, and that of other evaluations, in this book more meaningful through his able graphic assistance.

Aging Research Institute provided great assistance in locating valuable provider evaluators and in the process was struck by the importance of an ongoing post-occupancy initiative for environments for the aging. The future will be brighter because of their assistance.

All the evaluators listed in this book volunteered a great deal of time and financial resources to accomplish this feat. They did so without question and, more often than not, with an attitude that it was a privilege to help. They each contributed much to this effort, but each believes he or she has benefited more. To them goes the greatest praise; we have all been enriched by knowing them and from sharing a common experience with them. Thank you.

Lastly, there are three individuals who quietly shared in our journey, keeping each of us focused in their own ways, doing so not in concert with each other, but clearly in a unison that transcended their geographic remoteness. Linda, Richard, and Susie came along for that journey without being consulted at the beginning, but they saw it through with us to the end.

Introduction

This book, with its collection of post-occupancy evaluations, takes a look at a variety of long-term care environments in an effort to learn how residents and staff interact with the built environment. These projects, all constructed within the last 20 years, were chosen for their diversity so that we could document regional variances, local preferences, and the facilities' ability to provide a broad view of the state of the profession. While 21 American sites participated in the evaluation process, the evidence in its entirety is also an evaluation of the long-term care industry, and serves as a modern-day benchmark for aging in America.

Four projects from Scandinavia are also included, to provide the reader with a comparison of the approach to long-term elder care in these countries. The three Swedish evaluations were conducted using less rigorous criteria, whereas the one in Norway followed the protocol utilized in the United States.

Historically, most people have lived off the land and within extended nuclear families that maintained a geographic connection. Thus, the family could provide economic support to its elderly. However, this traditional system of economic security eroded in the United States in the 1880s as a result of the Industrial Revolution, the urbanization of America, the diminished importance of the extended family, and the increase in life expectancy. Subsequently, the mechanization of the remaining agrarian society, the rise of dual-income families, and the advent of Medicare and Medicaid further impacted care and support of older Americans. Interestingly, many less developed countries are just now beginning to experience these same changes within their borders.

U.S. Life expectancy in 1900 was 47 years of age. Three decades later, life expectancy had increased by 10 years, largely as a result of better sanitation and the introduction of public health programs. As able-bodied workers left their farms and rural communities to take industrial jobs in larger cities, grandparents were often left behind. By 1920, for the first time in our nation's history, more people were living in cities than on farms. By 1930, America was more urban, more industrial, and suddenly older. Those elderly citizens who were unable to care for themselves were sent to almshouses and poor farms.

The Social Security Act of 1935 provided old age assistance in the form of matching grants to each state. As a result, private old-age homes were established. Eleven years later, in 1946, the Hospital Survey and Construction Act provided funding for new hospitals, changing the public's perception of hospitals as places where poor people either recuperated or died. Indeed, hospitals became houses of hope.

In an effort to raise the quality of care, federal law provided grants for the construction of nursing homes "in conjunction with a hospital," resulting in the medical model of design and architecture of the 1950s. In 1965, President Johnson's new Medicare social insurance program extended health care coverage to almost all Americans aged 65 or older. As a result, the nursing home industry emerged and exploded with the construction of facilities nationwide.

For the next 25 years, although regulations affecting the operations of the nursing home industry were introduced (and some later repealed), the care model continued to embrace:

- An institutional design that served many in the same economically efficient way, resulting in dehumanizing the resident experience
- A medical model of service that provided room, board, and nursing care but only limited social services, activities, or community contact
- A culture of dependency promoting the institutional concept of "we take care of you by making all your decisions for you"
- A management philosophy of command and control involving all aspects of the resident's life

Then, in the late 1980s, a funny thing happened on the way to the nursing home. Assisted living, featuring the resident's ability to choose from a menu of services to accommodate a lifestyle need, was introduced and was rapidly embraced as an alternative to the nursing home.

With further refinements in programming and design, assisted living made it possible to merge individualized care with residentially inspired interior environments and architecture.

For earlier generations, perceptions of retirement's "golden years" corresponded directly to increases in leisure time, life expectancy, and retirement income. What baby-boomers will expect from their golden years will be remarkably different from their predecessors. Design responses are already addressing resident-centered care, but succeeding generations will continue to challenge the senior housing industry. Residents *will* rule, and future trends will include private rooms, residential neighborhoods, customized services, and access to technology, wellness, work, and community.

The continuing transition of aging in America inspired the Design for Aging Knowledge Community of the American Institute of Architects to embark upon a series of post-occupancy evaluations in order to document this culture change and to provide guidance for future care providers and designers. After 16 years of juried competitions known as the *Design for Aging Review,* which awarded citations to the "best of the best" in senior housing, a compilation of post-occupancy evaluations could actually compare the submissions of photographs, plans, and descriptive objectives with the reality of day-to-day operations and quality-of-life issues. Two-day evaluations, which examined issues of design, architectural details, programming, workplace conditions, and life-enhancing environments, were conducted at 21 American sites.

Site Selection

Being selected as one of the communities included in this first book does not make these projects better than their counterparts. However, selection does indicate that certain design features that advance the state of the art of senior living design are present and can be evaluated. The approach to site selection was as follows:

- Projects had to have been completed by 2005, with their innovative designs recognized by *Design for Aging Review* citation and/or publication, or by extensive publication and/or presentation at American Association of Homes and Services for the Aging, or other senior living industry forums
- Projects had to have been open for a minimum of one year, with stable management, operations, and occupancy
- Projects in total had to represent a diversity of senior housing types

- Projects in total had to represent a diversity of geographic locations
- Projects in total had to represent a diversity of sponsor types

A number of selected sites, when contacted, refused to allow the evaluation team to review their environments and operations. Sadly, the majority of these sites indicated that the primary reason for refusal was that they could not comprehend the benefit of such an evaluation and thus felt it would be an imposition on the staff and residents of the campus.

The authors gratefully acknowledge those sites that eagerly agreed to participate in this evaluation process; we recognize the time and effort expended in arranging tours, staff and resident interviews, and access to statistical data. Without their cooperation, and without their understanding that the information obtained would be of benefit to all, this book would still be nothing more than a dream.

Evaluation Criteria

Starting with the *Design for Aging Review,* each project's floor plans, original stated objectives from the owner and designer, and other data already on hand were reviewed in conjunction with the three parts of the creation process: design, construction, and operations.

The evaluation process intentionally did not include discussions with the designers; evaluations were based on the stated objectives and architect's statements presented during the submittal process for *Design for Aging Review.* Unique building program parameters, if not included in the submission information, were not considered. Additionally, unique design and operations characteristics that appeared as a result of local or state regulatory compliance, or modifications in operations due to diversity in state licensing requirements, may be noted but were not examined in detail.

With an average of two days per site, an enhanced, indicative evaluation was performed, with emphasis on the following topics:

- Degree of integration between the built environment, care program, and resident lifestyle
- Impact of spatial layout and design on staff function and resident social interaction
- How the environment overcame obstacles to innovation, including jurisdictional code requirements
- Specific features, including lessons learned that can be built upon and enhanced in future projects

- Selection of finish materials, colors, and patterns as enhancements to the built environment

Interview subjects fell primarily into five categories:

- Top management (CEO, board member, community component director)
- Front-line staff (CNA, nurse, activity director, therapist, social worker)
- Support staff (dietary, housekeeping, building and grounds maintenance)
- Residents (usually two)
- Family members (if possible)

The Evaluation Team

All members volunteered their time and, as part of the selection process, submitted their qualifications, including background and relevant experience in the design or operation of senior living environments. While in many cases team members did not know each other, each shared a common passion for good design and the delivery of exceptional care. This common bond served to unite the team and, in many instances, to forge new friendships. For each site evaluation, there were generally five evaluators, but often there was opportunity to include more than this basic core.

The five-member evaluation teams were comprised of:

- Two members from the design community, including at least one architect and, if possible, a landscape architect or interior designer
- Two members from provider organizations with considerable experience in direct operations
- One member from the Design for Aging Knowledge Community Advisory Group to coordinate and facilitate the evaluation

The Evaluation Chapter Layout

Each of the evaluated projects fell into one of seven categories:

- Independent living apartments
- Continuing care retirement communities, either with or without nursing care
- Assisted living
- Assisted living for those with dementia
- Skilled nursing, or simply nursing care
- Stand-alone elderly adult day care

- Special evaluations that include Scandinavian elderly facilities for comparisons

For convenience of the reader and ease of comparison, the chapters that relate to each category are grouped together. Each chapter contains "Data Points" at the beginning of the chapter so that readers can quickly get a sense of the project's scope. Following this are the architect's design objectives and responses submitted as part of the *Design for Aging Review* process. The POE team's evaluation of these objectives and responses are next followed by a more in-depth discussion focused on the following themes:

- Creating community
- Making a home
- Regional/Cultural design
- Environmental therapy
- Outdoor environment
- Quality of workplace and the physical plant

Each chapter concludes with operator perspectives gleaned from on-site interviews with the administrative personnel. At the end of each chapter, there is more detailed project data, obtained from both author research and information submitted to *Design for Aging Review.*

The Importance of Post-Occupancy Evaluations

Post-occupancy evaluations have many benefits for providers, staff, residents, and designers.

As structured hindsight, the review and critique of the design and operation of senior living communities can be extremely beneficial. Upon completion and after a period of stabilization, there is a unique opportunity to review the design team's assumptions about how environments will be used and assess whether design, operational or social goals have been met.

Post-occupancy evaluations can promote understanding between staff, administration, and residents as to the design intent of a specific room or feature, or a function that may not be readily evident to those who were not involved in the planning process.

Post-occupancy evaluations can be used to promote quality assurance, documenting which features facilitate tasks; or as a marketing tool, to demonstrate to prospective residents and staff the environment's unique contribution to quality of care.

Post-occupancy evaluations can be a time-saving resource for providers and designers contemplating new construction or renovation, offering lessons learned to avoid repetition of often costly mistakes and to improve the state of the art.

In recognition of the number of senior housing options already in place, and with the continuous construction of new facilities, there is much hands-on, experiential data available that is not documented. Too often these unique approaches to design and care for the aging remain unshared. Full utilization of post-occupancy evaluations and the distribution of those results will provide an immeasurable amount of useful data and information that ultimately will advance the art and science of environmental design for the aging and its relationship to the care provider and resident.

Part I

Independent Living Apartments

"Middle age is when you've met so many people that every new person you meet reminds you of someone else."

OGDEN NASH, 1902–1971

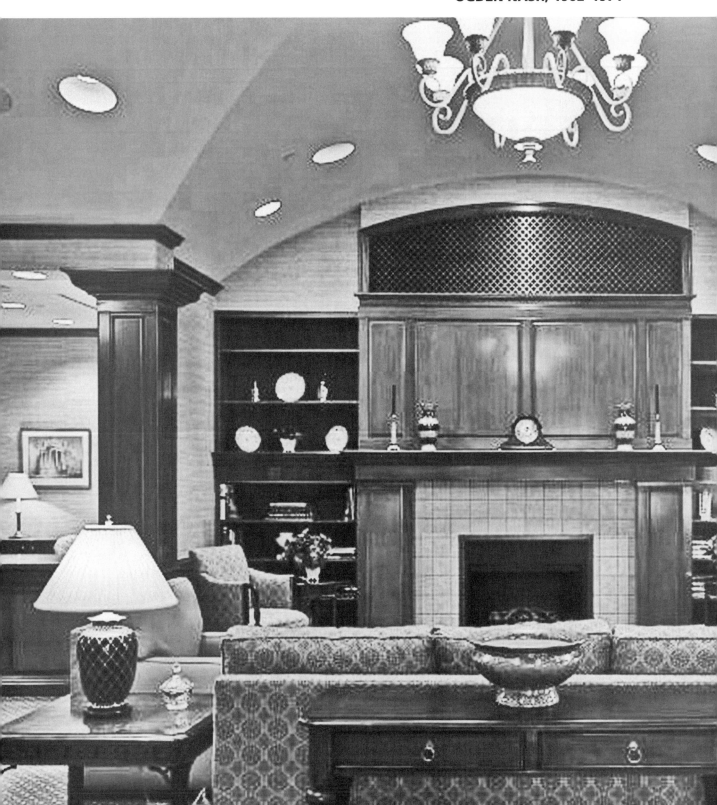

Chapter 1

Parkview at Asbury Methodist Village

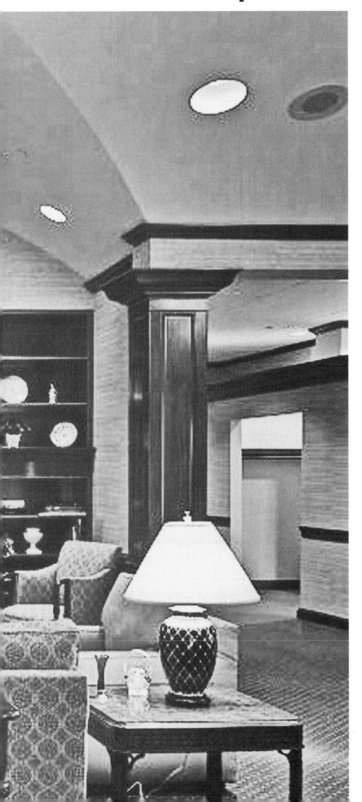

EVALUATION SITE: Parkview at Asbury Methodist Village

COMMUNITY TYPE: Independent Living Apartments
• 65 independent living apartments

REGION: Mid-Atlantic

ARCHITECT: Cochran, Stephenson & Donkervoet, Inc.

OWNER: Asbury Methodist Village, Inc.

DATA POINTS: Resident Apartment: 1,055–2,585 gsf
Total Area: 2,387.69 gsf/apartment
Total Area: 155,200 gsf
Project Cost: $175.38/gsf
Total Project Cost: $27,218,995
Investment/apartment: $418,753.77
Occupancy: 99% as of May 2006

FIRST OCCUPANCY: October 2005

DATE OF EVALUATION: May 2006

EVALUATION TEAM: Rich Compton; Eleanor Alvarez; Eileen Nacht, AIA; Ingrid Fraley, ASID

FIG. 1-1 This warm and welcoming view of the lobby upon entry minimizes the connection to the remote receptionist
Photo by Alain Jaramillo

Introduction

For more than 80 years, Asbury Methodist Village has provided services to the elderly on a sprawling 130-acre campus located in Gaithersburg, Maryland, a suburb of Washington, D.C. Mission-driven and spiritually based, Asbury's reputation for excellence is well known.

Over the years, this continuing care retirement community (CCRC) has evolved not only in the construction of housing and related services, but also in the development of unique educational, wellness, and cultural programs to support a comprehensive retirement lifestyle. The Rosborough Cultural Arts and Wellness Center offers an Olympic-size pool, personal fitness trainers, a 350-seat theater for regional and community productions, and the AVTV Asbury Village private television station. The Keese School of Continuing Education offers a wide range of lectures, classes, and educational tours during its academic year, which runs from September through May.

The many buildings on the campus include independent living cottages and apartments, assisted living, skilled nursing, adult day care, outpatient services, care management, pharmacy, rehabilitation, and community services, all supporting a population of 1,300 residents, 850 associates, and 1,600 volunteers. Walking paths, community gardens, putting greens, tennis courts, the pond, and surrounding woods create an outdoor environment that is scenic and therapeutic. Residents are connected not only by roads and walkways, but also by the lifestyle and community amenities that encourage total involvement in campus life.

The subject of this evaluation is one specific building, which represents the challenges and decision process that many owners and operators face when an existing building has aged and no longer serves its original purpose.

The "211 Building" was constructed in 1991 as a seven-story, apartment-style building to serve 192 assisted living residents. The resident floors were designed with traditional double-loaded corridors and small efficiency-style units. Resident common space consisted of a dining room, living room, and club room, located on the second floor of the terrace level. In addition, a large chapel located on the first floor provided religious services for all residents of the Asbury campus.

As residents continued to age in place, the day-to-day logistics of moving all 192 residents, utilizing only two elevators for meals and activities, became overwhelming. Reality dictated that once residents were moved to the terrace level, they remained there and did not return to their apartments until the end of the day.

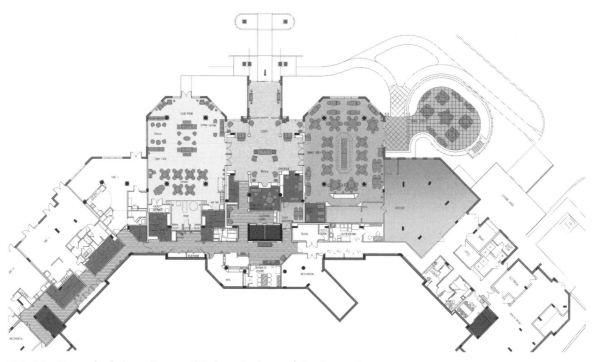

FIG. 1-2   Terrace-level plan   *Courtesy of Cochran, Stephenson & Donkervoet, Inc.*

Congestion increased and the common spaces could no longer function for their intended purposes. Operational inefficiencies rose, as did costs associated with these inefficiencies.

AUTHOR'S NOTE: *The remainder of this post-occupancy evaluation differs in format from its companion chapters. The original assisted living building was submitted to the "Design for Aging Review" in 1992. The transformation of the building into The Parkview Apartments has not been submitted to the "Design for Aging Review," but this story in itself is a post-occupancy evaluation of the original design. This transformation process is therefore worthy of discussion but uses a slightly different format. Within the following content, the owner's objectives and the architect's responses for that transformation process are clearly demonstrated and the results of the evaluation are documented.*

Master Planning

The master planning process consisted of a building and programming analysis to assess existing conditions and determine desired changes. The "211 Building" had to change from a high-occupancy, high-service, complex operational entity to a "highest and best use" product that minimized reuse complications.

To that end, the Asbury organization engaged in an extensive planning process that was thorough, research-based, inclusive, and highly communicative. Participants in this process included long-term care staff, industry experts, and consumer advocates who were able to identify a needed service gap on the campus, determine a viable financial plan, and review the staffing requirements for this new entity.

The conversion required thoughtful decisions at strategic points, but above all, team members had to keep their eyes on the big picture. At the same time, staying on track also required flexibility in overcoming unforeseen obstacles. They fixed what they could, converted some challenges into opportunities, and accepted those things that could not be changed. Even in the face of two critical issues that had severe financial consequences, the team demonstrated the courage to make difficult and important decisions under pressure, to the benefit of the finished product.

With a waiting list of 400 and a pent-up demand for larger apartments, the design team determined that the best use of the "211 Building" would be for independent living apartments, designed to appeal specifically to the active senior 60 years of age or older. With that demographic, these units would also appeal to cou-

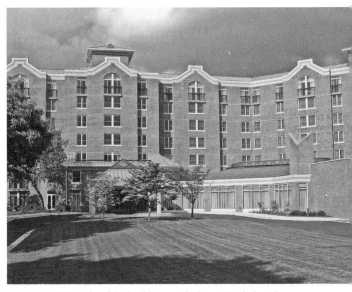

FIG. 1-3 This side of the building, with the original chapel on the right, was reconstructed to mimic the original façade, but created some confusion as to which entry is the main one *Photograph by Richard Compton*

ples. The resulting "Programming Document," used as a checklist by the design team, included the following information:

- Function of every space
- When spaces would be utilized
- Required adjacencies
- Décor of the spaces
- List of finishes
- Consideration of maintenance issues, aesthetics, and acoustics
- Furniture, fixtures, and equipment
- Other design criteria

It should be noted that, unlike most renovation projects, this community did not have to deal with the challenges of renovating an occupied building. In conjunction with the decision to move toward independent living, the completion of a new assisted living building solved the problem of what to do with the existing population.

Design Challenges

During the life of the "211 Building," water problems and leaks were not unusual. As part of the design program, a forensic study was conducted to determine the cause of water penetration through the existing façade. The findings indicated that the original brick cavity wall had not been properly constructed. Therefore, the decision was made to remove the exterior skin of the building. Only the building infrastructure was salvaged, including columns, floor slabs, elevator and stair shafts, and mechanical chases. At this point in the process, implosion of the original building was discussed, but a savings of $20 per square foot was estimated if the new unit layouts could be designed around the existing structural elements. Considering the unanticipated expense of removing the outer wall, this cost savings was a welcome addition to an escalating budget.

The main chapel, with its strong history and connection to the community, had to be preserved, and thus this space was not significantly changed during construction.

In addition, the façade on this side of the building was rebuilt to match the original design, to minimize the city review process. More aggressive bay projections were added to the other sides of the building to improve the layout of the units and to establish a new building image.

Large, "high-end" units were required to meet consumer demands. The existing floor-to-floor height of eight feet challenged the designers to minimize the visual impact of low ceilings. Coffered tray ceilings were incorporated and bay projections with higher windows maximized the amount of natural light and framed outdoor views to the park. To avoid extensive duct work and the resulting bulkheads, fan coil units were incorporated, sometimes with great frequency, in the individual units.

The number of apartments created was not based on a marketing study, but solely on the capacity of the existing footprint of the building's floors. Corridors are now single loaded, forcing all available square footage into the apartment units. The result is a total of 65 apartments with 13 different unit types, mixing one-bedroom, two-bedroom, and two-bedroom-with-den units. Units range in size from 1,030 square feet to 2,590 square feet. As a point of comparison, only 40% of the existing 745 independent living apartments on campus are larger than 1,000 square feet. The new common spaces on the main level include a dining room, club room, library, and main entry lobby.

Of particular interest is the attempt to reorient the entry to the apartment building to take advantage of the wooded views, with the accompanying new building name of "Parkview." This required a new entry with a new porte cochere to anchor the new entrance on the side of the building opposite the original entrance. The old entrance remains, primarily to serve the main chapel.

A new three-level parking garage, with a covered space for each of the 65 residents, was also constructed. It included 35 additional uncovered spaces on the top deck. Assigned parking is important to this active adult population, many of whom are still working.

Entry/Commons

The shift in the entry sequence poses an interesting dilemma. Although the redesign succeeded in moving the building focus and main entry to the "park" side of the site, the original approach, with its circular driveway and chapel entry, remains off Russell Avenue, which is the main street of the campus. This causes some confusion for the first-time visitor in finding the appropriate entrance to the building.

The road eventually leads one past the newly constructed garage and loading dock, past a massively screened generator, to a final arrival at the new porte cochere. Visitor parking is not clearly delineated, nor is it convenient to this front entry.

The reception desk is located in a discrete corner of the lobby, making it difficult for the receptionist to visually control the entry. From the visitors' approach, the receptionist is not in the direct line of sight, and the sense of confusion is immediate upon entry. However, upon the evaluation team's arrival, the receptionist was quick to leave the remote desk and provide assistance.

The lobby features a nicely designed fireplace surrounded by a furniture grouping in a transitional style. To the right is the club room, the main community space, used primarily for planned events and rarely for informal socialization. Changes from its original configuration within the assisted living building design were

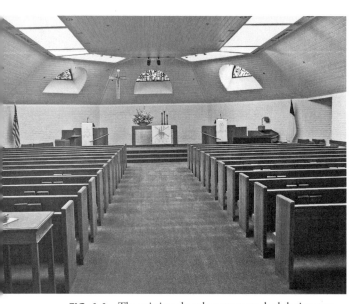

FIG. 1-4   The existing chapel was not touched during construction, and remains a landmark for campus residents
Photograph by Richard Compton

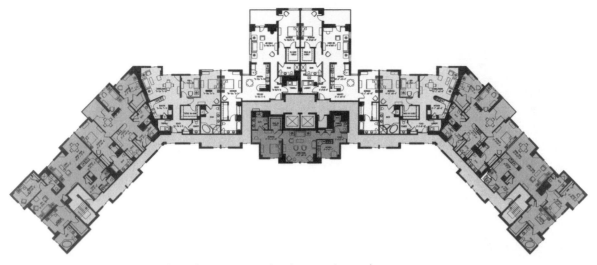

FIG. 1-5 Typical apartment-level floor plan   *Courtesy of Cochran, Stephenson & Donkervoet, Inc.*

minimal but included the addition of an accessible ramp to the raised podium area, a beverage/kitchen area to accommodate catered events, and an extremely large television.

Bible study, bridge club, and the Tuesday dance are some of the resident-initiated activities. The furnishings are senior-friendly, with moisture-proof fabrics that seem somewhat at odds with the intended focus on a younger population.

Dining

The dining room, to the left of the lobby, has a multi-purpose appearance, as opposed to perhaps a more logical upscale restaurant image. At the time of the evaluation, only one meal was offered and only on limited days: buffet on Wednesday; dinner on Thursday, Friday, and Saturday; and brunch on Sunday.

Some confusion has arisen about what the theme of the dining service should be, with two points of view expressed. One opinion is that the dining program should be another venue on campus with the same level of service, to avoid creating a perception that the Parkview dining experience is better. The second opinion is that this dining room has an opportunity to provide an upscale dining experience that is currently missing from the campus. Without full definition by operations, it is not surprising that only limited dining opportunity is available.

Parkview considers itself a restaurant, with surf-and-turf, display cooking, and upscale brunch service. Parkview residents have a point-of-service card for din-

ing, which records charges based on their use of any of the dining rooms on campus. The remaining campus residents prepay for meals and costs are deducted; though they are encouraged to visit the new Parkview dining room, they must pay an additional fee at this venue. Meal costs are higher in this dining room because of the higher quality of food and service. However, residents believe that they are not necessarily seeing this value, and consider other options both on and off campus to be more affordable or desirable.

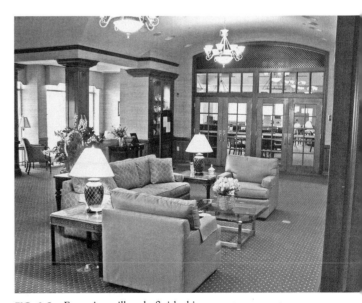

FIG. 1-6 Extensive millwork, finished in warm tones, creates a welcoming feeling for the lobby and dining room beyond
Photograph by Richard Compton

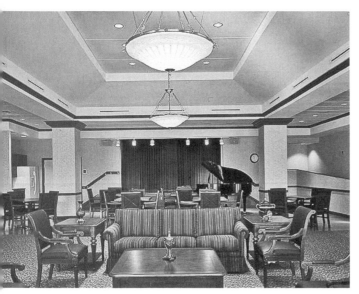

FIG. 1-7 The multipurpose room was part of the original configuration and required minimal renovation for the new independent population *Photograph by Richard Compton*

Parkview is also one of two dining rooms on campus where alcohol is served. Currently, residents bring their own alcohol and are free to serve themselves. Although some residents disapprove of this policy and refuse to eat in the dining room, Parkview would like to obtain a liquor license and provide spirits as a part of its standard service.

The outdoor dining experience is disappointing as a result of the change in the main orientation of the building. On what is now the back side of the building there is a wonderful patio, complete with outdoor dining furniture located adjacent to the loading dock, massive generator, and parking garage. Although screening has been added, this function at this location seems misplaced and inconvenient.

Commercial Kitchen

The original renovation plan included preservation of the original kitchen. As a result of the "ravages of construction," maintaining this objective was the second challenge for the design team. It became evident that the existing kitchen equipment was not usable, as it was of an "old school" health care design. Late in the construction process, the kitchen was gutted and all the equipment replaced, resulting in a delayed building opening.

Housekeeping and Maintenance

All of the housekeeping services provided in the resident apartments are at additional cost to the resident. A minimum of three hours of cleaning per apartment unit is required if a resident desires any cleaning service. Fifty percent of the residents contract for this service on a weekly or biweekly basis.

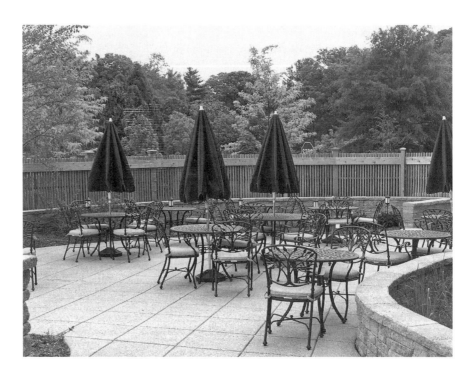

FIG. 1-8 The terrace extension of the dining room is located between the lobby and the loading dock *Photograph by Richard Compton*

One full-time maintenance person is assigned to the building to provide preventative as well as emergency maintenance services. Residents can receive additional services for small projects at a cost of $30.50 per hour. Larger projects are addressed by a list of approved contractors who are allowed to work in the units and understand the scope of services and expectations of quality.

The trash removal system is through the use of trash chutes, available on each of the floors, which connect to a large dumpster located in the main trash room at grade. This dumpster is then rolled down a hallway to the loading dock area, where it awaits pickup. Issues of pest and infection control are not foremost in the operator's mind at the moment, although a summer's assortment of flies, pests, and rodents may warrant reconsideration.

Corridors and Apartments

The single-loaded corridors allow natural light penetration and should provide some amount of orientation. However, the narrow four-foot-wide corridors do not allow residents to stop, rest, and orient to the outdoors. With the addition of many 90-degree bends, the vistas are compromised, so orientation by object, such as a prominent grandfather clock, is more likely to be of value.

Narrowness of corridors and excessive turns also affect the safe use of wheelchairs and motorized wheelchairs; turning around while in one would certainly be a challenge. Housekeeping reported difficulty in using wider vacuum cleaners in these limited spaces.

The operator has developed a system to turn off many of the corridor lights during the day, leaving the perception of burnt-out light bulbs that need to be replaced. Hallways may have been overlit or perhaps not well thought through for energy efficiency.

Elevators, although totally refurbished, are sized to the original assisted living building design. Because there is no freight elevator, deliveries and move-in processes are challenged by the shortened height and fast-closing doors of the elevator system. Another challenge is the location of the parking garage, which is not connected to this main set of elevators. A circuitous route is required to access a second set of elevators at the opposite end of the building.

Apartment designs were masterfully planned to accommodate odd spaces that resulted from the constraints posed by existing building structure. Large windows and coffered tray ceilings were incorporated to minimize the perception of low ceilings. Unconventional apartment arrangements were addressed by the

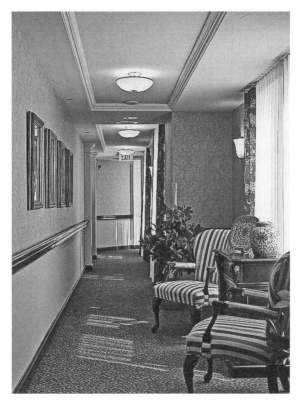

FIG. 1-9 Single-loaded apartment corridors are designed with strategically placed seating alcoves to minimize the impact of the four-foot-wide corridors   *Photo by Alain Jaramillo*

operator's provision of interior design services to help residents visualize the best use of their apartments.

Although units had some universal design features, such as lever handles on the doors, single-lever faucets, wire pulls, raised electrical outlets, and ranges with front controls, other aging-in-place features were not included. Grab bars in the showers, though not initially planned for, have now been added; shower enclosures have thresholds that would require a more extensive retrofit to create a roll-in shower; lighting over the vanities features exposed bulbs; all bathroom surfaces are white and lack contrast for residents with vision impairments; dishwashers are not raised and microwaves are located above the range. Because residents are allowed to stay in their apartments as their care needs progress, attention to these basic design conveniences would be beneficial. It should be noted that aging in place is approved only with the appropriate caregiver support, which is coordinated through Asbury's care management department. Although home health agency services are used and encouraged in the apartments, a care manager for the resident must be identified as the person who will

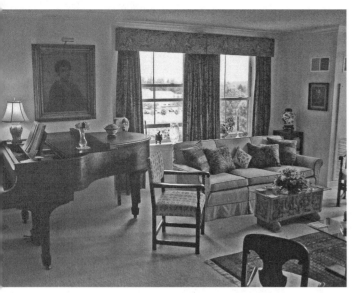

FIG. 1-10 Residents are able to furnish their unusual apartment layouts with the assistance of the project designer
Photograph by Richard Compton

ensure that all the required services are provided in a consistent manner.

Operator Perspectives

This organization engaged in an excellent planning process that embraced the mission "to promote relationships that celebrate a balanced and fulfilling lifestyle" for Parkview residents and the entire Asbury Methodist campus. The staff that worked on this project seemed to be handpicked with the common threads of experience, proven ability to work well with residents, and commitment to the vision of a new building on campus.

Parkview is also evidence of the power of a good idea. The administrator, at the time of critical decision making, took a careful view of the future needs of this community and led the way. Even with changes in key leadership positions during the planning and construction process, the solidity of the plan allowed the project to move forward and reach its goal.

Design consultants incorporated resident and staff input through the establishment of the Partnership Advisory Group. Draft plans were presented to all stakeholders and frequent marketing meetings reinforced the commitment to the plan. As the project went to construction, leadership became proactive and incoming residents were engaged in the planning process. Multiple special events were planned prior to, during, and after opening to solicit opinions and maintain strong lines of open communication.

The move-in process was well considered and well organized. Each day started with a clear idea of the goals and objectives to be met, as well as a review of the issues and successes from the prior day. Inaugural residents included former board members and others close to the Asbury organization, so standards of service were high and the team exceeded expectations. The resident satisfaction rate of 98% can only be attributed to this intense communication process. As a result, the famous "Parkview Team Approach" is now used as a model for other new openings within the organization.

When the Parkview Apartments opened, the occupancy goals were quickly exceeded, and at the time of the evaluation stood at a 99% occupancy level.

General Project Information

PROJECT ADDRESS
Asbury Methodist Village
211 Russell Avenue
Gaithersburg, MD 20877

PROJECT DESIGN TEAM
Architect: Cochran, Stephenson & Donkervoet, Inc.
Interior Designer: Partners in Planning
Landscape Architect: Cochran, Stephenson & Donkervoet, Inc.
Structural Engineer: Morabito Consultants, Inc.
Mechanical Engineer: James Posey Associates, Inc.
Electrical Engineer: James Posey Associates, Inc.
Civil Engineer: RBA Group
Dining Consultant: N/A

Gerontologist: N/A
Management/Development: N/A
Contractor: Donohoe Construction

PROJECT STATUS
Completion date: October 2005

OCCUPANCY LEVELS
At facility opening date: 91%
At time of evaluation: 99%

RESIDENT AGE (YRS)
At facility opening date: 77
At time of evaluation: 77

RESIDENTIAL FACILITIES

Project Element	No.	Apartments Typical Size (GSF)	Size Range (GSF)
One-bedroom units	8	1,055	1,055–1,490
One-bedroom with den units	7	1,340	1,340
Two-bedroom units	40	1,685	1,335–1,685
Two-bedroom with den units	8	1,490	1,490–2,585
Three-bedroom with den units	2	2,535	2,535
Total (all units)	65	98,625	GSF
Residents' social areas (lounges, dining, and spaces)		16,683	GSF
Medical/health/fitness and activities areas		0	GSF
Administrative, public, and ancillary support service areas		514	GSF
Service, maintenance, and mechanical areas		39,378	GSF
Total gross area		155,200	GSF
Total net usable area (per space program)		115,822	NSF
Overall gross/net factor (ratio of gross area/net useable area)		1.34	

SITE AND PARKING

SITE LOCATION
Suburban

SITE SIZE
Part of a larger CCRC campus, site area for this specific project not calculated.

PARKING

Type of Parking	For This Facility Residents	Staff	Visitors	Totals
Open surface lot(s)	0	16	22	38
Parking structure	100	0	0	100
Totals	100	16	22	138

CONSTRUCTION COSTS

SOURCE OF COST DATA
Final construction cost as of October 2005

SOFT COSTS

Land cost or value	N/A
All permit and other entitlement fees	Included in below
Legal and professional fees	Included in below
Appraisals	N/A
Marketing and preopening	Included in below
Other fees	Included in below
Total soft costs	$1,661,015

BUILDING COSTS

New construction except FF&E, special finishes, floor and window coverings, HVAC and electrical	$14,255,168
Renovations except FF&E, special finishes, floor and window coverings, HVAC and electrical	Included in above
FF&E and small wares	Included in above
Floor coverings	Included in above
Window coverings	Included in above
HVAC	$5,340,464
Electrical	$2,059,353
Parking garage	$1,625,758
Total building costs	$23,280,743

SITE COSTS
Total site costs, including demolition costs: $2,277,237

TOTAL PROJECT COSTS
Total project costs: $27,218,995

FINANCING SOURCES
Unknown

"The secret to staying young is to live honestly, eat slowly, and lie about your age."

LUCILLE BALL, 1911–1989

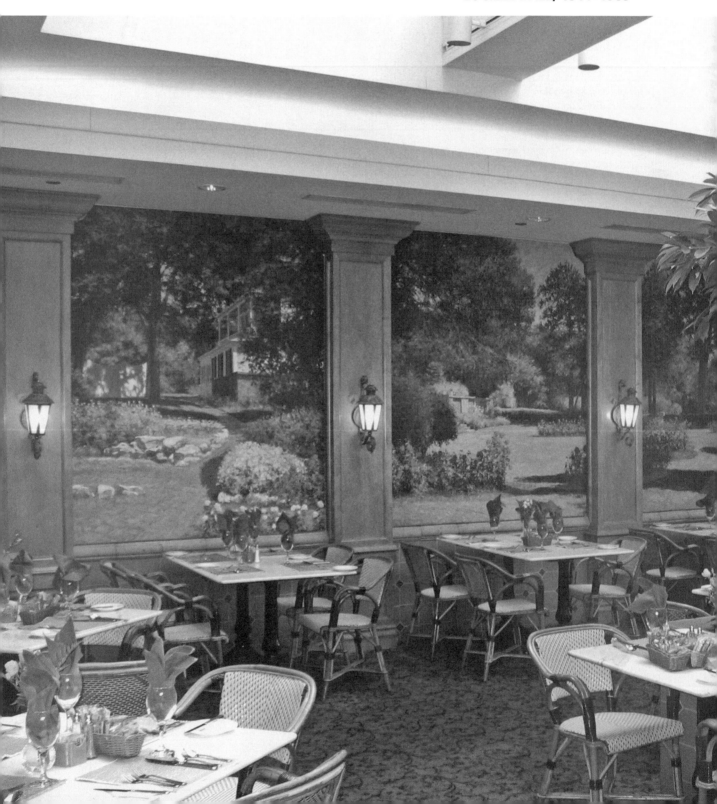

Chapter 2   The Hallmark

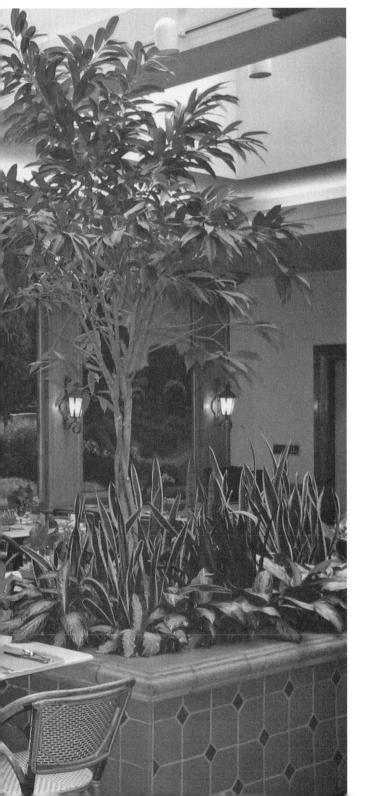

EVALUATION SITE: The Hallmark

COMMUNITY TYPE: Independent Retirement Apartments
- 341 independent living apartments

REGION: Midwest Urban

ARCHITECT: John Macsai & Associates

OWNER: Brookdale Living Communities, Inc.
(Original owner: The Prime Group)

DATA POINTS:
Resident Apartment:	630–1,646 gsf
Total Area:	1,411.09 gsf/apartment
Total Area:	481,180 gsf
Project Cost:	$72.21/gsf
Total Project Cost:	$34,747,000
Investment/apartment:	$101,897.36
Occupancy:	withheld at owner's request

PROJECT COMPLETED: 1990

DATE OF EVALUATION: May 2006

EVALUATION TEAM: Loretta Seidl, RDH, MHS; David Slack; Brenda Kessler, ASID; Robert Pfauth, AIA; Jeffrey Anderzhon, AIA

FIG. 2-1 The garden café offers residents a casual dining atmosphere filled with natural light from the skylight above
Photograph by Jeffrey Anderzhon

Introduction

The Lincoln Park area of Chicago offers spectacular vistas of Lake Michigan to the east, and provides an urban vibrancy and diversity that would attract anyone with a connection to this "Second City." This is an area of high-rise apartments overlooking the pastoral setting of Lincoln Park and the calming waters of the lake, a view that is visually interrupted only by Lake Shore Drive, which compensates for this interruption by providing easy access to the Loop. Most of these apartments are homes for individuals whose income can support the rents demanded by this area of lake vistas. Some of these individuals are elderly, and many buildings have thus become naturally occurring retirement communities simply because of the demographics of the residents.

It is not surprising, then, that The Hallmark takes its place among these high-rises as the only proclaimed retirement apartment community along Lincoln Park's "Gold Coast." The 341-apartment-unit, 37-story building sits at the end of Lincoln Park, anchoring this park entrance guarding its north side. Although distinctive in design, it blends well with its neighbors and can perhaps even be lost in the visually homogenous milieu that quickly swallows up the surrounding skyline. (See Figure 1 in the color insert.)

The main tower is placed on the south portion of a three-story lower building plinth, leaving the north half fully and forever free of adjacent visual blocking of views to the lake. This device also provides a somewhat more limited guarantee of visual access to the lake from the southern apartments, as the site is bounded on this side by a city street.

The community was designed in the early 1990s for upper-income residents who fit into the socioeconomic trend that is prevalent elsewhere in the neighborhood. Apartment sizes reflect that design parameter, ranging from a 630-square-foot, one-bedroom unit to a 1,024-square-foot, two-bedroom unit, and even a 1,646-square-foot, three-bedroom penthouse unit. The building amenities also reflect the intended clientele and include a full-time doorman and concierge, elegant entry lobby, a refined library and club room, and a full restaurant-style dining room complete with the requirement of seating reservations.

What the designers accomplished in siting and resident amenities, however, is offset by lack of vision and understanding that, once ensconced in their apartments with their magnificent views, the residents would never want to leave, regardless of an increase in frailty and the need for care. Aging in place was not a part of the build-

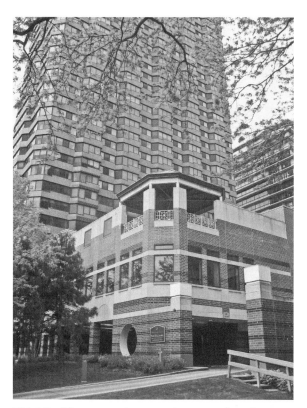

FIG. 2-2 The porte cochere entry is set away from the street and incorporated into the building design with roof terrace and gazebo above *Photograph by Jeffrey Anderzhon*

ing program, and over the past decade the operation of the building has both suffered and adapted.

As residents have aged in place—an event bound to occur—the resident floor corridors and standard apartment door widths have become more difficult to navigate with walkers and wheelchairs, and the dining rooms have become more crowded because of the use of these devices (as one might expect). The lighting throughout the building, which was once viewed as elegant and subdued, is now, to an older eye, inefficient and inadequate. Likewise, the furniture selected for visual appeal and contribution to ambience is now difficult for an older population to use with comfort.

Most critically, the elevators have become a major issue for several reasons, all related to aging in place. The door operators have been set on a longer time sequence to accommodate individuals who ambulate more slowly or who need wheelchairs. This, in turn, means that the traffic flow of the elevators is slowed significantly, and wait times become almost unbearable for the residents. This is further exacerbated by a need to accommodate

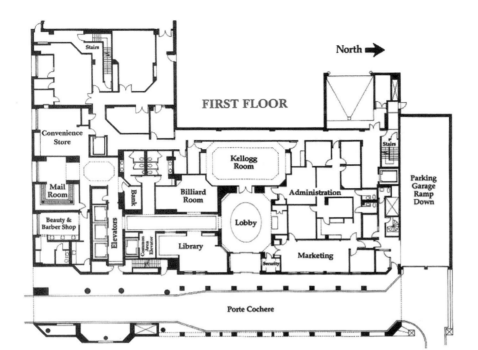

FIG. 2-3 Entry-level floor plan *Courtesy of The Hallmark*

FIRST FLOOR

North ➡

Stairs

Convenience Store

Kellogg Room

Stairs

Mail Room

Bank

Billiard Room

Administration

Parking Garage Ramp Down

Beauty & Barber Shop

Elevators

Common Area Elevator

Lobby

Library

Security

Marketing

Porte Cochere

---

walkers and wheelchairs, and thus fewer people, with each elevator trip.

Because of the aging building population, and not insignificantly their wealth, there are a considerable number of full-time, live-in, nonrelated care providers. These private care providers represent approximately 25% of the total population of the building and place an added burden on the building's spaces and services, including the elevator system, that was unforeseen at the time the design was being developed.

Originally constructed as an entry fee model by a Chicago developer, the development was purchased by Brookdale Living Communities in 1995 and converted to a straight monthly rental fee model that includes two daily meals. In the intervening years, the operator has added a fitness and physical rehabilitation center and an on-site wellness clinic, where community doctors, dentists, and other medical professionals hold periodic office hours and where a home health agency's offices are located, complete with 24-hour nurse aides.

Architect's Statement

AUTHOR'S NOTE: *The architect's statements for this evaluation were written by the authors but were derived from publications in which the architects discussed the design,* *interviews with the architects, and periodical articles in which the architects discussed the design.*

The 37-story tower of this luxurious congregate housing for the elderly provides each apartment with a magnificent view of Lincoln Park and Lake Michigan. Each living room has a bay window with a partially lowered sill to enhance easy and comfortable viewing, even for those in wheelchairs. The generously and richly furnished common areas are housed in the three-story base of the building.

Designers' and Owners' Stated Objectives and Responses

OBJECTIVE: Take advantage of the spectacular views to Lake Michigan and Lincoln Park.

DESIGN INTENT: The building is situated on the site to take full advantage of views along three sides of the highrise. Placing the vertical portion of the building along the south street and continuing the common area plinth to the north assures the maximum number of residents an uninterrupted view. In addition, the introduction of angled windows and lowered window sills maximizes the residential views even when an individual is seated in the apartment or using a wheelchair.

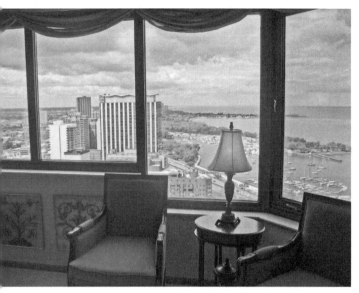

FIG. 2-4   Apartments feature lowered windowsills to enhance spectacular views toward Lake Michigan
Photograph by Jeffrey Anderzhon

OBJECTIVE: Maximize usage of the limited site, but provide a comfortable and protected entry sequence for both automobile and pedestrian.

DESIGN INTENT: By placing the porte cochere below the building's community plinth and raising the floor to floor height here, the use of site for this purpose is minimized, but the design allows a larger area for resident drop-off. Integrating the porte cochere into the building design, rather than making it a simple add-on, further draws the eye to the overall design rather than to the porte cochere itself.

OBJECTIVE: Minimize view obstruction of neighboring structures.

DESIGN INTENT: By lowering the original-design building height by five full floors and massing the bulk of the tower to the south side of the property, the majority of views from neighboring buildings were maintained. This also allowed increased visual access to Lake Michigan and Lincoln Park by the furthest west apartments within the tower.

Field Observations: Meeting the Objectives

OBJECTIVE: Take advantage of the spectacular views to Lake Michigan and Lincoln Park.

FIELD OBSERVATIONS: Utilizing generous expanses of glass provides very good visual access to the lake and park views, as well as views that become varied and interesting with the angled window placement in each apartment. By lowering a portion of this window expanse in each apartment room, the design does allow residents to access those views while seated. The apartments present an open feeling, and there is generous natural light that enters all but the most remote apartment entry hall.

The location of the high-rise portion of the building along the south street is a conscious design decision that both enhances the available views to the lake and park by the residents, and also maintains maximized visual access by neighboring buildings, particularly to the west of this project. This design decision also provided a very comfortable and inviting third-floor roof garden that is well protected from a relentless summer sun by both the building bulk and creative structural elements, including a shading trellis and covered "gazebo." This exterior space is protected from the famous Chicago wind by an east wall that adds to the entry façade; this wall is punched with "windows" that are glazed for wind protection but still allow visual access to the nearby park.

The architect's statement demonstrates obvious pride in the consideration given so that individuals in wheelchairs may access the views to the exterior. It is thus a little disconcerting that this design feature seems to be the only consideration given to individuals in wheelchairs. Though the building was designed and completed just prior to the enactment of the Americans with Disabilities Act, the designers certainly had knowledge of basic accessibility requirements and of the population for which the building was being designed. It is disappointing that the simple design consideration of wider, wheelchair-accessible doors into the apartment bathrooms was not included, even though the design predates ADA. In fact, when first opened, this community did not allow residents who required the use of either canes or wheelchairs to occupy the apartments.

OBJECTIVE: Maximize usage of the limited site, but provide a comfortable and protected entry sequence for both automobile and pedestrian.

FIELD OBSERVATIONS: Prior to approval of construction of this project, there was a good deal of opposition from neighboring building owners and tenants on the grounds that it would limit their visual access to the lake and park. Compromises were struck in the form of a lower building than originally envisioned and a very extensively landscaped area between the building and the east street. This portion of the property has a very strong

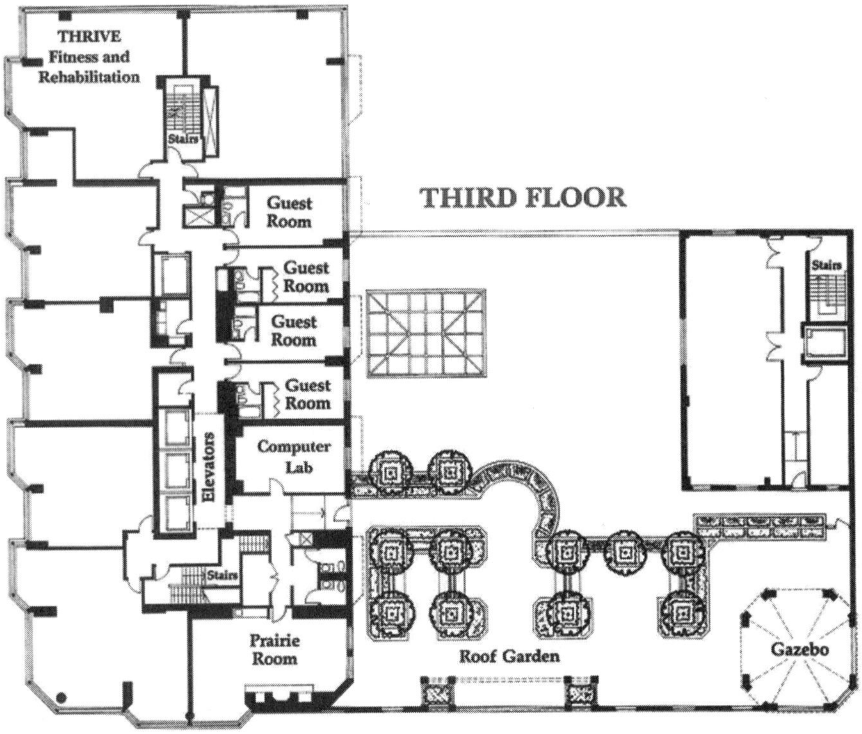

FIG. 2-5 Third-floor plan; terrace with gazebo *Courtesy of John Macsai & Associates*

connection to the park directly across the street; from a pedestrian perspective, it feels as though one is in the midst of a carefully tended garden rather than at the entry of an urban high-rise structure.

The automobile entry drive at the extreme northeast corner of the property is unassuming and minimized, but leads to a covered drive extending nearly the complete north-south length of the property created by the overhanging structure. This element could have been very confining, but the treatment feels open and provides more than adequate space for extended drop-off periods or facility bus loading for off-site activities. The drive exit is to the south street and thus does not impose on the park side of the property.

OBJECTIVE: Minimize view obstruction of neighboring structures.

FIELD OBSERVATIONS: Through a combination of intense zoning hearings and neighborhood objections, the original building design was adjusted to ameliorate the concerns of very vocal neighboring property owners. These design modifications included a reduction in the building height (and thus a reduction in the number of apartments) and placement of the tower on the south portion of the property, where it would minimize the visual blocking effect of the development. In addition, the building was set back from the east street that fronts on

Lincoln Park, per a planning restriction that was connected to the park.

Simple modifications could have been incorporated into the design as a compromise and the project would have been allowed to proceed. However, the design modifications allowed the building not only to be a good neighbor, but also to be an improved environment for residents. By shifting the building to the south, a third-level roof garden was created that gives residents a private exterior space. The compromises also allow a vehicular and pedestrian entry that does not dominate the street-level façade, as occurs in so many similar projects.

Field Observations: Themes and Hypotheses

Creating Community

If The Hallmark had not been developed specifically as a retirement apartment community, an apartment building would almost certainly have been constructed on this highly desirable site. The end result of this would have been be a naturally occurring retirement community not unlike so many other high-rise apartment buildings neighboring The Hallmark. There is, however, a sense of

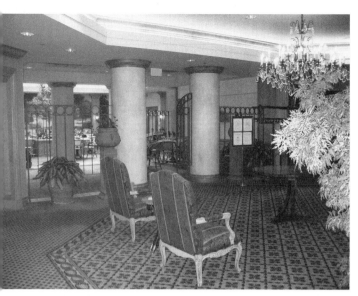

FIG. 2-6 Dining bistro lobby at the second floor with the casual café beyond *Photograph by Jeffrey Anderzhon*

community about this building that is both intuitive and somewhat evident as one enters the facility.

Unlike a typical apartment building, the main entry floor of The Hallmark contains rooms that are intended for social interaction, and these are placed so that they are visible immediately upon entry. In addition, the main building entry lobby is clearly a gathering place for residents before they leave on shopping trips or excursions into the Loop. This is where the residents converse with the concierge and with each other as they wait for the facility transportation. This is a busy gathering place also for residents just before they move into the Jefferson Room, a medium-sized multipurpose space, for a discussion on current events or a session of low-impact chair aerobics. This is the intersection of the building community and the neighborhood outside of the building.

On the second level, the dining rooms dominate resident activity. A skylit dining café is available for casual dining, while a more formal dining room, complete with maitre d', provides residents with an upper-class restaurant experience. Both areas are adjacent to the "Club Room," where residents can have a pre-dinner glass of wine as they wait to be seated. At mealtime, all of these areas are abuzz with the conversation of a connected community citizenry.

The convenience store, located on the first floor adjacent to the mailroom and barber and beauty shop, provides a sort of mini-main street to which residents travel each day, intermingling and sharing with others in a casual social atmosphere. Adjacent to the dining areas,

there is a more formal living area, complete with wine bar, where more structured socialization takes place at the regular meal intervals and, on occasion, over a glass of wine or cocktail.

On the east side of the building, on the uppermost floor, an apartment-sized social space has been reserved for family parties, resident get-togethers, or activities that involve small discussion groups or lectures. All of these spaces have been thoughtfully put together to provide a framework for resident community building. Although this does in fact happen, it is diminished to some extent by the fact that the building is a straight rental apartment model, as opposed to a shared equity model; thus, the residents have an understanding, however subtle, that a neighbor could depart at any time. This promotes, to some degree, a feeling of transience, and thus each resident may not be as anxious to develop deeper relationships within a community setting.

Making a Home

As noted earlier, the architect's statement shows obvious pride in the consideration given so that individuals in wheelchairs may access the views to the exterior. Unfor-

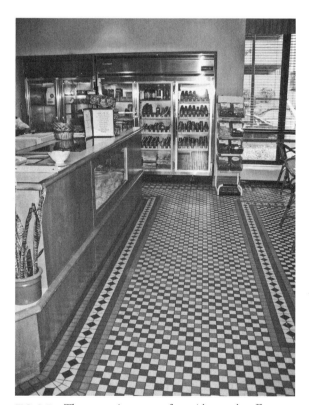

FIG. 2-7 The convenience store for resident and staff use on the first floor *Photograph by Jeffrey Anderzhon*

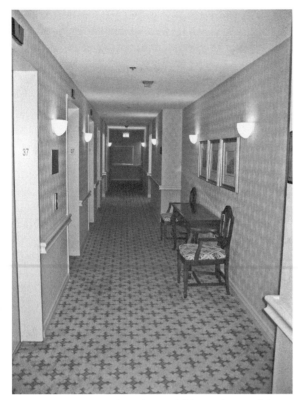

FIG. 2-8 Apartment-floor elevator lobby *Photograph by Jeffrey Anderzhon*

tunately, this design feature seems to be the only such consideration. Certainly, wheelchair access is vital to resident independence and dignity, and an important part of feeling at home in the environment. Though the building was not subject to the Americans with Disabilities Act, one would have expected the designers to pay more attention to basic accessibility requirements, given the population for which the building was being designed. For example, the lack of wider, wheelchair-accessible doors into the apartment bathrooms is disappointing. (As noted previously, the design predates ADA, and this community initially did not allow residents who used either canes or wheelchairs.)

Regional and Cultural Design

The exterior building design and interior spaces could fit into the urban fabric of nearly any city. There is nothing regionally distinctive in the design, nor is there anything offensively out of place. It does not follow the International Style of architecture that the city of Chicago made famous, but alternatively, it is not a completely cold rendering of an architect's imagination. It is clearly residen-

tial in feel and pays some homage to a residential context by its use of a masonry exterior finish.

The building clientele are individuals with some amount of wealth, and the lushly finished and detailed first three floor levels certainly play to that audience. The short and narrow corridors on the apartment floors are somewhat more muted in finish but not sparse, making the statement that these areas should be traversed as quickly as possible so that residents can either revel in the magnificent views from their apartments or the sumptuous finishes of the more public spaces.

Environmental Therapy

As originally conceived, The Hallmark was simply an age-restricted apartment building, with community space and dining facilities that would serve the closed community. Little or no thought was given to the need for therapies within the building, because of the belief that the younger, active elderly residents would seek these services within the broader community in the manner they had before moving in. Of course, the inevitable aging in place of the residents increasingly demanded closer attention to residents' care needs. Though it was always envisioned that a home health agency would occupy the second-level offices, it was not intended that these be anything more than merely offices—certainly not the exam rooms they have become. Additionally, a revenue-producing apartment has been converted to a rehabilitation and wellness center, where residents now visit following any medical procedure that prescribes therapy.

The building continues to adapt to resident-driven needs. As this evaluation took place, plans were being completed to turn the 17th and 18th floors into licensed assisted living apartments. This modification moves the project a step closer to becoming a continuing care campus, and is a manifestation of the operator's recognition of the continuing aging-in-place phenomenon. It is also a testament by residents that they have chosen a living location from which they do not want to move.

Outdoor Environment

The siting of the building has enabled the development of a nicely landscaped entry sequence from the east. This area provides a more formal transition from public space to building space. It distracts one's attention from the fact that this high-rise could be imposing, and draws one's attention to a more natural place. This transition is also helped by the fact that the building entry is set

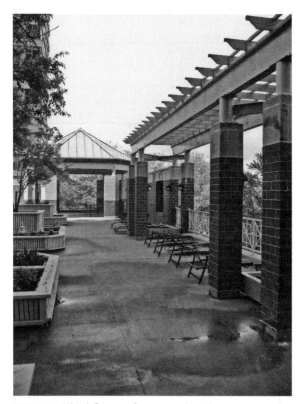

FIG. 2-9 Third-floor roof terrace and gazebo are protected from lake winds, providing opportunities for sun and shade
Photograph by Jeffrey Anderzhon

about six feet higher than the street level, thus providing a sort of vertical buffer. The resulting, and necessary, circuitous walk from the street level up to the entry level leads one through the annuals and perennials that provide continuous color and variety. It is a very pleasant journey and is a pleasant counterpoint for the hard surfaces of the building.

By placing the tower to the south of the site, the design allowed an opportunity to provide exterior space on the north side of the site. A roof garden, accessible from the building's third floor, was developed with a pleasant combination of both hard and planted surfaces and protected and open spaces. The east building façade continues along the face of this area to provide both visual protection and protection from the sometimes ferocious winds off the lake. Punched openings in this wall draw the viewer along the wall and provide teasing and varied glimpses to the park across the street, as well as to the lake beyond.

At the northeast corner of the roof garden, a large gazebo was constructed that protects occupants from the hot Chicago summer sun as well as from rain. Though large, this gazebo is detailed in a way that keeps it from

being overwhelming, so it provides an inviting destination that draws one from the garden entry through the planting areas to the end of the roof garden opposite its entry. This sequence serves to enhance the garden experience, which combines an intuitive sense of safety and security with a feeling that one is indeed in a garden rather than simply a contrived series of planters on a roof.

Quality of Workplace and the Physical Plant

Because The Hallmark was conceived as an independent living apartment facility, the staff originally consisted primarily of individuals in the dietary and housekeeping departments. With the aging in place that has occurred, the numbers of care providers (primarily private, live-in care providers) has increased significantly, to the point where nearly 25% of the residents of the building are these care providers. Clearly the complexion of the staff, either employed by The Hallmark or who work in The Hallmark, has shifted from service orientation to care orientation. This will change again when the facility fully completes its plans to convert two floors of apartments to licensed assisted living.

The most critical issue with the quality of workplace at The Hallmark is the vertical transportation system. The additional full-time care providers, privately hired by residents, have placed an unforeseen burden on the elevator system. While this is not the only portion of the infrastructure that has been tested, it is the most affected, particularly when combined with the modifications in door closure time necessary for the aging residents and in the decline in passenger capacity per trip that has resulted from the increasingly prevalent use of additional ambulation assistance devices.

The environment of the building provides an ambience, however, that is beneficial to the staff. The office area is functional, nicely appointed, and with enough space to be comfortable. The support spaces were planned with hospitality functionality and are organized and well suited for this purpose, flowing in a manner that allows efficiency in all aspects, from delivery from vendors to interface with residents.

Operator Perspectives

The Hallmark is viewed by Brookdale Living Communities, Inc., as its flagship property. As such, it is where the highest quality of staff migrates, and the property is maintained in a manner to retain its reputation as a showplace. Given these facts, the operator's perspective can only be expected to be enthusiastic and prideful.

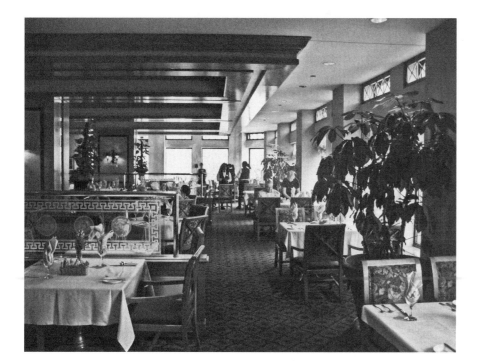

This pride and enthusiasm were certainly conveyed during each interview with staff, but were genuine and not simply parroting of the "company line." Interviewees were also frank in their discussion regarding areas of the environment in which there was disappointment. Certainly the elevator efficiency was one such area: the operator perspective was both disappointment in the current situation and frustration in the notion that very little can be done to rectify it. A concern was also expressed about operation of the building regarding individuals who are direct employees of the residents: How does an operator provide a consistent framework of overall operations when there is no direct control of the individuals who work within the building?

Understanding that plans are under way to convert two floors of the building to assisted living, the operators of the building are very cognizant of the advancing frailty of the residents and are approaching this issue with a generally positive solution. This solution, of course, has its own set of ramifications; however, The Hallmark believes that the environment is versatile enough to adapt to what is an increasingly evident future.

General Project Information

PROJECT ADDRESS
The Hallmark
2960 North Lake Shore Drive
Chicago, IL 60657

PROJECT DESIGN TEAM
Architect: John Macsai & Associates
Landscape Architects: Joe Karr Associates
Structural Engineer: Beer Gorski Graff, Ltd.
Mechanical Engineer: Environmental Systems Design, Inc.
Electrical Engineer: Consolidated Engineers
Food Service Consultant: Post Miller & Associates

PROJECT STATUS
Completion date: 1990

OCCUPANCY LEVELS
At facility opening date: 45%
At date of evaluation: withheld at owner's request

RESIDENT AGE (YRS)
At time of project completion: 71
At date of evaluation: 85
Average length of resident stay: 7 yrs.

PROJECT AREAS

INDEPENDENT LIVING RETIREMENT APARTMENTS

Project Element	New Construction No. Units in Building	Typical Size
Studio units (short-term stay/hotel units)	4	510 GSF
One-bedroom units	175	630–711 GSF
One-bedroom with den	69	780–960 GSF
Two-bedroom units	89	1,016–1,096 GSF
Three-bedroom (penthouse) units	4	1,646 GSF
Total (all units)	341	330,098 GSF
Residents' social areas (lounges, dining, and recreation spaces)		18,901 GSF
Medical, health care, therapies, and activities spaces		3,366 GSF
Administrative, public, and ancillary support services		3,069 GSF
Service, maintenance, covered parking, and mechanical areas		125,746 GSF
Total gross area		481,180 GSF
Total net usable area (per space program)		355,434 NSF
Overall gross/net factor (ratio of gross area/net usable area)		1.35

SITE AND PARKING

SITE LOCATION
Urban

SITE SIZE
Acres: 0.93
Square feet: 40,610

PARKING

Type of Parking	For This Facility Residents	Staff	Leased to Nonresidents	Totals
Under-building garage	20	56	75	151

CONSTRUCTION COSTS

AUTHOR'S NOTE: *At the time this project was submitted for the "Design for Aging Review" in 1994, detailed cost data was not required. The cost data presented here is from several sources, including the original designer and the operator.*

SOURCE OF COST DATA
Project completion dated: 1990

SOFT COSTS
Total soft costs: Unknown

BUILDING COSTS
Total building costs: $34,747,000
A detailed breakdown of building, site, and costs was not available for this project.

SITE COSTS
Total site costs: Unknown

TOTAL PROJECT COSTS
Total project costs: Unknown

FINANCING SOURCES
Private financing

Part II

Continuing Care Retirement Communities

"If you survive long enough, you're revered—rather like an old building."

KATHERINE HEPBURN, 1907–2003

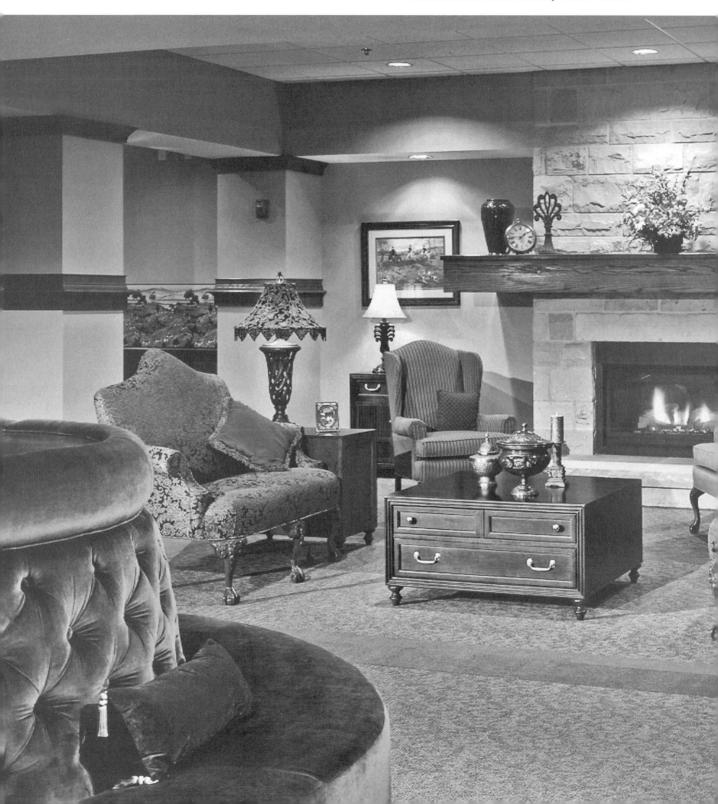

Chapter 3   Avalon Square

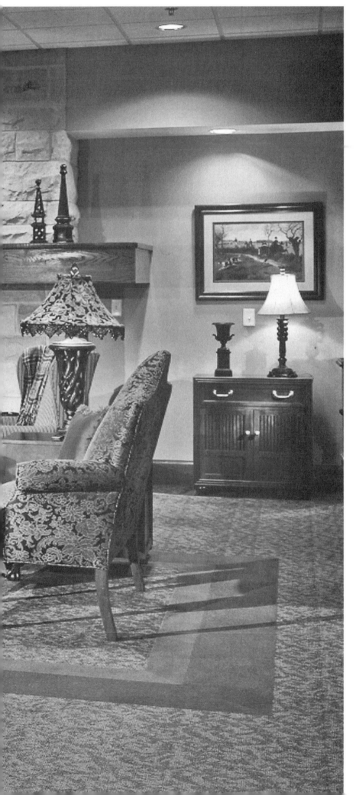

EVALUATION SITE: Avalon Square

COMMUNITY TYPE: Continuing Care Retirement Community
- 68 independent living apartments
- 52 assisted living apartments
- 27 assisted living apartments for those with dementia
- No licensed nursing care

REGION: Northern Midwest

ARCHITECT: KKE Architects, Inc.

OWNER: Presbyterian Homes of Wisconsin

DATA POINTS: Resident Room: 300–1,027 gsf
(assisted living)
675–1,700 gsf (independent living)
Total Area: 43,607 gsf (assisted living)
Total Area: 552 gsf/resident (assisted living)
Total Area: 105,731 gsf (independent living)
Total Area: 1,555 gsf/apartment (independent living)
Overall Total Area: 188,810 gsf
Project Cost: $120.99/gsf
Total Project Cost: $22,845,794
Investment/resident: $155,413.56
Staffing: 3.57 care hours/resident/day (assisted living)
Occupancy: 90% (assisted living) as of December 2005
100% (independent apartments) as of
December 2005

FIRST OCCUPANCY: August 2003

DATE OF EVALUATION: December 2005

EVALUATION TEAM: Margaret Calkins, PhD; Robert Pfauth, AIA; Shari McCabe; David Slack; Jeffrey Anderzhon, AIA; David Fulcher (observer)

FIG. 3-1   Lobby opposite dining room where residents congregate before meals   *Courtesy KKE\Phillip Prowse Photography*

Introduction

Waukesha, Wisconsin, began as a thriving community in the mid-1800s, a time when nearby Milwaukee was just beginning to establish itself. Waukesha, which is located on the Fox River, quickly became an industrial center, with the first sawmill beginning operations in 1837. However, the city's mineral springs quickly took center stage as promoters hawked the water's healing powers. The attraction of the springs spawned a burgeoning tourist trade complete with three different railroad lines bringing tourists from Milwaukee to the city's numerous hotels.

Over the years, Waukesha has been folded into the sprawling suburbs of Milwaukee, but has retained much of the urban character it originally established on its own, particularly in its downtown district. Perhaps it is fitting that Presbyterian Homes of Wisconsin chose to construct this continuing care retirement community of 68 independent living apartments, 52 assisted living apartments, and 27 assisted living apartments for those with dementia so near the healing waters of the springs.

Architect's Statement

This urban infill continuing care retirement community represents the client's desire to expand the spectrum of senior living and care environments they already offer.

Partnering with the city for the additional property acquisition, the campus occupies one square city block fronting Main Street in the downtown area. Integrating the existing 1928 five-story building with an 1871 hotel on the historic registry presented a major design challenge.

Avalon Square is a vertically integrated senior community and mixed-use development offering independent living, assisted living, and a specialty-care residence with an emphasis on memory care programming. A full range of opportunities for social, spiritual, and personal activities are offered in the ground-level town center. Residents have access to a chapel, library, museum and art gallery, café deli, convenience store, restaurant-style dining, private dining, computer networked activity learning center, barber/beauty salon, fitness center, lounges, and a secure, landscaped courtyard.

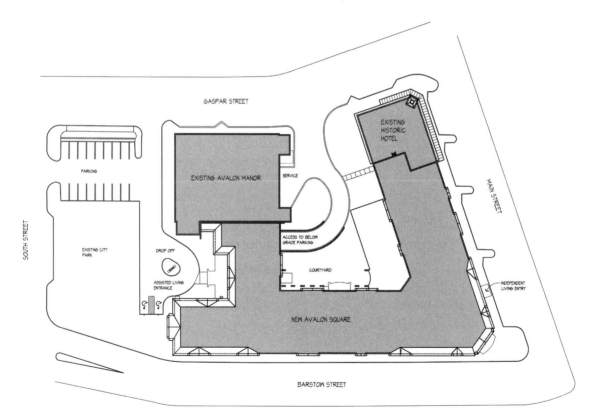

SITE PLAN
NORTH

FIG. 3-2 Site plan *Courtesy KKE Architects, Inc.*

Viable retail space created on Main Street offers immediate access to additional goods and services and enhances the existing urban fabric. The project's scale and use of materials were carefully developed to be sensitive to and compatible with the context of the historic downtown. (See Figure 2 in the color insert.)

Designers' and Owners' Stated Objectives and Responses

OBJECTIVE: Revitalize a blighted downtown Main Street location.

DESIGN INTENT: Retail space was provided along Main Street. Articulated storefronts, awnings, signage, lighting, hardscape features, landscaping, and the re-created hotel loggia all were designed to create pedestrian activity and revitalize the street. The library, with a visible fireplace and large arched windows, allow views into the commons as well as of the activity on Main Street and at the intersection.

OBJECTIVE: Maintain and integrate the historic 1871 hotel.

DESIGN INTENT: A requirement of the development was for the historic hotel to remain and undergo restoration. To begin, the dilapidated and structurally unsound building was taken down stone by stone. The stone was stockpiled off-site and then the building was reconstructed with a historically accurate façade and original stone. Research was done to accurately re-create the cupola that had been lost over the years and large, market-rate independent units were designed to work with the building fenestration. A ground-level retail space is accessible from Main Street via a loggia that reinforces pedestrian scale along the street.

OBJECTIVE: Create a viable, market-rate independent senior living environment in the same building that houses assisted living residents requiring assistance and care.

DESIGN INTENT: There are separate entrances for assisted living and independent resident populations. The site topography falls roughly four feet from Park Place to Main Street, where the designated entry for independent living leads to a gracious stairway up to the elevated lobby and town center. There is also elevator access to the upper floors from the independent living entry. The assisted living entrance is located on the south side of the building facing Park Place, adjacent to a small city park

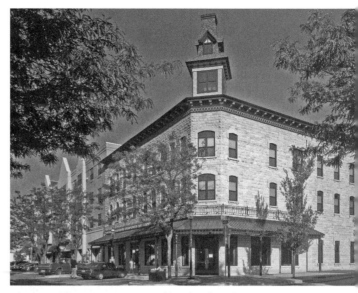

FIG. 3-3 The 1871 reconstructed hotel and retail space on the grade level   *Courtesy KKE\Phillip Prowse Photography*

and fountain, and includes a vehicular drop-off. Elevator cores for both resident populations are accessible from respective areas in the below-grade parking garage. Spacious apartment floor plans include amenities such as washer/dryers, eat-in kitchens, large closets, storage areas, individually controlled heat and central air conditioning, and high-speed Internet access. Many of the apartments have gas fireplaces.

OBJECTIVE: Integrate the existing Avalon Manor Hotel into the new CCRC.

DESIGN INTENT: The existing 1928 Avalon Manor Hotel was completely renovated. All units were redesigned to provide accessibility, appropriate lighting, and current design features while respecting the integrity of the building façade.

OBJECTIVE: Create a design that is responsive to the multifaceted aesthetics of the site context.

DESIGN INTENT: The scale of the building is sensitive to the surrounding structures, and the design of the south side of the project takes its cues from the existing 1928 Avalon Manor Hotel. Similar forms, fenestration, brick, and precast create referential imagery that is sensitive and complementary to the existing building. Additionally, the design for Main Street focused on creating a street façade consistent with the existing street edge. Brick, stucco, and stone, coupled with variations in form, break the mass of the project and imply the presence of several buildings rather than one.

Field Observations: Meeting the Objectives

OBJECTIVE: Revitalize a blighted downtown Main Street location.

FIELD OBSERVATIONS: The choice of location for this community certainly took some courage. There were issues of contiguous site agglomeration from a variety of owners—including an automobile service station with anticipated environmental issues—and the matter of incorporating the design of one historic building as well as another with somewhat less historic value but of great community recognition value. Although "blighted" is a subjective description of the location, there is probably little argument that the development contributed to a revitalization of the downtown area. The commercial space on the lower level of the building introduced occupied, quality retail space that was not previously present. This development was followed by several others in the downtown area, including at least one market-rate apartment project that has helped to bring additional residents to the Main Street area.

OBJECTIVE: Maintain and integrate the historic 1871 hotel.

FIELD OBSERVATIONS: The 1871 hotel, on the corner of Main and Gaspar Streets, and the former Avalon Manor Hotel have direct relationships with the mineral spring spa era of Waukesha's history. There is no doubt that had the building been razed, there would have been an outpouring of community protest. From an architectural and marketing perspective, retaining and integrating the hotel's façade was admirable. Luckily, the cost of doing so was manageable as well.

The integration retains the character of the hotel façade, and the diversity it offers to the street is refreshing. The new portion of the street façade complements the historic building without being at all derivative; much effort was expended to successfully conform the new floor plates to the existing hotel façade.

OBJECTIVE: Create a viable, market-rate independent senior living environment in the same building that houses assisted living residents requiring assistance and care.

FIELD OBSERVATIONS: Ordinarily, the creation of a variety of spaces or apartments within a single structure is not an overly difficult task. That is not the case when integrating the living space of residents requiring varying care levels. Building and health care regulations require a

division between the independent senior living and the assisted living areas, and Avalon Square was not immune to the challenges of this regulation. Although barriers such as this tend to limit resident travel in many facilities, there seem to be elements in the design and layout of Avalon Square that accentuate the division environmentally and socially. Each component is a viable environment on its own, but the facility struggles when trying to operate as one community.

During the evaluation interviews, the administration members said they consider Avalon Square a "mini-CCRC" because there is not a full nursing component within the development. However, they consider the assisted living component to be the heavier health care component, and in fact indicated their desire to consciously adjust the acuity level of the assisted living residents for heavier care.

OBJECTIVE: Integrate the existing Avalon Manor Hotel into the new CCRC.

FIELD OBSERVATIONS: Prior to project start, the owner managed an assisted living operation in the 1928 Avalon Manor Hotel building. Whether for budgetary reasons or to minimize the disruption of construction in the assisted living areas, the renovations to Avalon Manor were minimal compared to the newer parts of the CCRC. The varying quality of the construction in the assisted living versus independent living areas creates a subliminal caste structure that relates to the portion of the building (old or new) in which one resides.

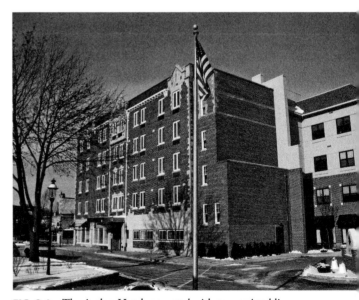

FIG. 3-4 The Avalon Hotel renovated with new assisted living construction connection *Photograph by Jeffrey Anderzhon*

Although the assisted living apartments and social spaces in this portion of the project are certainly nice, they do not compare favorably with those in the newly constructed part of the building. A very long corridor with little relief connects the two areas on the upper residential floors. On the lower level, the social spaces include a large library with ample lounge area, the segregated assisted living/dining room, some administrative offices, and an entry and elevator lobby. The renovation work that went into these areas is quite noticeably not as refined as the new construction. However, the exterior of Avalon Manor retains its original character, provides visual variety, and balances the façade of the 1871 hotel; using it helped the owner avoid creating a massive construction site in the downtown area.

The existing Avalon Manor has indeed been integrated physically into the CCRC, but it appears that this integration was completed with a decreased finishes budget and seems somewhat forced.

OBJECTIVE: Create a design that is responsive to the multifaceted aesthetics of the site context.

FIELD OBSERVATIONS: There can be little argument that the design approach to Avalon Square was sensitive to the site context. Integrating two historic icons into the project was valuable from a public relations standpoint, but it was also important to Waukesha residents. The site plan takes into account all the functions of the CCRC, clearly delineating public and delivery fenestrations. For the most part, the building relates well to its neighbors and fits into its environs.

The north side of the building, which faces Main Street and contains the retail spaces, relates well to the commercial aspects of the avenue. Because of the street angles, the building takes on an almost flat-iron feeling, calling out for the entry to be on the acute angle of the building. Instead, this important building juncture is devoted to an apartment social space that is quite nice, but places somewhat of a barrier between the communities inside and outside of the building. The main independent living entry west of this corner is lost among the start of the retail spaces and the streetscape.

The design of the east side of the building ignores the facing street altogether; though a number of the most popular social spaces are on this first level, the design did not include windows that showcase the street activity. Several chairs have been moved to a short corridor that contains the only windows of any significance (thus allowing residents to keep watch on the activity in the street). Certainly this adjustment is a testament to the residents' desire to engage in and experience the bustle of the downtown streets.

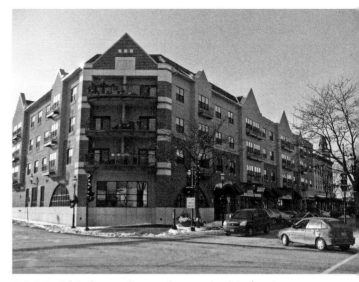

FIG. 3-5 Main Street at Barstow Street, an intuitive location for the front door, rather than the location to the right, below an understated canopy *Photograph by Jeffrey Anderzhon*

On the south façade of the building, the main entry to the CCRC is tucked into a recess created by the back wall of Avalon Manor and a short wing of the new construction. This entry is directly opposite a small city park and its vehicular cul-de-sac creates a pleasant entry experience. Finding this entry can be problematic, though, particularly when one intuitively perceives the flat-iron angle of the building as a natural entrance.

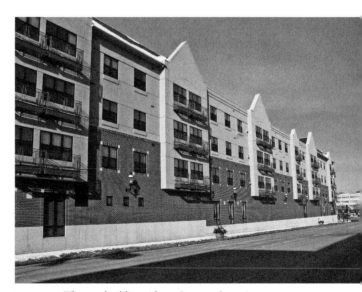

FIG. 3-6 The east building side on Barstow Street is a missed opportunity to provide visual access to the street for residents on the community level *Photograph by Jeffrey Anderzhon*

Field Observations: Themes and Hypotheses

Creating Community

Avalon Square is a very good example of what may well be an increasing trend in continuing care retirement community development: an urban, vertically oriented, single-structure facility. When development takes place in an established and arguably vibrant setting, the facility must integrate into the community rather than create it. In that regard, Avalon Square does well on several counts. It successfully utilizes two well-known structures, integrates the façades into the new project, and provides a design that complements the established urban architecture.

Avalon Square also integrates itself into the community through its retail space. These spaces serve both the larger community, via street access, and, to a lesser extent, the community within the development. Additionally, the wellness center located near the retail spaces provides residents and some 75 members from the larger community an opportunity to participate in structured exercise programs and to use fitness equipment.

Creating a community within the walls of the CCRC is as important as joining with and enhancing the community outside the facility. The CCRC must cross care provision barriers as seamlessly as possible and provide all residents with a sense of belonging to and ownership of the whole. At first blush, the design of Avalon Square appears to provide continuity between the independent living apartments and the assisted living areas. The exterior design neither overtly nor covertly segregates the two levels of elder care provided, but a clear delineation and segregation exists between the two populations, and the interior seems to exacerbate that division. Despite the physical environment's attempts to blend the two populations, the psychological separation between the communities is a powerful barrier and difficult to overcome.

The physical separation of the assisted living and apartment dining areas, as well as the disparate finish

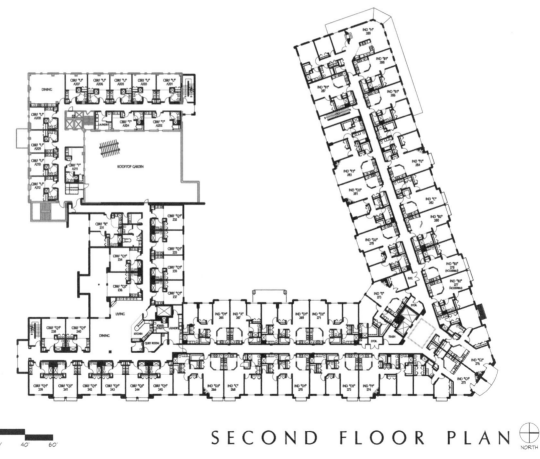

SECOND FLOOR PLAN

NORTH

0' 10' 20'   40'   60'

FIG. 3-7 Second-floor plan, independent and assisted living   *Courtesy KKE Architects, Inc.*

levels in each space, highlights the separation. Other social spaces, including the soda fountain, the "English Room," the "Museum," and the multipurpose room/chapel located at the intersection between assisted living and independent living apartments serve both populations, and do provide venues where some interaction between residents occurs. The design—whether intentional or not—also provides each population with an equal number of social spaces, including the library/lounge area in the Avalon Manor conversion and the upper-level social areas for assisted living. The independent living residents can enjoy the billiards room, card room, and formal library on the main level.

Making a Home

Renovating two recognizable historic buildings certainly provided a familiar home for the residents of Avalon Square. The buildings' history may also engender a certain amount of pride in the residents who call a well-known and well-loved community icon home.

The facility has many useful common areas, such as the soda fountain, billiards room, and libraries, which one hopes provide the residents with a homelike experience and diminish any institutional feel. The disparate finish levels are unfortunate and are not conducive to building a home that everyone feels a part of. Despite some of the design inequalities, the residents enjoy large, well-appointed apartments and lovely, interesting social spaces.

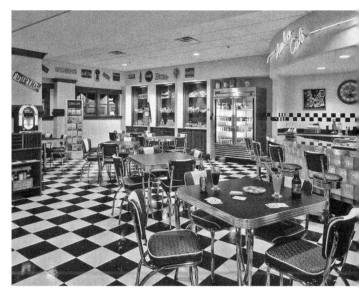

FIG. 3-9 The soda fountain design is taken directly from a community icon that was located in the Avalon Hotel *Courtesy KKE \ Phillip Prowse Photography*

Regional/Cultural Design

Integration of the 1871 hotel façade and the 1928 Avalon Manor Hotel building into the design of this CCRC created a structure that directly addresses the design of the region. The newer portions of the building complement the existing design fabric of the community without appearing overpowering or derivative. The structure definitely feels at home in its location.

The interior designs of the soda fountain and English Room pay tribute to two established community cultural icons, but unfortunately the rooms are generally restricted to apartment residents and cannot be widely enjoyed by all. Both draw their design inspiration directly from spaces original to the Avalon Manor Hotel.

Environmental Therapy

The environment appears to provide a fulfilling and comfortable quality of life for the independent living and assisted living residents. The location of Avalon Square continually provides residents with vicarious interactions and views of the surrounding city. Participation with the neighborhood would have been enhanced, or at least emphasized, with additional street-level windows. The facility design and layout provide adequate formal and informal and private and shared social spaces. The various areas support the lifestyles of the residents and at least provide alternatives to simply spending all of one's time in an apartment.

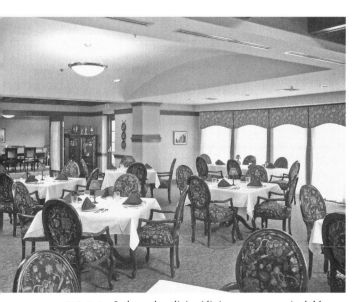

FIG. 3-8 Independent living/dining room opposite lobby shown in Fig. 3-1 *Courtesy KKE \ Phillip Prowse Photography*

Outdoor Environment

The building site is both urban and restricted. Providing appropriate entries for the public, for active independent residents, and for service deliveries leaves little site space for effective exterior environmental development. Although small, the courtyard accessed from the apartment dining room and the entry gallery is attractive and inviting.

On the second level of the Avalon Manor portion of the structure, there is a rooftop garden designed primarily for assisted living residents with memory impairment. Access to this area is difficult and probably not possible without staff supervision. The garden is secured by a high wooden fencing system that restricts visual access to the rest of the property. It does appear to be well used, particularly for structured outdoor activities, and it logically fills the need for exterior environments on a tight building site.

Quality of Workplace and the Physical Plant

The communication problems inherent in a vertically oriented CCRC affect both residents and staff. Administrative offices are centralized near the main entry on the lower level. Although this layout may promote broader communication among area leaders, it translates into cumbersome travel distances for staff and consequently less time devoted to actual care provision. Similarly, the separation of the dining rooms creates a somewhat problematic approach to the service of resident meals. The commercial kitchen is directly adjacent to the assisted living/dining room, but is some distance from the apartment dining room. Prepared foods must be carted across the main entry gallery into a secondary, well-equipped "pantry" and then into the apartment dining room. This creates a rather convoluted and lengthy path.

Operator Perspectives

Presbyterian Homes of Wisconsin made a conscious commitment to the community when it selected the downtown location for Avalon Square. There were numerous obstacles to overcome for its success, many of which had little or nothing to do with the physical design of the structure. Given the myriad of unmovable parameters, the operator is generally pleased with the result, but it also readily admits that a series of compromises was made during the course of construction. Achieving a higher level of social interaction between the two distinct populations within the facility is of paramount concern to the operator. Pursuing the objective of adjusting the acuity level of the assisted living residents will make a solution to this problem all the more difficult to achieve.

Presbyterian Homes is very aware of the problems that arise when operating a vertically oriented CCRC, which are exacerbated in this case by the distance from one end of the building to the other created by the U-shaped floor plate. However, we observed during our visit that the quality of care has not diminished as a result of the physical restrictions of the facility, and the residents we interviewed wholeheartedly consider Avalon Square their home.

General Project Information

PROJECT ADDRESS
Avalon Square
222 Park Place
Waukesha, WI 53186-4815

PROJECT DESIGN TEAM
Architect: KKE Architects, Inc.
Interior Designer: Encompass Interiors
Landscape Architect: None; landscaping by owner
Structural Engineer: Pierce Engineers, Inc.
Mechanical Engineer: Design/build contractor
Electrical Engineer: Design/build contractor
Civil Engineer: Jahnke & Jahnke Associates, Inc.
Contractor: The Jansen Group, Inc.

PROJECT STATUS
Completion date: August 2003

OCCUPANCY LEVELS
At facility opening date: 90% (independent apartments)
                              40% (assisted living)
At time of evaluation: 100% (independent apartments)
                              90% (assisted living)

RESIDENT AGE (YRS)
At facility opening date: 79 (independent apartments)
                              84 (assisted living)
At time of evaluation: 82.5 (independent apartments)
                              88.3 (assisted living)

PROJECT AREAS

Project Element	Units, Beds, or Clients	New GSF	Renovated GSF	Total Gross Area	Total on Site or Served by Project
		Included in This Project			
Independent living apartments (units)	68	79,046	0	79,046	79,046
Assisted living (units)	52	22,036	20,526	42,562	42,562
Assisted living for dementia (units)	27	11,018	6,842	17,860	17,860
Common social areas (people)	181	22,000	8,166	30,166	30,166
Kitchen (daily meals served)	215	504	2,254	2,758	2,758
Elder outreach/home health (clients)	120	600	0	600	600
Retail space (shops/restaurants, etc.)	5 spaces	12,606	0	12,606	12,606
Fitness/rehab/wellness (daily visits)	35	3,212	0	3,212	3,212
Total		**151,022**	**37,788**		**188,810**

INDEPENDENT LIVING RETIREMENT APARTMENTS

Project Element	No.	Size Range
	Apartments	
One-bedroom units	24	675–807 GSF
One-bedroom/den units	27	929–1,091 GSF
Two-bedroom units	15	1,157–1,216 GSF
Two-bedroom plus den units	2	1,700 GSF
Total (all units)	68	66,565 GSF
Residents' social areas (lounges, dining, and spaces)		27,560 GSF
Medical/health/fitness and activities areas		3,776 GSF
Administrative, public, and ancillary support service areas		425 GSF
Service, maintenance, and mechanical areas		3,580 GSF
Total gross area		105,731 GSF
Total net usable area (per space program)		87,600 NSF
Overall gross/net factor (ratio of gross area/net usable area)		1.21

ASSISTED LIVING

Project Element	New Construction No. Units	New Construction Typical Size	Renovations No. Units	Renovations Typical Size
Studio units		GSF	27	415 GSF
One-bedroom units	20	697 GSF	3	680 GSF
Two-bedroom units	2	1,027 GSF		0 GSF
Total (all units)	52	15,994 GSF		13,245 GSF
Residents' social areas (lounges, dining, and recreation spaces)				785 GSF
Medical, health care, therapy, and activities spaces				0 GSF
Administrative, public, and ancillary support services				880 GSF
Service, maintenance, and mechanical areas				0 GSF
Total gross area				30,904 GSF
Total net usable area (per space program)				30,024 NSF
Overall gross/net factor (ratio of gross area/net usable area)				1.03

DEMENTIA-SPECIFIC ASSISTED LIVING

Project Element	New Construction		Renovations	
	No. Units	Typical Size	No. Units	Typical Size
Studio units	14	428 GSF	12	300 GSF
One-bedroom units	1	575 GSF		0 GSF
Total (all units)	27	6,567 GSF		3,600 GSF
Residents' social areas (lounges, dining, and recreation spaces)				2,081 GSF
Medical, health care, therapy, and activities spaces				GSF
Administrative, public, and ancillary support services				
On floor				455 GSF
Service, maintenance, and mechanical areas				0 GSF
Total gross area				12,703 GSF
Total net usable area (per space program)				12,248 NSF
Overall gross/net factor (ratio of gross area/net usable area)				1.04

OTHER FACILITIES

Project Element	New Construction	
	No.	Size
Wellness/fitness center	1	3,212 GSF

SITE AND PARKING

SITE SIZE
Acres: 1.83
Square feet: 80,000

PARKING

Type of Parking	For This Facility			
	Residents	Staff	Visitors	Totals
Open surface lot(s)			18	18
Underground garage	90			90
Totals	90		18	108

CONSTRUCTION COSTS

SOURCE OF COST DATA
Final construction cost as of August 25, 2003

SOFT COSTS

Land cost or value:	$394,712
All permit and other entitlement fees: Included in contract for construction	
Legal and professional fees:	$490,000
Appraisals:	Included in finance fee
Marketing and preopening:	$407,000
Total soft costs:	$6,761,642*

*Included capital interest, working capital finance, development fee, and FF&E.

BUILDING COSTS

New construction except FF&E, special finishes, floor and window coverings, HVAC, and electrical:	$9,810,747
Renovations except FF&E, special finishes, floor and window coverings, HVAC, and electrical:	$2,400,000
FF&E and small wares:	$450,000
Floor coverings:	$410,820
Window coverings:	$26,039
HVAC:	$1,912,116
Electrical:	$1,074,430
Medical equipment costs:	N/A
Total building costs:	$16,084,152

SITE COSTS

New on-site:	$1,112,284
New off-site:	N/A
Renovation on-site:	N/A
Renovation off-site:	N/A
Landscape:	N/A
Special site features or amenities:	N/A
Total site costs:	$1,112,284

TOTAL PROJECT COSTS

(Includes all fees and costs, except financing)

Total project costs: $22,845,794

FINANCING SOURCES

501c(3) Housing & Urban Development guaranteed bonds and owner equity

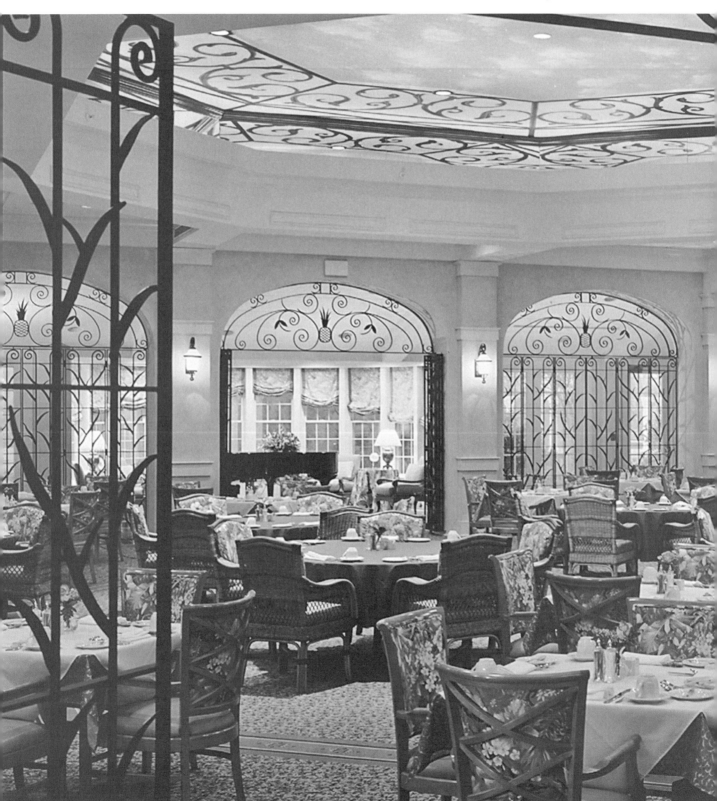

"My health is good; it's my age that's bad."

ROY ACUFF AT AGE 83, 1903–1992

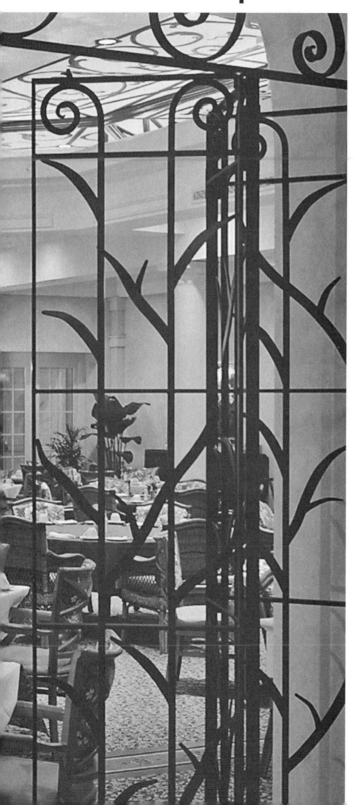

Chapter 4

Bishop Gadsden Episcopal Retirement Community

EVALUATION SITE: Bishop Gadsden Episcopal Retirement Community

COMMUNITY TYPE: Continuing Care Retirement Community
- 56 villas for retirement
- 98 independent living apartments
- 8 nursing care beds

AUTHOR'S NOTE: *Since the project was originally submitted, 84 assisted living apartments and 19 assisted living apartments for those with dementia have been added to the 42 nursing care beds on this campus. The data for these additions is not included here.*

REGION: Mid-South

ARCHITECT: Cochran, Stephenson & Donkervoet, Inc.

OWNER: Bishop Gadsden Episcopal Retirement Community

DATA POINTS: Resident Room: 1,915–2,135 gsf (villas)
995–1,550 gsf (independent living)
260 gsf (nursing)
Total Area: 112,315 gsf (villas)
Total Area: 2,005.63 gsf/unit (villas)
Total Area: 194,360 gsf (independent living)
Total Area: 1,222.39 gsf/apartment (independent living)
Total Area: 7,400 gsf (nursing)
Total Area: 925 gsf/resident (nursing)
Overall Total Area: 446,025 gsf
Project Cost: $108.74/gsf
Total Project Cost: $48,500,000
Investment/resident: $299,382.71
Staffing: 3.21 care hours/resident/day (nursing care)
Occupancy: 95% (nursing) as of April 2006
100% (villas and independent apartments) as of April 2006

FIG. 4-1 Main dining room with wrought iron work reminiscent of vintage iron work in Charleston *Photo by Rion Rizzo, Creative Sources Photography*

FIRST OCCUPANCY: April 1999

DATE OF EVALUATION: April 2006

EVALUATION TEAM: Terri Sherman; Karen Hodge; Thomas Hauer; Eric McRoberts, AIA; Jeffrey Anderzhon, AIA

Introduction

Bishop Gadsden has grown over the past 21 years from an assisted living and nursing facility into a full CCRC that includes independent living apartments and cottages, and a shared space called the Commons. Bishop Gadsden draws upon the regional style and southern charm of nearby Charleston, South Carolina, for its architectural style and character. The use of exterior materials such as brick, stucco, and wrought iron, along with courtyard-centered building planning, clearly make this project at home in its setting. A tree-lined and heavily landscaped entry drive, along with a strategically placed new chapel, reinforces Bishop Gadsden's southern roots and religious affiliation.

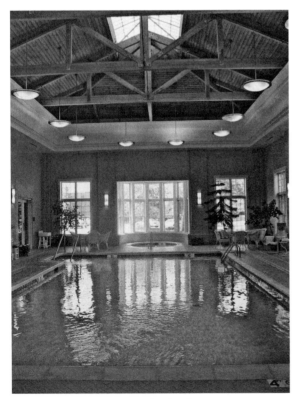

FIG. 4-2 The swimming pool and wellness center
Photograph by Jeffrey Anderzhon

The campus houses 159 residents in independent living apartments, 56 residents in independent living cottages, and 84 assisted living residents in studios and one- and two-bedroom apartments. A memory support unit for 19 residents and 50 skilled beds round out the CCRC.

The entry experience is comfortable and welcoming, reminiscent of a large southern home with a series of linked rooms or parlors that are on an axis with and lead to a large landscaped courtyard. In an effort to attract younger seniors, the new apartments and cottages are spacious, and the Commons extensive. Linked by an enclosed, daylit promenade, the new Commons area includes multiple dining venues, a pub, an auditorium, an indoor pool and fitness center, a clinic/pharmacy, a business center, and a beautiful new chapel.

Our short visit made it apparent that Bishop Gadsden embodies the notion of southern hospitality. In its buildings, grounds, and people, it offers not only a high quality of southern living for residents, but also a wonderful work environment for staff.

Designers' and Operators' Stated Objectives and Responses

OBJECTIVE: Convert a successful assisted living and nursing center into a full CCRC.

DESIGN INTENT: Add new Commons, independent living apartments, and cottages to existing campus.

OBJECTIVE: Attract younger, more active seniors.

DESIGN INTENT: The designers aimed to provide larger-than-average unit plans and to incorporate features found in "empty nester" communities. The Commons are equipped with a range of active adult amenities, including a pool, fitness center, café, shops, and business center, as well as extensive nature trails for outdoor activities.

OBJECTIVE: Develop a strong Charlestonian character and image.

DESIGN INTENT: The facilities were planned—inside and out—to conjure the images of Charleston: lushly landscaped courtyards, and large and small Georgian architectural designs that have been adapted to the country lifestyle. The cottages look like many typical homes in Charleston, complete with a side porch entrance facing a street façade.

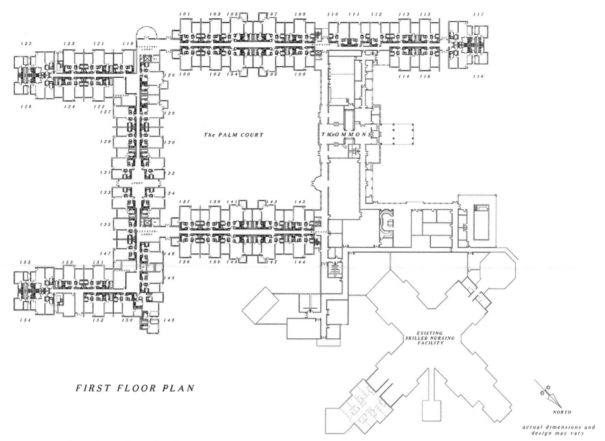

The PALM COURT

THE COMMONS

EXISTING SKILLED NURSING FACILITY

NORTH

actual dimensions and design may vary

FIRST FLOOR PLAN

FIG. 4-3 Floor plan, independent living and community center *Courtesy of Cochran, Stephenson & Donkervoet, Inc.*

OBJECTIVE: Create a new identity for the community that is accessible to all residents.

DESIGN INTENT: Provide direct, convenient, indoor access for residents of assisted living and nursing to the informal activity areas of the Commons, which provide wellness, optional activities, and alternative dining opportunities.

OBJECTIVE: Allow each level of care to have its own identity.

DESIGN INTENT: Each building group retains its own entrance, with convenient, fully accessible parking and common areas.

OBJECTIVE: Give independent living residents options for aging in place.

DESIGN INTENT: All of the units include a customary range of accessibility features and are fully adaptable to wheelchair usage. The apartment building and Commons have electric cart parking areas, and specific valet parking areas within the Commons encourage the residents in the cottages to use their golf carts to visit other areas of the campus. There are golf cart parking areas at all cottages as well.

OBJECTIVE: Preserve the natural beauty of the site.

DESIGN INTENT: The cottages and apartments are designed around lovely, landscaped ponds and gardens. Additionally, the design team placed cottages and buildings throughout the campus in locations that did not disrupt the stately live oak trees growing on the property.

OBJECTIVE: Create a design that helps to maximize operational efficiency.

DESIGN INTENT: The back-of-the-house functions were relocated to the new Commons areas to deliver service seamlessly and more efficiently to all parts of the campus. The move was undertaken to benefit and improve service to all three levels of care.

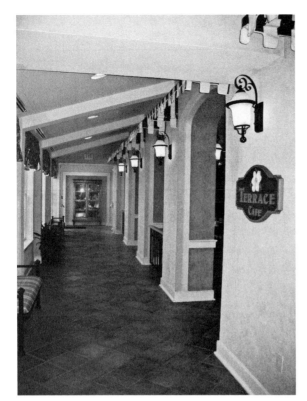

FIG. 4-4 "Main Street" access to café and other community center amenities. A single-loaded corridor with natural light that penetrates into the building *Photograph by Jeffrey Anderzhon*

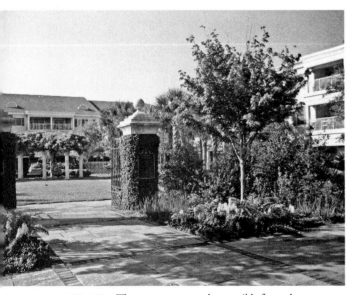

FIG. 4-5 The center courtyard, accessible from the community center and apartments, has seating areas, open spaces, sun and shade *Photograph by Jeffrey Anderzhon*

OBJECTIVE: Meet special care needs of residents.

DESIGN INTENT: An eight-unit memory care unit was included in the work when the assisted living addition was constructed, to further improve aging-in-place options. The unit has its own wanderers' path, secure outdoor garden, and family living areas.

Field Observations: Meeting the Objectives

OBJECTIVE: Convert a successful assisted living and nursing center into a full CCRC.

FIELD OBSERVATIONS: Although the original assisted living and nursing center were designed in keeping with the traditional medical model, the cottages, independent living apartments, and Commons area have transformed the campus into a showpiece for southern retirement living. Bishop Gadsden now offers the full continuum of care, including independent cottages, apartment independent living, assisted living, assisted living memory support, and skilled nursing care. The recent renovations and additions to the assisted living and nursing center, as well as a new centerpiece chapel, created a more consistent interior architecture throughout the CCRC.

Financially, Bishop Gadsden is a very sound and market-desirable CCRC with three- and five-year waiting lists for the apartments and cottages, respectively. The new cottages and apartments are spacious and offer many attractive amenities for residents. The approach, entry, and Commons also make a great first impression that is carried throughout the entire CCRC.

OBJECTIVE: Attract younger, more active seniors.

FIELD OBSERVATIONS: The scale, layout, and "Charleston" character of the new Commons should certainly appeal to younger seniors. Reminiscent of a fine southern resort, Bishop Gadsden includes a pool and fitness area, formal dining room, informal café, pub/lounge, auditorium, business center, beauty shop, and pharmacy.

Most of the amenities are connected through daylit walkways with a strong visual connection to the well-landscaped courtyards that draw inspiration from the gardens of Charleston. Bishop Gadsden's strong affiliation to the Citadel and the College of Charleston, as well as convenience to downtown Charleston's rich cultural heritage, also appeal to younger seniors.

OBJECTIVE: Develop a strong Charlestonian character and image.

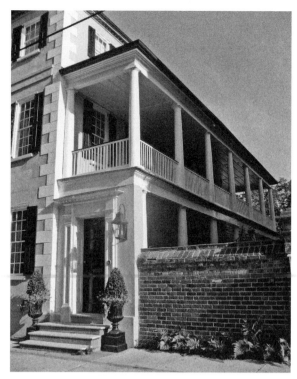

FIG. 4-6 A typical Charleston house with a "shotgun porch" entry *Photograph by Jeffrey Anderzhon*

FIELD OBSERVATIONS: The initial approach down Bishop Gadsden's tree-lined drive to the entry lobby and Commons showcases the landscaped courtyards and brick and stucco façade that exude Charlestonian charm and character. The new apartments, cottages, and Commons

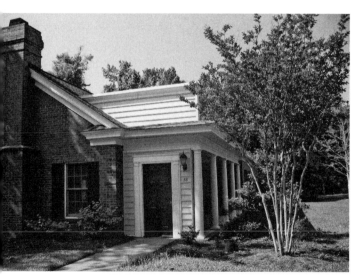

FIG. 4-7 A Bishop Gadsden cottage with a "shotgun porch" entry *Photograph by Jeffrey Anderzhon*

area are organized around heavily landscaped courtyards enhanced by native plants and typical southern garden amenities. Wrought iron, a popular material in Charleston's many gardens, is not only found throughout the courtyards, but also serves as internal room dividers and a mural motif in the dining areas.

The interiors are comfortable, with a warm color palette to complement the white wood detailing at doors and entrances. Period furniture pieces are situated throughout, as is artwork from local artists, mostly depicting scenes of Charleston. (See Figure 3 in color insert.) The shotgun side porches, with an entry door at the front, are part of an interesting cottage design that reflects one of Charleston's signature details.

OBJECTIVE: Create a new identity for the community that is accessible to all residents.

FIELD OBSERVATIONS: The new Charlestonian entry and the Commons are the hubs of activity for the community. All levels of housing and care, except the cottages, have interior connections to the Commons area. As is often the case with large CCRCs, the travel distance to and from the Commons is excessive for the apartment residents and might deter participation in activities. Connections to the Commons from the assisted living and skilled care areas were long and a bit circuitous, minimizing their contribution to the vitality of the Commons areas.

The new chapel, though beautiful, is located at the front entrance to the community and is a great distance from the Commons. It is accessible to independent living residents externally or by traversing through the health center. A more central location for the chapel might have provided better access to all residents on campus.

OBJECTIVE: Allow each level of care to have its own identity.

FIELD OBSERVATIONS: With the exception of the new assisted living memory support neighborhood, each level of care retains its own entry, and this delineates one from the other. The skilled care and assisted living memory support units are clearly defined, self-contained areas. The memory support area was recently renovated and the skilled care will soon be upgraded from its medical-model layout.

The recent demolition of 26 smaller assisted living studios and subsequent construction of 40 new one- and two-bedroom assisted living apartments brought the total number of assisted living units to 84. The changing layout drew a line between the old and the new. The separation has affected not only residents but also staff assigned to their respective areas. Little socializing occurs between the two groups.

OBJECTIVE: Give independent living residents options for aging in place.

FIELD OBSERVATIONS: Bishop Gadsden has taken into account the fact that as independent living apartment residents age and become less mobile, they may need mobility devices such as golf carts, electric carts, or wheelchairs. There are spaces throughout the campus and cottages allotted for mobility devices. These parking spaces are well conceived, and hidden so as to not hinder marketing efforts. In the cottages, a small, covered breezeway area allows convenient golf cart storage. Strategically placed hallway niches in the independent living areas provide ample space for parking electric carts.

It is not clear how difficult it would be to convert an independent living apartment for the accessibility required for an aging-in-place resident. Bishop Gadsden does not have a strong philosophy or history of aging in place, but hopes that the strong residential character at all levels of care will help comfort residents who are moving through the continuum.

OBJECTIVE: Preserve the natural beauty of the site.

FIELD OBSERVATIONS: During the planning stages, the community took obvious care to work around existing mature trees. Because of this, Bishop Gadsden gives the overall impression of an older, well-established CCRC. The entrance drive and cottages take advantage of natural ponds, which also allow the growth of adjacent vegetation consistent with the geographical area.

The courtyards, which are so much a part of the

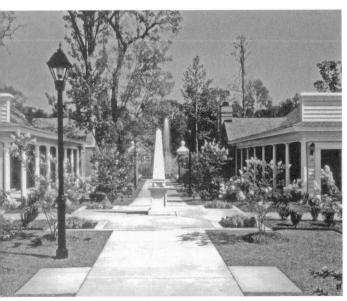

FIG. 4-8 The cottage courtyard provides a sense of order to the campus plan *Photo by Dickson Dunlap*

character and fabric of Charleston, are well defined and beautifully landscaped, but provide few shaded areas or opportunities for outdoor activities. The courtyards tend to be visual amenities rather than sites of activity, particularly in the warmest South Carolina weather. Residents would also like to have more opportunities for gardening and a central pavilion for large outdoor gatherings.

OBJECTIVE: Create a design that helps to maximize operational efficiency.

FIELD OBSERVATIONS: Although designers hoped that the new Commons would improve deficiencies in service and operations, many issues remain. A single loading dock provides shipping and receiving for all food, medical supplies, paper products, and trash, which creates problems with overlapping services.

Two separate preparation kitchens necessitate redundancy in equipment as well as transportation of food supplies. Food in bulk must traverse the skilled care dining room to access the serving pantry. A few corridors that were designated for service and finished accordingly have become common corridors for residents and staff to access various portions of the building. The serving line in the café is inefficient and a primary concern for residents.

OBJECTIVE: Meet special care needs of residents.

FIELD OBSERVATIONS: The "Arcadia" memory support area includes eight new private rooms that were added to 11 existing rooms. These 19 beds constitute the assisted living memory support area, a secured unit with looped corridor design that allows residents to wander freely by eliminating any dead-end corridors.

Commons and activity areas include a living room, residential activity kitchen, and casual seating area, which are all well utilized and create a social environment. The dining room is separated from the other activity areas so as to be less confusing to residents. The dining room is bright, with a view of a secured courtyard; however, the dining room is not large enough to accommodate visitors and the courtyard not large enough for any outdoor group activities. The resident rooms are all private and large, but not oriented with a view from the bed to the bathroom for cueing.

Field Observations: Themes and Hypotheses

Creating Community

Staff and residents agree that the spacious, beautifully designed Commons areas provide a wonderful setting for

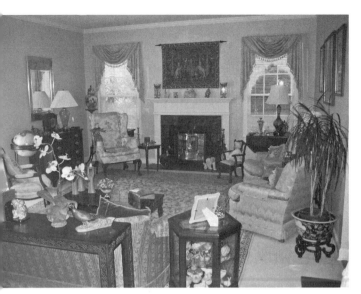

FIG. 4-9 A cottage living room made into a home by the residents *Photograph by Jeffrey Anderzhon*

gatherings and socialization and promote a strong sense of community at Bishop Gadsden. The strong Georgian appointments consistent with neighboring Charleston are warm and authentic and emulate the comfort of a large southern home. An energetic activities staff and programs at all levels of care, along with a new "Samaritan" program that allows independent living residents to volunteer in the assisted living and nursing units, help to knit the community together. The only barrier to community building is the difficulty between long-standing residents and new residents in the assisted living household.

Making a Home

The apartments toured were well organized and spacious, with high ceilings. Each apartment includes an exterior patio or balcony with lovely views to the heavily landscaped courtyards. Although the units themselves may appeal to a younger population, the apartment corridors were long and unbroken with fewer views, daylight, or connections to the outdoors.

The new cottages are distinctive in layout and character. Each a single unit, the cottages use the common Charleston "shotgun" porch to give them a contextual presence. They are spacious, with a glazed sunroom, often oriented toward a water feature, and all connected to one another as well as to the Commons through a landscaped, grid sidewalk system. Although the size, layout, and character of the cottages would have much appeal to a younger senior, the lack of storage—particularly in the bedrooms—was a concern noted by residents.

Regional/Cultural Design

Stately oaks, lush gardens, and brick façades lend Bishop Gadsden a charm and aesthetic inspired by the Georgian architecture of Charleston. Porches typical of the region, native plants, and other design details further enhance the Charlestonian character.

The community succeeds in developing a connection to the typical regional design and has executed that design with elegance and quality. The period furniture and artwork from local artists are warm reminders of the southern appeal of the Carolinas.

Environmental Therapy

The addition of cottages, apartments, the Commons area, and assisted living memory support complete the full continuum of care at Bishop Gadsden. The grounds, beautiful southern interiors, resident amenities, spacious apartments, and single cottages all have great market appeal and have put this facility on a strong financial base with a lengthy waiting list. The only inconsistency within the continuum of care apparent to the evaluators was the older assisted living and nursing center.

The community's commitment to aging in place has yet to be fully tested, but parts of the design do speak to that commitment. Parking for carts and motorized wheelchairs is an important feature to encourage independence and movement as residents age and experience

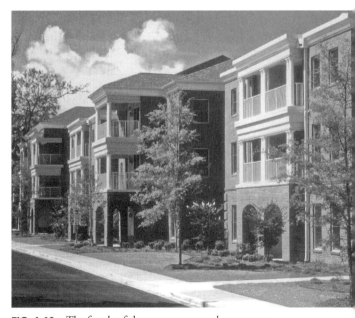

FIG. 4-10 The façade of the center courtyard apartments reflects the use of brick in a Charleston vernacular architectural style *Photo by Dickson Dunlap*

limited mobility. The outdoor spaces and Commons spaces also enhance the environment for residents.

The original assisted living portion is comprised mostly of studio units with tight bathrooms, making accessibility difficult. Interior finishes were recently upgraded in resident corridors, but still lack the spaciousness, connection to the outdoors, and charming southern character of the newer buildings.

The health center, which maintains a central nurses' station, lacks daylight and open spaces. The skilled care dining room also lacks the daylight and charm found in the other dining venues. Despite the few shortfalls, environment is only one part of the equation in a successful health center. The committed and energetic staff and activities programs were first rate and no doubt contribute to the health and well-being of residents.

Outdoor Environment

The grounds, from the entry to the numerous interior courtyards and gardens, are exquisite at Bishop Gadsden, and certainly part of its strong market appeal. The design of the hardscape and use of indigenous trees and plants are consistent with the Charleston motif and enhance the surrounding architecture. Interior spaces, particularly in the Commons areas, relate well to the exterior courtyards through glazed promenades.

The new independent living apartment corridors and original assisted living and nursing center are not as bright and well connected to the outdoors as other areas on the campus. The gardens and courtyards, though visually inviting, lack activity even on pleasant, sunny days like that of the evaluation. In general, the spaces do not offer opportunities for outside activities or shade from the hot southern sun.

Quality of Workplace and the Physical Plant

The beautiful environment of Bishop Gadsden benefits not only residents and families but also quality of work-place for staff. Staff were very energetic, upbeat, and consistently attested to their philosophy of providing resident-centered care. Based on the long tenure of most of the staff interviewed, Bishop Gadsden seems to be a pleasant place to work. Many programs and perks are in place for the 320 staff members, and they are encouraged to constantly improve knowledge, education, and training. Staff did consistently mention that a general lack of storage throughout the community and undersized employee break rooms are two of the campus' deficiencies as a work environment.

Operator Perspectives

Bishop Gadsden is delighted with the ambiance of the new apartments, cottages, and Commons, and feels that the recently completed chapel rounds out the elegant design of the campus. The operator is pleased with the ways the designers captured the Charleston vernacular in the interior and exterior architecture. Coupled with the high quality of care, these features have made Bishop Gadsden a community of choice. The proximity of Charleston is also a powerful draw for the community.

As with any newly completed, large project, in hindsight the owner would have changed several elements of the design. The café, a popular dining venue for residents, is not well planned and is congested by poor traffic flow. The Commons area provides residents with opportunities for small and large group activities, but lacks intermediate-sized spaces. They would also have preferred a day spa area near the pool and fitness areas to provide a central wellness hub.

The owner clearly understands that the older assisted living and nursing center spaces must be renovated to compete with the interior design and spatial quality of the newer housing areas and the Commons. The owner intends to address these and other design issues in a subsequent phase of development.

General Project Information

PROJECT ADDRESS
Bishop Gadsden Episcopal Retirement Community
1 Bishop Gadsden Way
Charleston, SC 29412

PROJECT DESIGN TEAM
Architect: Cochran, Stephenson & Donkervoet, Inc.
Associate Architects: Steven Goggans & Associates, Inc.
  Cummings & McCrady, Inc.
Interior Designer: GMK Associates, Inc.
Landscape Architect: Charleston Design Group
Structural Engineer: Kyzer & Timmerman
Mechanical Engineer: McKnight-Smith-Ward-Griffin
  Engineers, Inc.
Electrical Engineer: McKnight-Smith-Ward-Griffin
  Engineers, Inc.
Civil Engineer: Hussey, Gay, Bell & DeYoung, Inc.
Dining Consultant: Culinary Design Services, Inc.
Gerontologist: Lorraine Hiatt, Ph.D.
Management/Development: N/A
Contractor: McDevitt Street Bovis, Inc.

PROJECT STATUS
Completion date: April 1999

OCCUPANCY LEVELS
At facility opening date: Not available
At date of evaluation: 100% (villas and apartments)
95% (nursing)

RESIDENT AGE (YRS)
At facility opening date: 82
At date of evaluation: 84

PROJECT AREAS

		Included in This Project		
Project Element	Units, Beds, or Clients	New GSF	Total Gross Area	Total on Site or Served by Project
Apartments	159	263,700	263,700	159
Cottages/villas	56	151,000	151,000	56
Skilled nursing care	8	7,400	7,400	48
Common social areas	265	12,000	12,000	265
Kitchen	660	6,000	6,000	660
Retail space (shops/restaurants, etc.)	2 spaces	1,400	1,400	2 spaces
Fitness/rehabilitation/wellness (daily visits)	N/A	1,200	1,200	N/A
Pool(s) and related areas (users)	N/A	3,325	3,325	N/A

RESIDENTIAL FACILITIES

Project Element		Cottages			Apartments	
	No.	Typical Size (GSF)	Size Range (GSF)	No.	Typical Size (GSF)	Size Range (GSF)
Studio units				20	995	995
One-bedroom units				25	860	860
Two-bedroom units				62	1,230	1,225–1,370
Two-bedroom plus den units	56	2,005	1,915–2,135	52	1,550	1,405–1,550
Total (all units)	56	112,315	GSF	159	194,360 GSF	
Residents' social areas (lounges, dining, and spaces):					2,200 GSF	
Medical/health/fitness and activities areas:					0 GSF	
Administrative, public, and ancillary support service areas:					7,700 GSF	
Service, maintenance, and mechanical areas:					13,650 GSF	
Total gross area:					274,876 GSF	
Total net usable area (per space program):					217,910 NSF	
Overall gross/net factor (ratio of gross area/net usable area):					1.26	

SKILLED NURSING

Project Element	New Construction	
	No. Beds	Typical Room Size
Residents in one-bed/single rooms	8	260 GSF
Total	8	2,080 GSF
Social areas (lounges, dining, and recreation spaces)		1,025 GSF
Medical, health care, therapy, and activities spaces		255 GSF
Administrative, public, and ancillary support services		225 GSF
Service, maintenance, and mechanical areas		0 GSF
Total gross area:		7,400 GSF
Total net usable area (per space program):		3,585 NSF
Overall gross/net factor (ratio of gross area/net usable area):		2.06

OTHER FACILITIES—COMMUNITY CENTER

Project Element	New Construction
Social areas (lounges, dining, and recreation spaces)	18,900 GSF
Administrative, public, and ancillary support services	9,800 GSF
Service, maintenance, and mechanical areas	6,000 GSF
Total gross area	50,400 GSF
Total net usable area (per space program)	30,700 NSF
Overall gross/net factor (ratio of gross area/net usable area)	1.64

SITE AND PARKING

SITE LOCATION
Suburban

SITE SIZE
Acres: 52.8
Square feet: 2,299,968

PARKING

Type of Parking	For This Facility			
	Residents	Staff	Visitors	Totals
Open surface lot(s)	185	28	23	236
Carports or garages	100			100
Totals	285	28	23	336

CONSTRUCTION COSTS

SOURCE OF COST DATA
Final construction cost as of April 1999

SOFT COSTS
Land cost or value:	N/A
Basic architectural and engineering:	N/A
Expanded architectural and engineering:	N/A
All permit and other entitlement fees:	N/A
Legal:	N/A
Appraisals:	N/A
Marketing and pre-opening:	N/A
Total soft costs:	N/A

BUILDING COSTS
New construction except FF&E, special finishes, floor and window coverings, HVAC, and electrical and medical equipment:	$42,250,000
Renovations except FF&E, special finishes, floor and window coverings, HVAC, and electrical:	In above
FF&E and small wares:	In above
Floor coverings:	In above
Window coverings:	In above
HVAC, plumbing, fire protection:	In above
Electrical:	In above
Medical equipment costs:	In above
Total building costs:	$42,250,000

SITE COSTS
New on-site:	$6,250,000
New off-site:	N/A
Renovation on-site:	N/A
Renovation off-site:	N/A
Landscape:	In above
Special site features or amenities:	N/A
Total site costs:	$6,250,000

TOTAL PROJECT COSTS
(INCLUDE ALL FEES AND COSTS, EXCEPT FINANCING)
Total project costs: $48,500,000

FINANCING SOURCES
Nontaxable bonds through Charleston County Health Facility revenue bonds

CARE COMPARISONS

AUTHOR'S NOTE: *Bishop Gadsden does not participate in Medicare/Medicaid, thus care comparison data is not available.*

"The trouble with life in the fast lane is that you get to the other end in an awful hurry."

JOHN JENSEN, 1965–

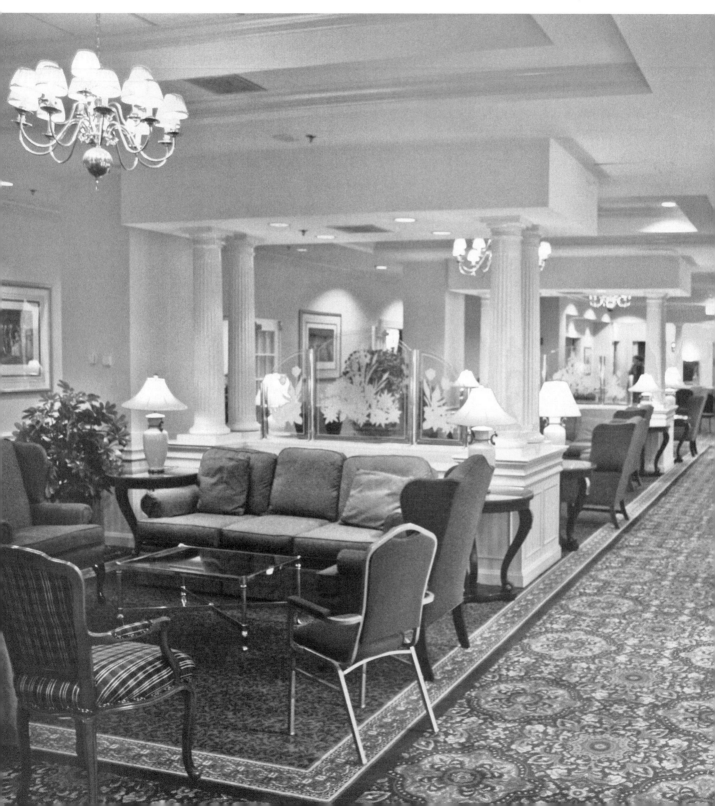

Chapter 5   The Jefferson

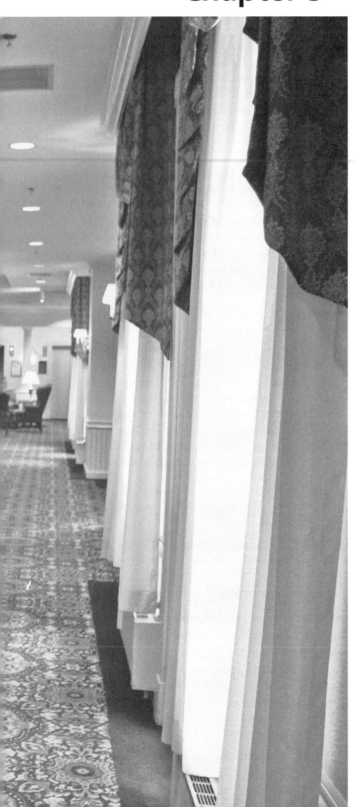

EVALUATION SITE: The Jefferson

COMMUNITY TYPE: Continuing Care Retirement Community
- 325 independent living apartments
- 39 assisted living apartments
- 30 assisted living for those with dementia
- 31 nursing care beds

REGION: Mid-Atlantic

ARCHITECT: Cochran, Stephenson & Donkervoet, Inc.

OWNER: Sunrise® Senior Living
(original owner was Marriott Corporation)

DATA POINTS:

Resident Room:	642–1,378 gsf (independent living)
	309–340 gsf (assisted living and assisted living for dementia)
	262–335 gsf (nursing care)
Total Area:	396,456 gsf (independent living)
Total Area:	1,219.86 gsf/apartment (independent living)
Total Area:	42,575 gsf (assisted living and assisted living for dementia)
Total Area:	617.03 gsf/resident (assisted living and assisted living for dementia)
Total Area:	13,497 gsf (nursing care)
Total Area:	435.39 gsf/resident (nursing care)
Total Project Area:	713,959 gsf
Project Cost:	$75.63/gsf
Total Project Cost:	$54,000,000
Investment/resident:	$127,358.49
Staffing:	3.71 care hours/resident/day (nursing care)
	2.5 care hours/resident/day (assisted living and assisted living for dementia)
Occupancy:	100%

FIRST OCCUPANCY: 1992

DATE OF EVALUATION: February 2006

EVALUATION TEAM: Debra Doyle; Marcia Price; Kevin Glover, AIA; Ingrid Fraley, ASID; Jeffrey Anderzhon, AIA

FIG. 5-1 This expansive lobby, the center of community life, supports many resident activities. Every morning house-keeping places furnishings in their original configuration
Photograph by Kevin Glover, AIA

Introduction

In the 1950s, Washington, D.C., and its suburban communities within Maryland and Virginia were connected by trolley lines. One such community, comprised predominantly of residential neighborhoods with modest single-family homes and small low-rise apartment buildings, was known as Parkington. The Parkington Shopping Center, anchored by a Sears, Roebuck & Company store, served the local community as well as those visitors who made the journey by car and trolley from Washington, D.C.

Parkington entered a period of severe decline in the 1960s and 1970s; it was not until the construction of the Washington Metro Rail system, and especially the opening of the Ballston Metro Station in 1979, that significant changes in real estate in this area occurred. This metro corridor is now home to tall, modern apartment complexes, condominiums, the Ballston Commons Mall, and many restaurants. A model of transit-oriented development and smart growth, today's Ballston is a "hot spot" in the greater D.C. area for 20-something professionals.

Ballston has also attracted commercial development and high-rise office towers housing several U.S. government agencies and organizations, including the National Science Foundation, the U.S. Fish and Wildlife Service, and the Office of Naval Research, and not-for-profit groups such as The Nature Conservancy. High-tech companies such as CACI and Qwest are also located in Ballston.

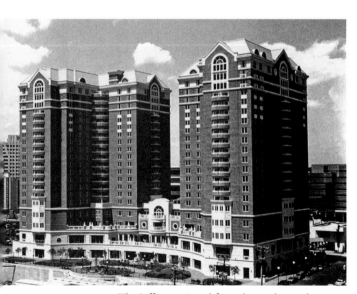

FIG. 5-2 The Jefferson viewed from the southeast, showing the south ellipse and the south roof terraces *Photo by Michael Dersin Photography*

With its close proximity to the nation's capital, the Marriott Corporation viewed the Ballston area as a prime location for retired military, and thus embarked upon the construction of a 20-story high-rise retirement community known as The Jefferson, which has 325 independent living apartments, 39 assisted living apartments, 30 assisted living beds for those with dementia, and 31 nursing care beds. The 1.5-acre site was part of a larger area of demolition, and 14 years ago this high-rise was the first of many buildings to be constructed just a block from the Ballston Commons Mall and the entrance to the Ballston Metro Station. It was the perfect location from which residents could enjoy a full range of intellectual, social, and cultural activities within their community as well as the entire Washington metro area.

Designer's and Operator's Stated Objectives and Responses

AUTHOR'S NOTE: *Because of the age of this facility, there was no recoverable record of stated design objectives or design intents. Those indicated here have been gleaned from articles and publications regarding The Jefferson by the design architect and others.*

OBJECTIVE: Design a continuing care retirement community to fit within the restrictions of a 1.5-acre urban building site.

DESIGN INTENT: To fit 700,000 square feet of living and facility space on a 1.5-acre urban site, twin residential towers were designed to link with a four-story community base. The towers house 325 independent living condominiums. The connecting base minimizes internal travel and provides access to nursing care, assisted living units, retail areas, community functions, and stacked parking.

OBJECTIVE: Provide a connection to the outdoor environment while separating the health care and independent living areas.

DESIGN INTENT: Sun-filled terraces at every floor embrace a grand elliptical plaza, providing safe outdoor access for residents and the public. Elevators segregate traffic by separately serving residential, nursing, and service areas.

OBJECTIVE: Design a building that sets the tone for the neighborhood and future construction.

DESIGN INTENT: Building materials and details convey an upscale residential image in a user-friendly environment filled with innovations for the elderly. The fully accessible facilities meet criteria under both the Fair Housing and Americans with Disabilities Acts.

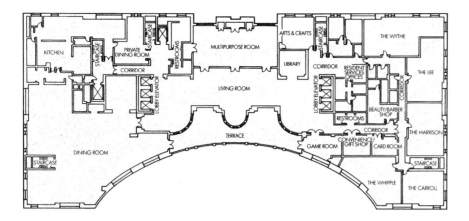

FIG. 5-3 Second-level floor plan *Courtesy of Cochran, Stephenson & Donkervoet, Inc.*

Field Observations: Meeting the Objectives

OBJECTIVE: Design a continuing care retirement community to fit within the restrictions of a 1.5-acre urban building site.

FIELD OBSERVATIONS: To comply with the owner's building program and to maximize the use of a small parcel of premium real estate, a high-rise solution was the obvious design direction. However, the clever use of a four-story building "plinth" on which to set two separated towers housing the apartments (thus maximizing the apartment yield), not only achieved the necessary yield of building area, but provided a more interesting visual appearance than a conventional rectangular box. Certainly, the restricted site raises design challenges, but also, when appropriately considered, stimulates very satisfying design solutions that a less restrictive site might not have engendered.

As with any urban setting, parking is always at a premium for residents and guests, as well as the 225 full- and part-time employees. With the addition of private duty aides, the building population easily surpasses 1,000 on a

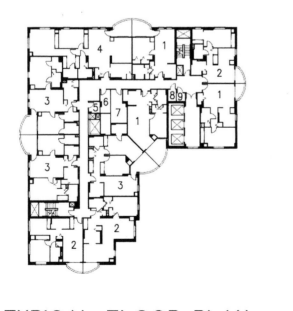

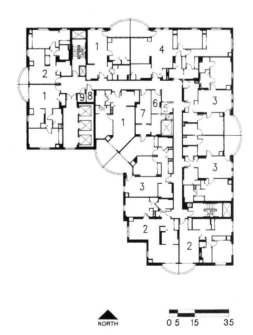

TYPICAL FLOOR PLAN

NORTH

0 5 15   35

FIG. 5-4 Typical apartment-level floor plan *Courtesy of Cochran, Stephenson & Donkervoet, Inc.*

daily basis. To address the needs of employees and outside staffers, creative uses of nonrevenue-producing spaces have resulted in closet-sized offices and reclamation of nonfunctional parking areas in the garage for departmental use. Training facilities, meeting spaces, and a larger employment/human resources department are on the wish list as additional operational space.

OBJECTIVE: Provide a connection to the outdoor environment while separating the health care and independent living areas.

FIELD OBSERVATIONS: The building's shape, along with the mandated urban planning for the entire area, provides a visually appealing ellipse that is open to the public on the south side of the building. A visitor who initially addresses the building from the north is naturally drawn to this open area through an entry court that provides an enticing view of it. This outdoor connection is further reinforced by the introduction of a series of rooftop terraces on both the second and third floors that overlook the ellipse and provide access to the exterior for residents of the health center.

Public entry to all portions of the building is off the grand ellipse into a small lobby controlled by reception. The elevators do not function without a resident access card or an override of the system by the front desk. This first level also houses the administrative support offices, resident mail, exercise room, pool, loading dock, and related back-of-the-house functions, including the employee lounge.

Residents requiring skilled nursing services or memory support are located on the third floor, whereas

assisted living residents are on the third and fourth floors, a part of the building that forms the plinth. Each floor acts as a self-contained community, with offices, dining, lounges, and large balconies to emphasize the connection to the outdoors. However, these health care floors are designed in a traditional medical-model mode, with primarily shared rooms in nursing and assisted living for those with dementia and studio assisted living units. Staff movement between floors is by stair rather than elevator, and communications is by portable phone, as each floor has its own hardwired system and is independent of the others. Management is in the process of renovating these floors, and may consider changes that include the introduction of a universal worker staffing concept.

OBJECTIVE: Design a building that sets the tone for the neighborhood and future construction.

FIELD OBSERVATIONS: Zoned for mixed use, the complex offers retail and commercial space on the first level, thereby helping to integrate the building with the city streetscape and to promote interaction between residents and the local business community. Entry is achieved at only a few points, creating a greater level of security and the sense that, while a part of the neighborhood, The Jefferson is also a private community.

The exterior façade is well done, blends easily into the surrounding neighborhood, and offers residents access to outdoor plaza areas. Similar buildings that have been constructed to the south of The Jefferson complement the building and finish the "enclosure" of the ellipse suggested by the original building construction.

Field Observations: Themes and Hypotheses

Creating Community

The second floor is the heart of the community (see Figure 4 in the color insert), featuring a grand lobby and dining rooms; private dining; multipurpose, arts and crafts, library, game, and card rooms; a country store; a beauty salon; and administrator's offices. This level connects the east and west towers and serves as the main street of the high-rise community.

The open design of the second floor, coupled with more intimate spaces, allows effective mixing of populations and related activities, broadening resident social connections and adding an attractive variety to life. Residents have formed clubs that encourage independence, celebrate individuality, and address the diverse interests of the community.

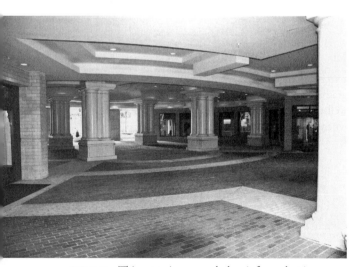

FIG. 5-5 This extensive covered plaza is for pedestrian use only to access the first-floor receptionist *Photograph by Kevin Glover, AIA*

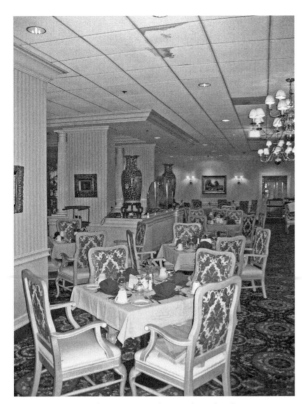

FIG. 5-6 Inspired by Marriott hospitality, the dining room is well appointed and incorporates smaller groupings of tables to diminish the vastness of the space *Photograph by Jeffrey Anderzhon*

Located on the third and fourth floors, each floor of the health center acts as its own contained community; there is little interaction with the remainder of the facility except for apartment resident visitors. Floors 5 through 21 are fee-simple condominiums, the only ones in Ballston. Ten different unit plans per floor include three one-bedroom units, three two-bedroom units, three one-bedroom den units, and one two-bedroom den unit. Although the condominiums are purchased and thus privately owned, the health care center is part of a real estate investment trust (REIT), with Sunrise Senior Living providing management services to both parts of the complex. For condominium residents, a lifestyle package based upon a monthly fee is offered by Sunrise; options include weekly housekeeping, maintenance of the common floors, transportation services, all activities, and a choice of meal plans.

The commercial kitchen does an outstanding job of providing service to all venues, including the health care floors, and operates efficiently in all areas of food preparation, despite design constraints that affect work processes and workflow. Though The Jefferson continues to thrive on the Marriott-driven philosophy of enhanced meal ser-

vice, planning for the future dietary needs of an upscale urban clientele is always a challenge.

An adequate fitness program is offered to residents despite the limitations in size and location of the pool and exercise room. By focusing on the promotion of personal training and other specialized exercise and therapy programs, staff has been able to work within the building constraints.

Many of the facility programs focus on culture, arts, and politics, and the suburban Washington, D.C., location provides an abundance of intellectual speakers from the community, addressing a variety of issues of interest to this population of retired military, government, and corporate officials. Many programs are offered on site, but transportation to off-site lectures and performances are also in demand, broadening the concept of community from just the residents of The Jefferson to the entire resident population of Washington, D.C.

Making a Home

The arrangement of the independent living apartments is constantly being challenged, as residents often purchase adjoining apartments when available and combine them with their own. The trend toward larger apartments has meant that 25 of the original condominium units have been "absorbed" in order to maximize the square footage of another apartment. Thus, there are technically only 300 apartments remaining in the building. However, as each original apartment has a separate fee simple title, 325 units continue to be listed on the tax rolls.

The urban location of The Jefferson affords residents more than just apartment living in the city. It also provides a lifestyle that unites neighbors with their common values and interests. Largely as a result of residents' military and government service, this home thrives on these common bonds, which are reflected in daily programs and activities. It would be hard to imagine these well-traveled and well-educated residents living anywhere else.

Regional/Cultural Design

This sophisticated urban population demands a higher level of service. It relied originally on the experience of the Marriott Corporation, and now, with the recent change in management duties, looks to Sunrise Senior Living to address all their requirements. Traditional furnishings are perfectly placed, and each morning housekeeping rearranges the furniture based upon plans to ensure exact placement. The choice of soft, rich, hospitality finishes results in a quiet, comfortable, and upscale environment accented by fresh flowers. However, with the change in management, the health care floors were redecorated to a "country" theme with less formal interior finishes that have not been well received by the community.

A part of the military culture, the men's breakfast club (with 36 attendees) opens Friday mornings with a veterans' color guard in attendance. The record of military service is one of the common themes drawing this community together and certainly drawing on the regional culture as the center of governmental business.

Environmental Therapy

Even within the constraints of this tight urban site, amenities that provide opportunities for physical and mental stimulation are included. The pool and exercise area, with personal fitness trainers and individualized exercise programs, are well received. The second-floor common areas support the many resident-inspired clubs as well as programmed activities.

The health center is currently under study for refurbishment, as the 1990s-inspired design of double-loaded corridors and isolated activity rooms would certainly benefit from reconfiguration and the introduction of true neighborhood concepts. The current arrival and departure sequence via the elevators cries out for improvement, as human contact with staff is completely missing and results in some confusion as to where to go and how to proceed.

Outdoor Environment

Though it may be somewhat counterintuitive that there can be a connection with the outdoors within a high-rise project, The Jefferson accomplishes this in very creative ways. The building setbacks provide rooftop patios that are inviting and well furnished, that take advantage of both sun and shade, and that present themselves as secure even as they rise above the surrounding grade.

The creation of essentially two towers above the fourth floor allows visual access for apartments from a variety of perspectives. These vistas, complemented by balconies for nearly every apartment, allow resident access to the exterior in several ways.

Quality of Workplace and the Physical Plant

Fair Housing and ADA regulations were met in 1992, but the consensus from operations is that the building lacks flexibility to accommodate social as well as technical changes. During the two-year fill-up process, the average

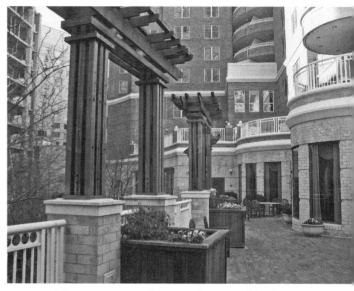

FIG. 5-7 The community roof terrace off the second-level lobby has limited views. Terraces for nursing and assisted living are above *Photograph by Jeffrey Anderzhon*

age upon entry was late 70s. Residents have aged in place, and the daily population of both towers increases dramatically with the presence of private duty aides. It should be noted that there is no contract to move to a higher level of care, so most residents continue to occupy their apartments regardless of their health status, and architectural changes to provide universal design features are made at the expense of the owner-resident.

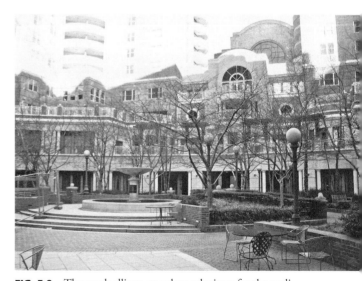

FIG. 5-8 The south ellipse, an urban substitute for the traditional courtyard, with the community roof terrace above *Photograph by Jeffrey Anderzhon*

Advancements in technology are also difficult to incorporate, as "maintain" rather than "retrofit" is management's current long-term view of the building. For example, the independent residents have to call an outside number to reach any administrative or support services, as there is no internal communication system. Wireless technology is nonexistent, although cable is present.

Of specific interest to the evaluation team was the unique approach to human resources in the form of the "Department of People and Culture." The employees of The Jefferson are diverse in their cultural backgrounds, and management has gone to great lengths to identify cultural differences and similarities that affect communication and work performance.

Extensive time and training are devoted to employees so that they can provide quality in the work environment. A hospitality-driven philosophy supports five-star food and service training to all levels. The workplace dynamic empowers people to "do the right thing" and to be innovators in service. Proper service, impeccable settings, military precision, and customized services are all expectations of the residents, and this staff is challenged every day to meet and exceed these expectations.

Operator Perspectives

As The Jefferson moves into the 21st century, a new reality of expectations is on the horizon, as baby boomers replace the war generation. In preparation for future residents, The Jefferson is extending its level of service to provide additional choices and to customize services. Under consideration is the addition of concierge services, as well as food and beverage deliveries to apartments, flexible round-the-clock dining options in formal and casual venues, and to-the-table food preparation carts in assisted living. Food trends, health trends, and personal trends are all under scrutiny and open for modification.

Current entry into the independent lifestyle of The Jefferson requires purchase of an apartment unit with all the associated costs of home ownership, including payments for mortgage, taxes, utilities, insurance, and con-

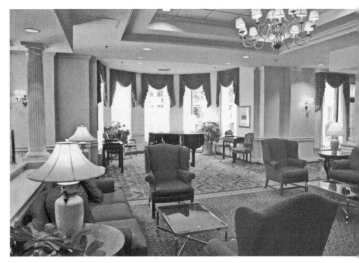

FIG. 5-9   The second-level community lobby, where residents congregate before meals and for community events
Photograph by Kevin Glover, AIA

dominium maintenance fees. This "lifestyle" package can be a significant monthly expenditure and requires sustained affluence. That, in combination with the trend to purchase two units and combine them into one large apartment, has management discussing the future affordability of The Jefferson and considering whether baby boomers will continue to purchase high-end real estate with a catered lifestyle package.

Although the condominium community thrives within its current context, dwindling resident population is anticipated. With the recent dramatic increases in real estate values, heirs are keeping the condominiums vacant, or using an option to rent units, hoping to experience further gains in real estate appreciation. What impact, if any, this will have on the vitality of the community has yet to be determined.

Finally, the transition of management is still being challenged to meld the "mansion mentality" of Sunrise Senior Living with the "hospitality philosophy" of Marriott. This has resulted in a unique management culture and supportive team effort that is a mixture of both and that is dedicated to preserving The Jefferson lifestyle.

General Project Information

PROJECT ADDRESS
The Jefferson
900 North Taylor Street
Arlington, Virginia 22203

PROJECT DESIGN TEAM
Architect: Cochran, Stephenson & Donkervoet, Inc.
Interior Designer: Marriott Corporation
Landscape Architect: Graham Landscape Architecture
Structural Engineer: George Evans Associates, Inc.
Mechanical Engineer: Henry Adams, Inc.
Electrical Engineer: Henry Adams, Inc.
Civil Engineer: Cook and Miller, Ltd.
Dining Consultant: Unknown
Gerontologist: N/A
Management/Development: N/A
Contractor: Marriott Corporation

PROJECT STATUS
Completion date: 1992

OCCUPANCY LEVELS
At facility opening date: Unknown
At time of evaluation: 100%—all levels of care

RESIDENT AGE (YRS)
At facility opening date: 70
At time of evaluation: 83

PROJECT AREAS

Project Element	Included in This Project	
	Units, Beds, or Clients	New GSF
Apartments (units)	325	396,456
Assisted living (beds)	39	27,828
Assisted living for those with dementia (beds)	30	14,747
Skilled nursing care (beds)	31	13,497
Common social areas (people)	750	37,991
Kitchen (daily meals served)	2,250	1,923
Retail space (shops/restaurants, etc.)	4	7,885
Fitness/rehabilitation/wellness (daily visits)	45	450
Pool(s) and related areas (users)	35	2,795
Parking under building (cars)	340	192,807
Mechanical and service areas	N/A	17,580
Totals		713,959

INDEPENDENT LIVING RETIREMENT APARTMENTS

Project Element	No.	Apartments Typical Size (GSF)	Apartments Size Range (GSF)
One-bedroom units	97	676	642–697
One-bedroom with den units	97	813	751–1,125
Two-bedroom units	98	1,009	984–1,051
Two-bedroom plus den units	33	1,378	1,378
Total (all units)	325	289,865 GSF	
Residents' social areas (lounges, dining, and recreation spaces):		64,787 GSF	
Medical/health/fitness and activities areas:		3,245 GSF	
Administrative, public, and ancillary support service areas:		3,329 GSF	
Service, maintenance, and mechanical areas:		35,230 GSF	
Total gross area:		396,456 GSF	
Total net usable area (per space program):		361,226 NSF	
Overall gross/net factor (ratio of gross area/net usable area):		1.10	

ASSISTED LIVING
(INCLUDING FOR THOSE WITH DEMENTIA)

Project Element	New Construction No. Units	New Construction Typical Size
Private bedroom units	11	309 GSF
Shared occupancy bedroom units	29	340 GSF
Total (all units)—69 residents	51	22,593 GSF
Residents' social areas (lounges, dining, and recreation spaces):		4,775 GSF
Medical, health care, therapy, and activities spaces:		972 GSF
Administrative, public, and ancillary support services:		329 GSF
Service, maintenance, and mechanical areas:		13,906 GSF
Total gross area:		42,575 GSF
Total net usable area (per space program):		28,669 NSF
Overall gross/net factor (ratio of gross area/net usable area):		1.48

SKILLED NURSING

Project Element	New Construction No.	New Construction Typical Room Size
One-bed/single rooms	3	262 GSF
Two-bed/double rooms	14	335 GSF
Total (all units)—31 residents	17	6,984 GSF
Social areas (lounges, dining, and recreation spaces):		1,850 GSF
Medical, health care, therapy, and activities spaces:		436 GSF
Administrative, public, and ancillary support services:		315 GSF
Service, maintenance, and mechanical areas:		3,912 GSF
Total gross area:		13,497 GSF
Total net usable area (per space program):		9,585 NSF
Overall gross/net factor (ratio of gross area/net usable area):		1.41

SITE AND PARKING

SITE LOCATION
Urban

SITE SIZE
Acres: 1.5
Square feet: 64,813

PARKING

Type of Parking	For This Facility			
	Residents	Staff	Visitors	Totals
Under building lot	310	20	10	340

CONSTRUCTION COSTS

AUTHOR'S NOTE: *At the time this project was submitted for the "Design for Aging Review" in 1992, detailed cost data was not required. The cost data presented here is from several sources, including the original designer and the operator.*

SOURCE OF COST DATA
Final construction cost as of 1992

SOFT COSTS
Land cost or value:	Unknown
All permit and other entitlement fees:	Unknown
Legal and professional fees:	Unknown
Appraisals:	Unknown
Marketing and preopening:	Unknown
Total soft costs:	Unknown

BUILDING COSTS
New construction except FF&E, special finishes, floor and window coverings, HVAC and electrical:	Unknown
Renovations except FF&E, special finishes, floor and window coverings, HVAC, and electrical:	Unknown
FF&E, and small wares:	Unknown
Floor coverings:	Unknown
Window coverings:	Unknown
HVAC:	Unknown
Electrical:	Unknown
Medical equipment costs:	Unknown
Total building costs:	$54,000,000

SITE COSTS
New on-site:	Unknown
New off-site:	Unknown
Landscape:	Unknown
Total site costs:	Unknown

TOTAL PROJECT COSTS
Total project costs: Unknown

FINANCING SOURCES
Private financing

CARE COMPARISON

(Nursing component only)
Source: www.medicare.gov—February 2006
SNF staffing: 3.71 care hours/resident/day
SNF occupancy: 31 of 31 = 100%

Hours per Resident per Day	The Jefferson	VA Average	National Average
Not-for-profit	No		
Multifacility	No		
Levels of care	SNF		
Medicare	Yes		
Medicaid	Yes		
Licensed #	31		
# residents	31	107.9	95.3
% occ this day	100%		
RNs	0.86	0.50	0.50
LPNs	0.63	0.90	0.70
RN + LPN	1.49	1.40	1.20
CNA	2.22	2.20	2.30
RN + LPN + CA	3.71	3.60	3.50

"I don't deserve this award, but I have arthritis and I don't deserve that either."

JACK BENNY, 1894–1974

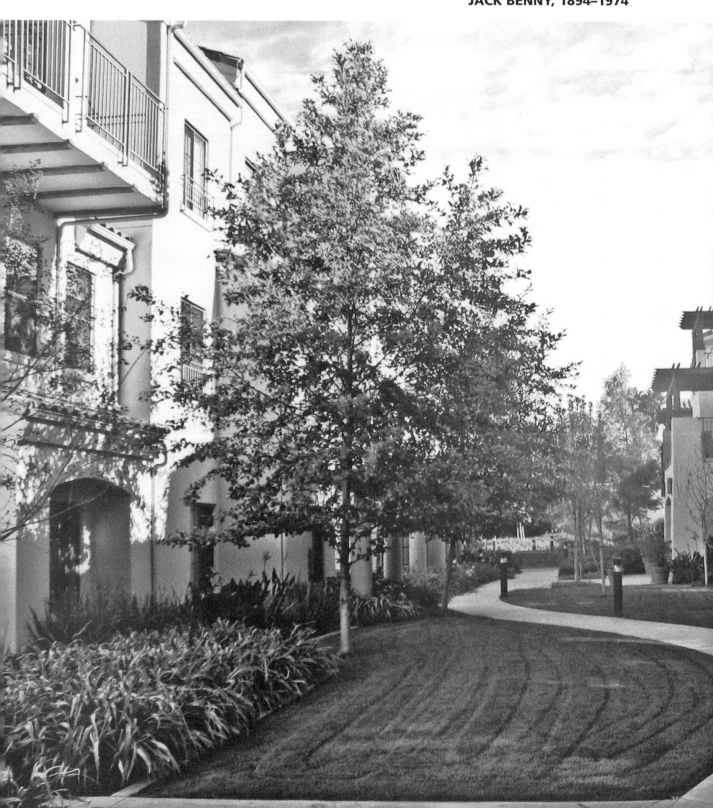

Chapter 6 La Vida Real

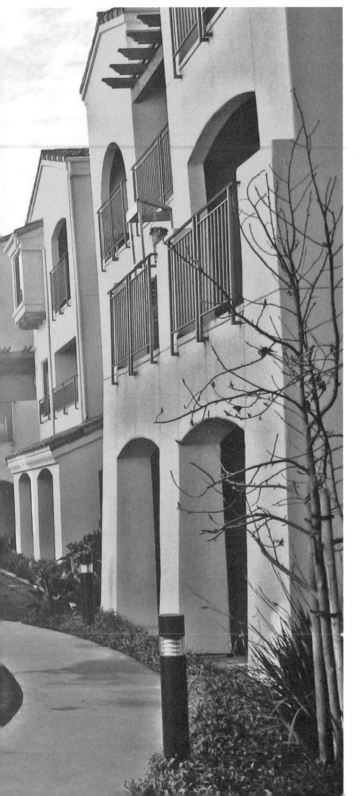

EVALUATION SITE: La Vida Real

COMMUNITY TYPE: Continuing Care Retirement Community
- 210 independent living apartments
- 98 assisted living apartments
- 14 assisted living apartments for those with dementia
- No licensed nursing care

REGION: West Coast

ARCHITECT: Mithun

OWNER: Senior Resource Group

DATA POINTS: Resident Room: 470–586 gsf (assisted living)

469–1,125 gsf (independent living)

Total Area: 103,274 gsf (assisted living)

Total Area: 922.09 gsf/resident (assisted living)

Total Area: 249,946 gsf (independent living)

Total Area: 1,190.22 gsf/apartment (independent living)

Overall Total Area: 353,220 gsf

Project Cost: $136.87/gsf

Total Project Cost: $48,346,099

Investment/resident: $150,143.16

Staffing: 1.65 care hours/resident/day (assisted living)

Occupancy: 100% (assisted living) as of April 2006

100% (independent apartments) as of April 2006

FIRST OCCUPANCY: September 2003

DATE OF EVALUATION: April 2006

EVALUATION TEAM: Mitch Green, AIA; Jeffrey Anderzhon, AIA; Joyce Polhamus, AIA; Eleanor Alvarez; Terri Sherman

FIG. 6-1 A nicely landscaped courtyard between two apartment wings reflects a Spanish colonial vernacular architectural style *Photograph by Jeffrey Anderzhon*

Introduction

Among the relatively new suburban sprawl in the foothills northwest of San Diego, La Vida Real itself spreads to nearly consume its 11-acre site. The buildings' Spanish vernacular structures blend into the neighborhood and at first glance are either unassuming or repetitive. This continuing care retirement community, containing 210 independent living apartment units, 98 assisted living apartments, and 14 assisted living apartments for residents suffering from dementia, contains four levels that take advantage of the gently rolling site. The floor area ratio is relatively high for a suburban site even on the land-cost sensitive West Coast, and creates significant density that most likely does not differ much from the surrounding multifamily residential and commercial properties.

Upon entering La Vida, the calming feel of the well-landscaped entry court awes visitors. Unfortunately, the entrance is somewhat confusing as well, because there appears to be actually two entries: one to the left, which leads into the apartment side of the campus, and one on the right, which leads to assisted living. This entry courtyard is the only connection between the two portions of the campus that is not restricted to staff, and it is an opening statement that distinctly delineates independent and assisted living.

In the face of the campus's density, the limited but extensively landscaped exterior spaces are refreshing, inviting, and provide an organic counterpoint to the stuccoed edifices. The exterior spaces take on their own spatial identities and easily combine with the structured environment, at times blurring the distinction between the two. The blurred lines create a dichotomy of environment in which interior and exterior merge, despite the conscious segregation of care levels.

The environmental design emanates a Southern California style (see Figure 5 in the color insert) that is intuitively expected and comforting in its conformance. Despite that conformity, the design asserts instances of

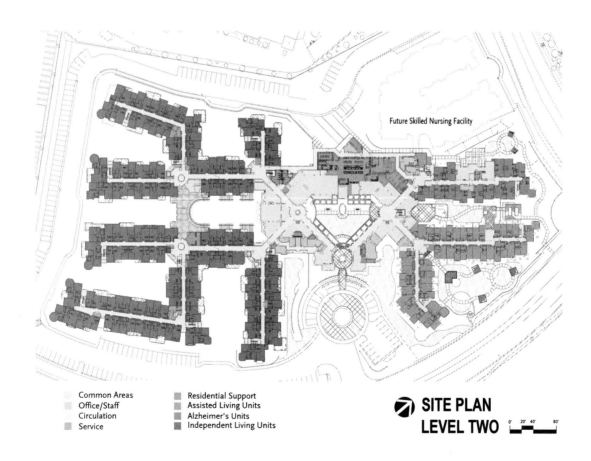

Common Areas
Office/Staff
Circulation
Service

Residential Support
Assisted Living Units
Alzheimer's Units
Independent Living Units

SITE PLAN LEVEL TWO 0' 20' 40' 80'

FIG. 6-2 Site plan, level two *Courtesy of Mithun*

creativity and reveals small design surprises that tease the eye and encourage visitors to look for more unique details. The design fits, but also states that it does not have to completely dismiss the Spanish colonial vernacular to avoid being boring. The senses begin to open further the more time one spends in this building, and soon visitors are immersed in this "new" Southern California design.

Designers' and Owners' Stated Objectives and Responses

OBJECTIVE: Design in a Spanish colonial style.

DESIGN INTENT: The Spanish colonial style is regionally appropriate for this Southern California community, and the architectural vernacular was selected based on the zoning criteria and design standards mandated by the municipality. In fact, the project evokes images of a Spanish hill town. The main entry courtyard is like a town center, with more civic or hospitality-inspired meeting spaces, and the residential wings appear to have been added to over time, just as in a town. The façade of the residential wings varies so that no two segments are exactly alike.

OBJECTIVE: Provide an intuitive sense of orientation when arriving and moving about the community.

DESIGN INTENT: Clearly marked paths and connectors help to guide circulation and define the public, semipublic, and private spaces. The circulation spaces do not appear as mere hallways or corridors, but instead become galleries, loggias, and edges of the prominent common spaces that are oriented to vistas of the landscaped outdoor courtyards. It is a classic interweaving of indoor space with outdoor space.

OBJECTIVE: Create a high-quality environment within a defined budget.

DESIGN INTENT: The level of detail and fine interior design varies throughout the facility, with the most refined and highest-quality finishes decorating common spaces. More moderate designs were used in the units.

OBJECTIVE: Include landscaping that supports the spirit of the new community.

DESIGN INTENT: The perimeter landscaping of the project blends with the landscape of the neighborhood, but also takes that landscaping to the next level. Designers included drought-resistant plant materials and worked to maintain indigenous species. The project's main entry

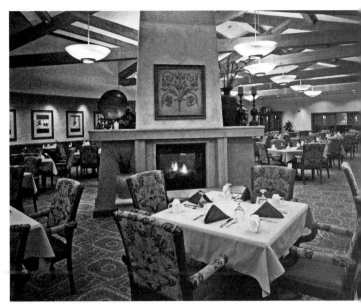

FIG. 6-3 A warm, inviting independent living/dining room includes areas for intimate dining within its open design
www.architecturephotoinc.com

is clearly defined from the street, with an elegant drop-off area, outdoor entry rotunda, enriched paving, trellises, pots, and colorful plant materials.

The courtyards are the heart of the project. Each individual courtyard has a unique character, with distinct paving, trellises, pavilions, and plant materials that complement the architecture. Many of the courtyards extend deep into the building, where they provide natural light and air, as well as important outdoor space adjacent to the common spaces and residential neighborhoods.

Field Observations: Meeting the Objectives

OBJECTIVE: Design in a Spanish colonial style.

FIELD OBSERVATIONS: The density of the site makes it difficult to get a sense of the scale of the building. Even though the building is large enough to replicate a Spanish village, the analogy is lost because the size and layout only allow the building to be seen a piece at a time. However, the design is indicative of the Spanish colonial style and is certainly appropriate given its location.

The main entrance leading to the courtyard is grand and inviting, and urges the visitor to move into the beautiful surroundings to discover what lies beyond. Although the courtyard does not resemble a town square or public meeting area, as the design objective had intended, it does succeed as a beautiful space lush with landscaping and is more akin to a private garden. Additionally, the lack of activity within the courtyard, and the tendency to use the space as a connector between independent and assisted living, further reduces the town-square quality of the space. Perhaps locating amenities such as the beauty salon, café, or library within the courtyard would have enhanced the atmosphere necessary for this objective to be met.

OBJECTIVE: Provide an intuitive sense of orientation when arriving and moving about the community.

FIELD OBSERVATIONS: The grand archway entrance opens to two distinct entrances on each side. One entry leads to the assisted living portion of the campus and common areas; the other side is the entry to the independent living portion of the campus. The two sides connect through the common areas in a triangular fashion and then join in the dining areas. This layout benefits only the staff, as no connection between the two areas is available to residents. The dining rooms are adjacent to each other and are backed by the common kitchen, which efficiently serves both venues.

This main entry sequence provides a strong sense of arrival, and the first circulation corridors into both assisted living and the independent apartments have visual access to the entry courtyard through large expanses of glass. The visual access orients visitors, but is immediately lost beyond the rotunda where the corridors terminate. Elsewhere on the campus, there is no visual access to the exterior to give visual orientation clues or provide relief from the continuous array of apartment doors and painted corridor walls.

Throughout the campus, rotundas define entrances and provide choices for wayfinding. These choices are not intuitive and are actually quite confusing, particularly for the visitor or new resident. Without distinct indication through design, wayfinding becomes an issue for staff during new resident orientation and for providing service workers adequate directions to individual apartments.

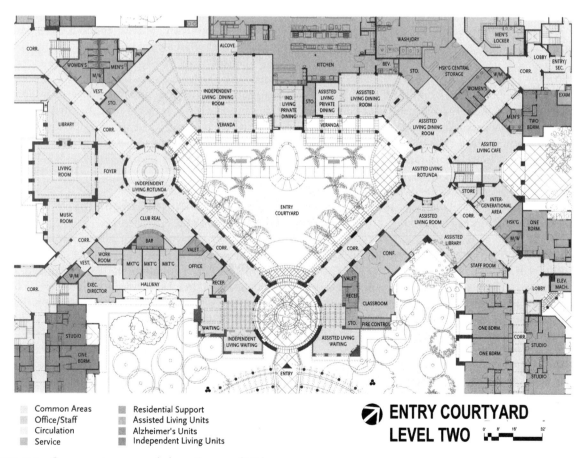

Common Areas · Office/Staff · Circulation · Service · Residential Support · Assisted Living Units · Alzheimer's Units · Independent Living Units

ENTRY COURTYARD LEVEL TWO

FIG. 6-4 Campus entry courtyard plan *Courtesy of Mithun*

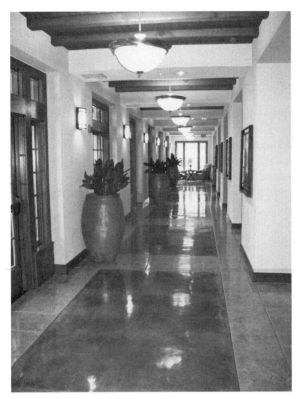

FIG. 6-5 A single-loaded assisted living corridor with natural light flowing into the space is adjacent to the entry courtyard *Photograph by Jeffrey Anderzhon*

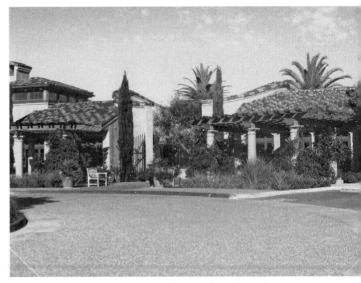

FIG. 6-6 Main entry with courtyard beyond is well landscaped and attractive *Photograph by Jeffrey Anderzhon*

OBJECTIVE: Create a high-quality environment within a defined budget.

FIELD OBSERVATIONS: Without question, the cost per square foot for La Vida Real is reasonable, particularly for Southern California. In addition, there is no noticeable difference in finishes or quality between the more lucrative independent living areas and the assisted living areas; both were treated with equal respect and attention to detail. This approach ameliorates the fact that there is a clear physical and psychological distinction between the two.

Within common and social spaces, there is a hierarchy of materials and finishes that work with the overall feel of the design. The finishes give a richness and depth of accommodation that both comfort and calm the residents. The memory care unit may be an exception to this level of attention, as it contains contrived wall features, is dark, and has no visual orientation to the outside.

OBJECTIVE: Include landscaping that supports the spirit of the new community.

FIELD OBSERVATIONS: Because of the size of the structure vis-à-vis the size of the lot, there are only small and dis- connected courtyards between wings of the building. These courtyards are extensively landscaped and contain a variety of resident choices for furniture and amenities. The courtyards, particularly the entry courtyard, blend into the surrounding structures and become rooms on their own. It is apparent that the landscape designer and architect collaborated closely to create interesting views and vistas, although the environs beyond the site are quite bland and nondescript.

Drought-resistant plant materials were selected because of the high probability of brush fires in the region. Nevertheless, the facility has three separate sprinkler systems running on a regular basis and a significant lawn area that requires watering as well. Landscaping overall was beautiful and tied into the décor well, and the courtyards do serve to break up building massing that would otherwise be confining. The additional attention and expense showered on these small courtyards help to draw the eye away from the repetitive form of the building.

Field Observations: Themes and Hypotheses

Creating Community

With 322 apartment units on campus that are physically connected, there are ample opportunities to create a cohesive community across disparate care-provision levels. To some extent, there was an attempt within the

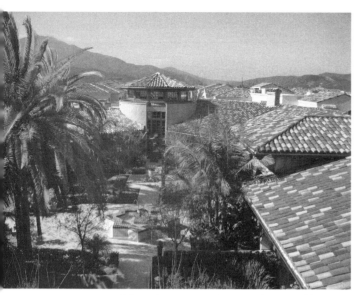

FIG. 6-7 The only connection between the assisted living and independent living portions of the campus is by way of this entry courtyard, as seen from above   *Photograph by Jeffrey Anderzhon*

design to create that community with the common entry courtyard and continuity in exterior design and interior fit and finish. Unfortunately, there is a disconnection between the more active independent living residents and the frailer assisted living residents, which is created by the design and reinforced by the attitude of the residents and administration. This distinction is especially disappointing when one spouse needs care support while the other remains living in the independent apartments.

Aside from the physical separation, however, the finer details of design do not treat the health care side of the campus differently from the independent living portion. The level of finishes and number and size of socialization spaces are not significantly different for either side of the community. These spaces include ample gathering rooms that serve large group functions, as well as small socialization areas where individuals can enjoy an intimate conversation with a neighbor. The community spaces on the assisted living side tend to be more activity oriented, whereas those on the independent living side tend to be more socially oriented.

Given that the independent living side of the campus has residents who are more active, and given that there are certainly more residents on this side of campus, there logically are more community spaces for their use. Among these is an Internet café with a coffee-house ambience and great views into a courtyard. A fully appointed theater, with comfortable, accessible seating, is another popular locale for residents. Just outside this theater is a "lobby"

that creatively provides space for pre- and post-movie discussions and socialization. Smaller gathering rooms allow card-club meetings and work as areas for individuals to gather for discussions.

Much of the community interaction occurs around meals. Both sides of the La Vida campus have well-appointed dining rooms that, although large, convey a sense of intimacy and fine restaurant dining in both their décor and their operation. Outside each dining area is a rotunda that serves as a social gathering space for pre-meal conversations. On the independent living side, the Club Real serves as additional space where residents can have a cocktail in a casual club setting.

The residents do share a sense of community, but that sense tends to be confined to one side of the campus and does not extend to the larger suburban community. The facts that this is a typical commuter suburb, where residents shy away from becoming too intimate with their neighbors, and that it is one of the newer suburbs of San Diego contribute to a lesser level of connection to the larger community. However, there are outreach efforts, including an intergenerational program allowing use of the swimming pool and cooperative programs with the local community college in such activities as tai chi, music, arts, and yoga.

Making a Home

The comfortable and familiar design of the facility helps residents to feel more at home in their surroundings, and the exceptional amenities, such as the swimming pool and lush gardens, also help residents to settle in and enjoy their new lifestyle.

The apartments all benefit from lovely design finishes and offer various choices and amenities to residents. The bathrooms are functional but not necessarily spacious, particularly for those in wheelchairs. Although the use of pocket doors for the bathrooms avoids door-swing interference with floor area, the fact that the doors recess completely into the wall becomes problematic for residents with limited or diminished use of their hands. Almost all of the apartments have their own balconies or patios, a feature that enhances residents' personal space and gives them their own independent access to the outdoors and enjoyment of the courtyards.

The separation between assisted living and the independent living quarters could be a downside for residents in the assisted living portion of the building. There are many emotional and psychological effects of aging in place and moving to a higher level of care: a design that counteracts the discomfort of this transition would help residents to relax and feel more at home at La Vida.

Regional/Cultural Design

Without question, the aesthetics of La Vida comport with the commonly held perspective of regional design in Southern California, tending toward a heavy Spanish colonial influence. The design does this, however, with some amount of refreshing variance from the typical stucco and tile roof typology. The landscape design and courtyard organization help the building to discover its own territory. It could be argued, however, that there is only a superficial cultural foundation, as the large majority of the residents within La Vida or the community of Rancho San Diego could not trace their roots back to a Spanish colonial heritage. The cultural influence stems almost entirely from a stereotypical geographic iconography that has come to pervade the regional architecture.

Regardless of its roots, this design is both accommodating to the surrounding regional vernacular and well done within a more contemporary context. It contains enough depth to be easily received and take on a character of its own. That depth also brings comfort to the resident and visitor and an intuitive understanding that the detailing and finishes are appropriate choices for the campus.

Environmental Therapy

La Vida is a comforting and welcoming environment that contains nicely detailed, well-furnished common spaces that are compatible with resident social interac-

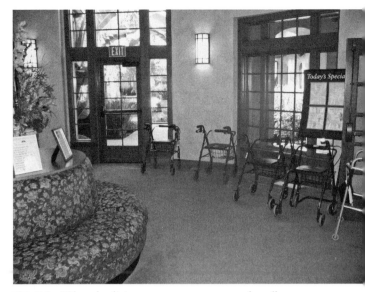

FIG. 6-9 When the dining room cannot accommodate all the walkers at lunch, the assisted living rotunda becomes a convenient storage spot *Photograph by Jeffrey Anderzhon*

tion. Residents indicated their general pleasure with the campus and with the support provided by the staff and administration on campus. However, little in the design overtly contributes to therapy for the residents; in fact, some elements seem to detract from effective therapy.

It could be argued that the length of the corridors and the travel distance from the furthest apartment to the central community spaces provide residents with daily exercise. Unfortunately, lengthy travel distances for residents also contribute to early use of motorized wheelchairs, which in turn requires spaces to park the vehicles and wider corridors to accommodate them. Neither was considered in the design of La Vida, and as apartment residents continue to age in place this issue will take on more prominence.

In the assisted living portion of the campus, the length of corridors is only slightly different but perhaps relatively more problematic. In fact, they are underlit and gloomy. The dementia assisted living apartments are all quite similar, and although consistency is important to appropriate care provision for residents who move into higher levels of care, lighting and connections to exterior spaces are sacrificed for consistency.

It is a difficult balance to achieve: creating a therapeutic environment on a continuing care campus that is consistent in design and feel but also benefits the care provision portion of the program. The design of La Vida accomplishes the consistency but unfortunately does not provide the most effective environment for the residents of the dementia unit.

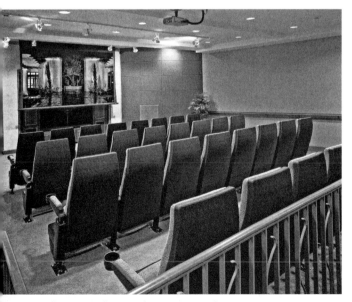

6-8 A well-appointed movie theater is a popular
ion for residents to spend the evening
architecturephotoinc.com

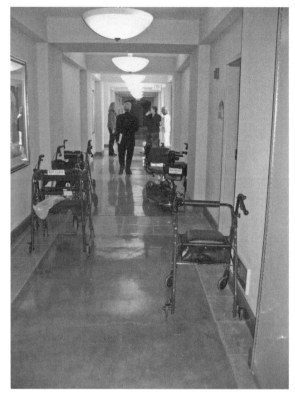

FIG. 6-10 Lengthy corridors contribute to resident use of ambulation assistive devices, as seen in this independent living corridor near an activity room *Photograph by Jeffrey Anderzhon*

Outdoor Environment

The courtyards created from the void spaces of the building are the only outdoor environments available to residents, visually and physically. These are difficult to locate from common spaces and are less utilized than hoped. However, the courtyards are attractive, well landscaped, separate the close-set apartment wings, and soften the scale of the project. With only a few exceptions, all the independent apartment units have either a balcony or a patio that takes full advantage of the courtyard vistas.

An attractive swimming pool with ample deck space for lounging is provided in the south courtyard below the living room in the independent living area. It is well shaded from the intense California sun, but is underused, perhaps because there is no adjacent dressing or locker room and residents must travel the long corridors in their swimming togs.

The memory garden adjacent to the dementia assisted living is attractive, but not easily accessible, and does not provide a great deal of natural light in the dementia unit. As this wing is on a level below grade, the

courtyard seems to be carved from the hill—it feels like sitting in a bowl. Despite the covered porch available for residents, the courtyard remains underutilized.

The extensive thought and consideration given to the outdoor environment are unfortunately diminished by a fairly significant disconnection with the building itself. The courtyards are inviting and luxurious, with areas of both shade and sun, but are difficult to reach. With the notable exception of the entry courtyard, none of the courtyards provides clues as to what portion of the campus is nearest.

Quality of Workplace and the Physical Plant

Staff efficiency, particularly of dietary and food service staff, is enhanced by the building design. The back-of-house functions of the campus are well organized and separate from resident and public functions, but remain connected at the most critical points.

The size of the campus and the fact that it is essentially one building are somewhat overwhelming to staff. As do residents, staff members say that wayfinding is a little difficult and that it is difficult for staff to be visible to residents at all times. However, the staff is dedicated to the service of the elderly and has been both capable and creative in overcoming detracting environmental issues.

Comfort and convenience of staff, however, have been considerations secondary to comfort and conven-

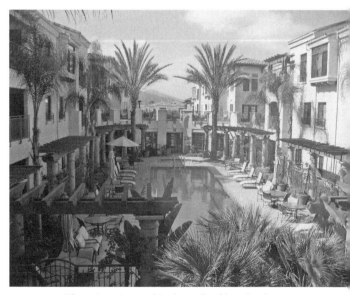

FIG. 6-11 The swimming pool is also utilized by a local community college for swimming lessons *Photograph by Jeffrey Anderzhon*

ience of residents. The tight site design minimized parking and relegated staff to the leftover spaces around the edge of the campus, primarily along the south and east perimeter. These spaces, all of which are uncovered, are for use by residents; there are a few at the entry for visitors. Staff are thus required to park on the street or in the parking lot of a retailer across the street from the campus—the opposite side of the campus from the staff entry.

It is rare that such a large and complex building can be completed without design issues that affect the operation of that building, and La Vida is no exception. With the large number of residents served at each meal, it is very unusual that there was not a computerized system in place from the beginning to track resident meal use. Instead, staff check off paper slips when residents enter the dining areas, and then the slips are gathered and tallied at the end of the day for input into the computerized billing system.

Other, small design problems include the location of the electrical panels and air conditioning units, both of which create difficulty in maintenance accessibility. The choice of finishes for wood trim in the corridors, combined with an increase in the number of ambulation assistance devices, has required the maintenance department to hire a full-time painter simply for touch-ups throughout the campus building. Additionally, the dryer vents are too close to the rooftop air conditioning units, so the filters must be changed more often than usual.

Operator Perspectives

La Vida Real was constructed as a new continuing care retirement campus in a relatively new community without the advantage of reputation or an established market for a retirement product. The administration has had to not only actively market the campus, but also has had to undertake an educational program that teaches the benefits of retirement campus life. To their credit, they have been very successful. It is not surprising that the operator is very positive about the success of the environment and the significant role it has played in the marketing successes.

General Project Information

PROJECT ADDRESS
La Vida Real
11588 Via Rancho San Diego
Rancho San Diego, CA 92019

PROJECT DESIGN TEAM
Architect: Mithun
Interior Designer: Martha Child Interiors
Landscape Architect: IVY Landscape Architects, Inc.
Structural Engineer: Putnam Collins & Scott Associates
Mechanical Engineer: HV Engineering
Electrical Engineer: Travis Fitzmaurice Associates
Civil Engineer: Stuart Engineering
Dining Consultant: N/A
Gerontologist: N/A
Management/Development: N/A
Contractor: Swinerton Builders

PROJECT STATUS
Completion date: September 2003

OCCUPANCY LEVELS
At facility opening date: 25%
At time of evaluation: 100%

RESIDENT AGE (YRS)
At facility opening date: 82
At time of evaluation: 85

PROJECT AREAS

Project Element	Units, Beds, or Clients	New GSF	Total Gross Area	Total on Site or Served by Project
	Included in This Project			
Apartments	210	166,328	166,328	210
Senior living/assisted living/personal care	98	64,458	64,458	98
Special care for persons with dementia	14	5,403	5,403	14
Common social areas (people)	480	19,724	19,724	480
Kitchen (daily meals served)	1440	36,985	36,985	1440
Fitness/rehab/wellness (daily visits)	N/A	913	913	N/A
Pool(s) and related areas (users)	N/A	6,643	6,643	N/A

INDEPENDENT LIVING RETIREMENT APARTMENTS

Project Element	No.	Typical Size (GSF)	Size Range (GSF)
	Apartments		
Studio units	14	469	457–499
One-bedroom units	105	669	669
Two-bedroom units	69	905	905–1057
Two-bedroom plus den units	22	1125	1126–1142
Total (all units)	210	166,328 GSF	
Residents' social areas (lounges, dining, and recreation spaces):		11,252 GSF	
Medical/health/fitness and activities areas:		5,684 GSF	
Administrative, public, and ancillary support service areas:		4,603 GSF	
Service, maintenance, and mechanical areas:		14,388 GSF	
Total gross area:		249,946 GSF	
Total net usable area (per space program):		187,867 NSF	
Overall gross/net factor (ratio of gross area/net usable area):		1.33	

ASSISTED LIVING

Project Element	No. Units	Typical Size
	New Construction	
Studio units	39	470 GSF
One-bedroom units	48	586 GSF
Total (all units)	98	64,458 GSF
Residents' social areas (lounges, dining, and recreation spaces):		6,905 GSF
Medical, health care, therapy, and activities spaces:		1,842 GSF
Administrative, public, and ancillary support services:		2,456 GSF
Service, maintenance, and mechanical areas:		1,580 GSF
Total gross area:		93,466 GSF
Total net usable area (per space program):		75,661 NSF
Overall gross/net factor (ratio of gross area/net usable area):		1.24

DEMENTIA-SPECIFIC ASSISTED LIVING

Project Element	New Construction	
	No. Units	Typical Size
Studio units	3	470 GSF
Two-room studio	11	481 GSF
Total (all units)	14	5,403 GSF
Residents' social areas (lounges, dining, and recreation spaces):		1,567 GSF
Medical, health care, therapy, and activities spaces:		65 GSF
Administrative, public, and ancillary support services:		288 GSF
Service, maintenance, and mechanical areas:		157 GSF
Total gross area:		9,808 GSF
Total net usable area (per space program):		7,323 NSF
Overall gross/net factor (ratio of gross area/net usable area):		1.34

SITE AND PARKING

SITE LOCATION
Suburban

SITE SIZE
Acres: 11
Square feet: 479,160

PARKING

Type of Parking	For This Facility			
	Residents	Staff	Visitors	Totals
Open surface lot(s)	79	26	21	126
Lot(s) under building(s)	51	—	—	51
Totals	130	26	21	177

CONSTRUCTION COSTS

SOURCE OF COST DATA
The following information is based on actual costs as of August 2003

SOFT COSTS

Land cost or value:	$5,225,000
Basic architectural and engineering:	$554,840
Expanded architectural and engineering:	N/A
All permit and other entitlement fees:	$1,416,982
Legal:	$220,932
Appraisals:	$12,500
Marketing and preopening:	$858,599
Total soft costs:	$8,288,853

BUILDING COSTS

New construction except FF&E, special finishes, floor and window coverings, HVAC, and electrical:	$37,017,679
Renovations except FF&E, special finishes, floor and window coverings, HVAC, and electrical:	N/A
FF&E and small wares:	$3,039,567
Floor coverings:	In above
Window coverings:	In above
HVAC:	In above
Electrical:	In above
Medical equipment costs:	In above
Total building costs:	$40,057,246

SITE COSTS
All site costs included in above building costs

TOTAL PROJECT COSTS
Total project costs: $48,346,099

FINANCING SOURCES
No information provided on financing sources

"My parents didn't want to move to Florida, but they turned sixty, and it was the law."

JERRY SEINFELD, 1954–

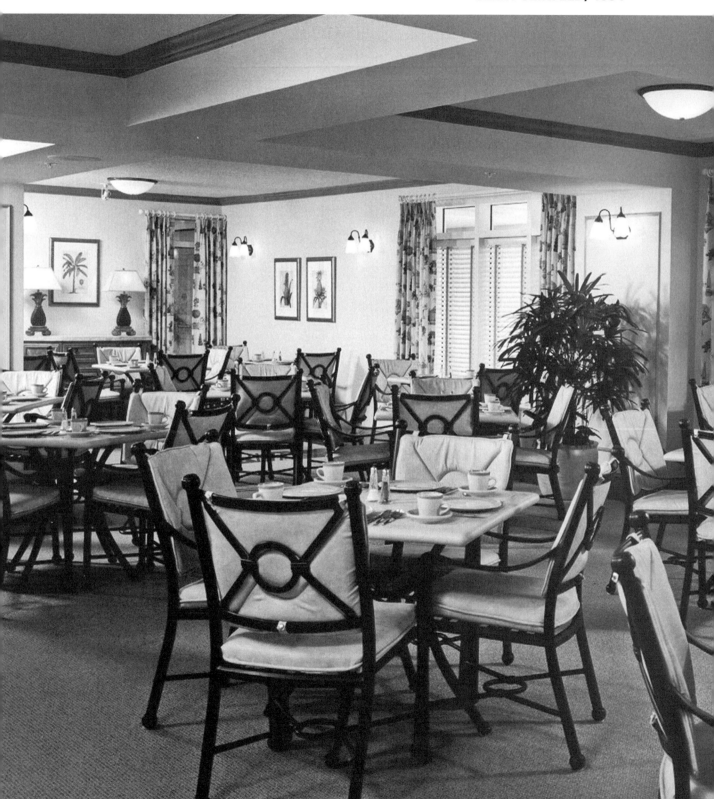

Chapter 7   McKeen Towers

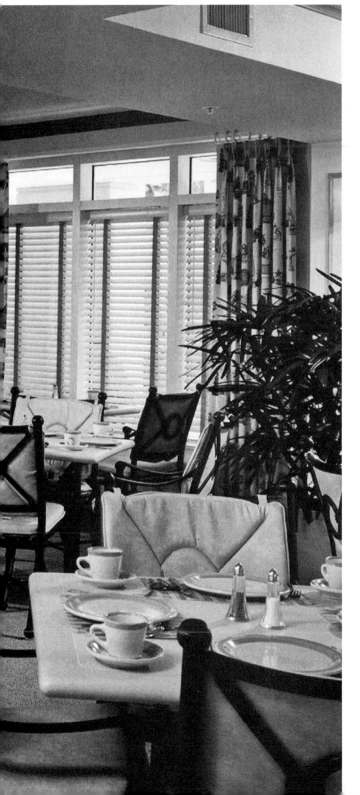

EVALUATION SITE: McKeen Towers

COMMUNITY TYPE: Continuing Care Retirement Community
- 69 independent living apartments
- 34 assisted living apartments
- 42 nursing care beds

REGION: Southeast

ARCHITECT: O'Keefe Architects, Inc.

OWNER: Carmelite Sisters for the Aged and Infirm

DATA POINTS: Resident Room: 450–1,652 gsf (independent living)
450–700 gsf (assisted living)
300–544 gsf (nursing care)
Total Area: 97,327 gsf (independent living)
Total Area: 1410.54 gsf/apartment (independent living)
Total Area: 33,999 gsf (assisted living)
Total Area: 999.97 gsf/apartment (assisted living)
Total Area: 34,858 gsf (nursing care)
Total Area: 829.95 gsf/resident (nursing care)
Overall Total Area: 166,184 gsf
Project Cost: $150.44/gsf
Total Project Cost: $25,000,000
Investment/resident: $172,413.79
Staffing: 4.33 care hours/resident/day (nursing care)
Occupancy: 95% as of January 2006 (independent living and assisted living)
98% as of January 2006 (nursing care)

FIRST OCCUPANCY: January 1998

DATE OF EVALUATION: January 2006

EVALUATION TEAM: Keith Kreidel; Nancy Perez-Miller, AIA; Mark Higgins, AIA; Ingrid Fraley, ASID

FIG. 7-1 Formal dinners are served at two seatings in designated sections of this second-floor dining room *Courtesy of O'Keefe Architects Inc.*

Introduction

The Carmelite Sisters for the Aged and Infirm are renowned in South Florida for their strong commitment to excellence and dedication to caring for the elderly. This Roman Catholic religious order of women was founded by Mother Angeline Teresa in 1929 with the approval and support of Patrick Cardinal Hayes, Archbishop of New York. Her vision of providing compassionate care with dignity and respect for the elderly in a home-like atmosphere is certainly the foundation of the Lourdes-Noreen McKeen Retirement Community.

In 1960, the Carmelite Sisters in West Palm Beach sponsored two facilities: one provided long-term care, and the other provided seasonal housing for the elderly. The latter, known as the Pennsylvania Hotel, accommodated "snowbirds," northern residents who spend only part of the year in Florida on a seasonal basis.

The Pennsylvania Hotel was designed by Addison Mizner, a prominent Florida architect, who practiced and lived in Palm Beach in the 1920s. To meet the changing and challenging needs of the elderly, the Pennsylvania Hotel was demolished and the Lourdes-McKeen Retirement Community was designed and subsequently constructed on the hotel site. Architectural details from the hotel, such as the original mailboxes, decorative lighting fixtures, and even stained-glass windows, were saved and incorporated into the new tower, which houses 69 independent retirement and 34 assisted living apartments along with 42 nursing beds that complement the 120 nursing beds that had already been constructed on the site. Although this contemporary high-rise building complements and blends into the Flagler Avenue neighborhood (see Figure 6 in the color insert), it should be noted that the demolition of the landmark hotel sparked heated debate and controversy between the Sisters, the city council, and historic preservationists.

McKeen Towers offers elegant living accommodations for the active retiree on a rental basis, with an array of stu-

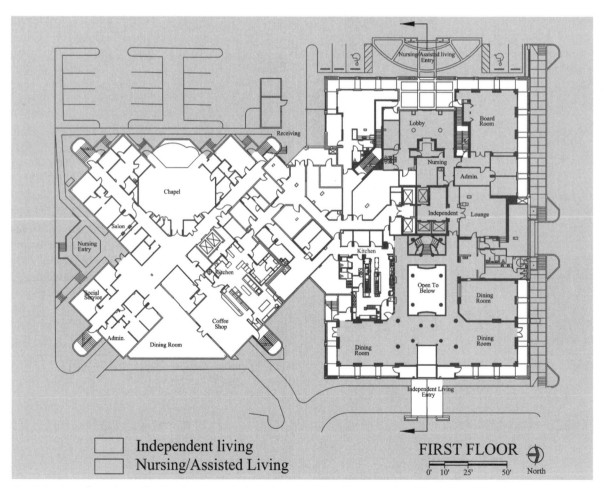

FIG. 7-2 First-floor plan indicating the separate independent and assisted living entries
Courtesy of O'Keefe Architects Inc.

dio, one-bedroom, and two-bedroom apartments featuring stunning views of downtown West Palm Beach or the intercoastal waterway and Atlantic Ocean. Twelve penthouse apartments are located on the top floor of the 13-story tower. While living on the waterfront in West Palm Beach, residents can stroll through familiar surroundings, dine at fine restaurants, shop in the boutiques at City Place, and enjoy the cultural programs at the Kravis Center.

For residents requiring personalized assistance and supportive services, the Lourdes Pavilion offers quality services and thoughtful amenities designed to support an assisted living lifestyle. Private apartments located on the fifth and sixth floors are accessed via wide corridors. These floors include well-appointed lounges and dining spaces that are finished and furnished similar to McKeen Towers, providing a seamless transition in décor and the physical environment between care levels.

The Lourdes-Noreen McKeen Residence provides long-term nursing care for the frail elderly. An earlier construction project (the data for which is not included in this evaluation), this facility provides 120 skilled nursing beds in a five-story building. With the construction of the Towers, an additional 21 beds of nursing care became available on each of the third and fourth floors.

Designer's and Operator's Stated Objectives and Responses

OBJECTIVE: Maintain one staff member for every seven skilled nursing residents.

DESIGN INTENT: The nursing portion of the project is designed with two 21-bed clusters, thus shortening travel distances for staff efficiency. The V-shaped wings and vertical design support operations' requirement of a universal worker. Staff can travel efficiently between different user groups to complete duties assigned throughout the facility.

OBJECTIVE: Provide rooms with a view to the water.

DESIGN INTENT: The site location on an intercoastal waterway offers a panoramic view of the Atlantic Ocean.

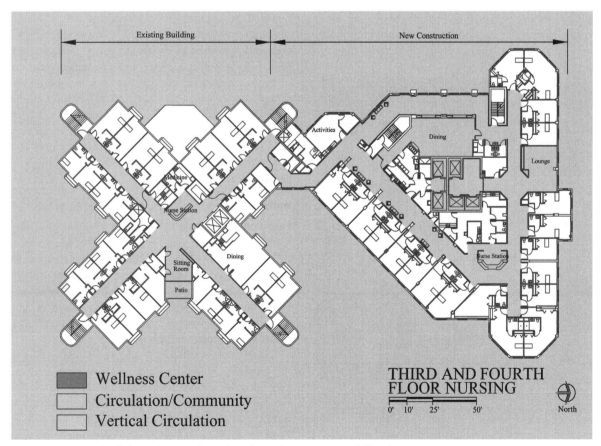

FIG. 7-3 Nursing-level plan indicating the V-shaped corridors *Courtesy of O'Keefe Architects Inc.*

The V-shaped design responds appropriately and offers views of the ocean to 95% of the units. The continuous-loop corridor and V-shaped design keep walking distance to a minimum, and decrease resident confusion and anxiety by eliminating dead-end corridors. Dining areas for fourth- and fifth-floor skilled nursing were opened up to surrounding corridors, with windows to allow views to the exterior and western sunsets.

OBJECTIVE: Respond to urban context and surrounding region.

DESIGN INTENT: The Mediterranean design responds to the regional climate and urban context. The arcade and terraces provide shade and shelter for residents to sit and enjoy the cultural events of the city. The urban setting of the CCRC allows residents to maintain their independence by being involved with the community outside their built environment. This environment, coupled with the caring spirit of the Carmelite community, enhances residents' quality of life both physically and psychologically.

OBJECTIVE: Separate assisted living and skilled nursing residents from independent residents.

DESIGN INTENT: A nine-foot slope in the site facilitated concealment of the parking garage under the building

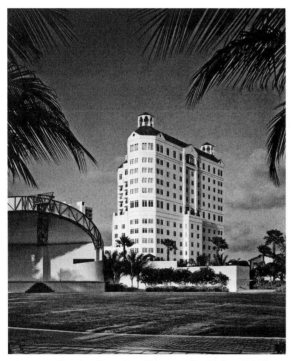

FIG. 7-4 Exterior from the adjacent park with band shell
Courtesy of O'Keefe Architects Inc.

while creating separate and unique entries for both user groups. The independent living residents enter the building at the ground level facing the intercoastal waterway, whereas nursing and assisted living residents enter one level above, on the opposite side of the building. Each group has its own lobby and elevator cores that service only the amenity areas intended for that particular group. The two groups never encounter each other, which was a major concern of the client.

OBJECTIVE: Design for sensory and mobility loss.

DESIGN INTENT: Extensive use of nongloss and nonglare surfaces, indirect lighting, and acoustical treatments throughout the building.

Field Observations: Meeting the Objectives

OBJECTIVE: Maintain one staff member for every seven skilled nursing residents.

FIELD OBSERVATIONS: The two skilled nursing floors were designed to accommodate 21 residents on each floor, thus supporting the staffing ratio of one to seven. However, each floor has to be treated as a separate staffing unit. After seven years of operation, operator consensus seems to be that 21 residents per floor are too few to achieve operational efficiency and to spread out the staffing overhead, especially the licensed nurses. The V design is awkward for maintaining visual access and supervising residents, and the location of the nurses' station at the point of the V is remote from the dining and activity areas.

OBJECTIVE: Provide rooms with a view to the water.

FIELD OBSERVATIONS: Although the initial planning featured the majority of apartments with water views, the construction of an unrelated building adjacent to McKeen Towers has reduced views of the water to just half of the apartments. Four days before the implementation of a new ordinance limiting the height of new construction on adjacent lots to four floors, a permit was issued for this adjacent high-rise.

Public spaces still have strong visual connections to the outdoors, including water and city views that are prominent focal points in lounges and dining areas. On the skilled nursing floors, the dining rooms are separated from the adjacent corridor only by a half-height wall, so views to the water are enjoyed by both diners and residents who may be out for a stroll.

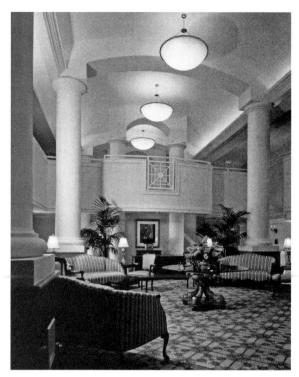

FIG. 7-5 The lobby entrance for the independent living residents has a grand staircase that leads to the second-level dining areas   *Courtesy of O'Keefe Architects Inc.*

The effort to minimize the distance from elevator to apartment, which is less than 100 feet, is certainly a benefit to both residents and staff, and is responsible for keeping the introduction of motorized wheelchairs to a minimum.

OBJECTIVE: Respond to urban context and surrounding region.

FIELD OBSERVATIONS: With the building's location on Flagler Avenue, adjacent to the city waterfront park, residents are treated to a variety of city-planned events that are just steps from their front door, including boat shows, fireworks displays, and the annual Komen Run. Just a few blocks away, City Place offers shopping and dining opportunities for every individual's taste, while the library and Meyer Amphitheater address cultural and educational desires. Lifestyle choices can vary from total independence to total pampering and indulgence through the services of the on-site facility concierge.

Architecture and interior design reflect the upscale trends of West Palm Beach, and the property is impeccably maintained. The Tower is well sited, with a strong presence and façade in keeping with its neighbors' upscale aesthetic.

OBJECTIVE: Separate assisted living and skilled nursing residents from independent residents.

FIELD OBSERVATIONS: The change in slope is cleverly used to create separate entrances for two different resident populations. The entry to the Towers that faces the water is a glamorous showcase worthy of inclusion in *Architectural Digest.* The two-story lobby is light, airy, well appointed, and immaculately maintained, resulting in a delightful interior experience.

At the opposite building side and one story up, the entrance to the Lourdes Pavillion loses some of the glitz, as it is located off the rear parking lot rather than the waterfront. Although interior finishes and furnishings are of equal quality and decorative appeal, the security station and smaller lobby size impart a bit of a predictable senior residence aesthetic. Further separation is ensured by the restriction of the elevator cabs to only assisted living and skilled nursing floors.

OBJECTIVE: Design for sensory and mobility loss.

FIELD OBSERVATIONS: Many accommodations are made to enhance sensory experiences and promote mobility. The water views undeniably have an uplifting and sensory calming effect. Leaning rails are used extensively, instead of more institutional handrail designs, and travel distances are limited to a maximum of 100 feet from the elevator. The V-shaped building does indeed avoid dead-end corridors, and eases circulation throughout each floor. Interior signage was purposefully downplayed to enhance the residential ambience. However, the lack of signage increases initial confusion; orientation is difficult until the plan of the building is experienced and well understood.

Lighting is well considered and illumination levels are increased by the lighter and more reflective color schemes that prevail. Multiple layers of lighting are used throughout and certainly add a dramatic effect, particularly in the main entry lobby, although the resulting numerous lamp types are a bit overwhelming for maintenance and pose inventory challenges.

Acoustical ceiling tiles are placed well in the public areas to support those with hearing loss, and the four decorative styles did not seem to be a maintenance issue. However, acoustics are disappointing in the chapel, where the sound system is outdated. The chapel in the original nursing building unfortunately suffers from the same lack of acoustical integrity, making it difficult for the religious residents and visitors to completely enjoy either of these beautiful spaces.

Field Observations: Themes and Hypotheses

Creating Community

Residents of the Lourdes-Noreen McKeen Retirement Community are drawn here for a variety of reasons. The location speaks volumes about integrating senior housing within the context of an urban setting and the inherent commingling of city-sponsored cultural events, close proximity to businesses and shops that address daily necessities, and of course, the beauty of the surrounding natural features.

The Carmelite Sisters' reputation for excellence is based upon their respect for quality of life in all its stages, as well as their passion for caregiving. A satisfying lifestyle is achieved through a blending of physical and spiritual needs across a broad spectrum of residents with diverse financial capabilities. Whether it is residents in Medicaid beds in skilled nursing or residents in penthouse suites in the Tower, all the residents and the surrounding community benefit from the dedication of these Sisters to serving the elderly. Although admission rules and regulations are in place, the Sisters also work from the heart, and are willing to try to meet a person's needs when other area "competitors" have refused accommodation.

Architecturally, the building supports the original program, separating two distinct groups of residents through exclusive entrances and elevators. However, McKeen Towers is also an example of the "power of the people" and their determination to use a building for their convenience regardless of its original intent.

Though the waterfront entrance to the Tower is the "wow" factor for the community, it is seldom used. Other than a small number of metered parking spaces owned by the city to support the waterfront park, there is no parking on this side for residents, family members, or guests. All above-ground parking occurs at the entrance to the Lourdes Pavilion on the back side of the building. Additional off-site parking in public garages is located nearby. This sets the pattern for residents, staff, and guests to use the entrance to the assisted living building and subsequently use the interior corridors and stairways to cross into the independent living areas.

As Tower residents age in place, some of their resistance to the assisted living and skilled nursing components within the building has lessened. In addition, the older Lourdes-Noreen McKeen Residence has two functions that encourage independent residents to cross over into this area of the facility. Although the Tower offers breakfast and dinner in separate dining rooms, lunch is

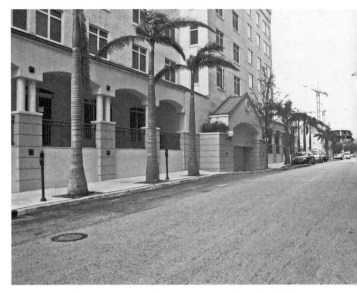

FIG. 7-6   A change in grade assists in the separation of building entrances, with the independent living on a lower level from the assisted living entrance   *Photograph by Mark J. Higgins, AIA*

available only in the Terrace Café, located in the older building. Additionally, with the loss of the Tower's full-time chaplain, the main chapel, again in the older building, is the focus for religious services and daily Mass. Thus, residents and staff find themselves utilizing a back corridor and its service elevators as the main means of getting around between areas of the facility. This route affords the most direct access to the places that residents want to visit. It is the route most traveled by all, yet it is the narrowest corridor, has the plainest of finishes, and even intersects with the back of the loading dock. Aware of this developed traffic pattern, the Sisters have wisely installed a handrail for resident use and safety.

Making a Home

With the focus of the evaluation on the facilities, staffing, and residents, it can be reiterated that McKeen Towers and the adjoining Lourdes Pavilion provide immaculate surroundings embracing upscale residential décor. Public areas are well proportioned, with human scale in mind, and support a variety of social activities that are well attended. It should also be noted that as a result of residents and staff working around the physical separation of the health care levels, Lourdes-McKeen has extended its notion of family, eased transitions to different care levels, and become "one big house."

The concierge, who is well known in the community from previous management duties at hotels and social clubs, has known some of the residents for years. He lives in one of the apartments in the tower and has the confidence of residents and family members. In addition, seven Carmelite Sisters and one priest live in the Towers, and their presence ensures that the day-to-day operations are well executed. However, it is their unique and personal investment in the lives and happiness of each resident that contributes to the feeling of home.

Regional/Cultural Design

While the skilled nursing and assisted living portions of the community have enjoyed high occupancy, the Towers languished in unacceptable ranges of occupancy below 80% for more than four years. Feedback from the marketplace revealed that the predominance of one-bedroom units was undesirable; the apparent demand for two-bedroom, two-bathroom apartments was totally unforeseen.

Stabilization at 95% occupancy was achieved by utilizing strategies that worked in concert. A change in the marketing director provided a new personality whose marketing approach is full of warmth, vitality, information, and respect. This, in conjunction with a change in marketing philosophy to emphasize the selling of a lifestyle, seemed to refocus consumer attention away from the perceived limitations of the apartment offerings and toward the lifestyle of this community.

Another component was the psychological impact on seniors living in the West Palm Beach community who did not want to face the possibility of going through another hurricane season alone. In this regard, the design features of the building—which include hurricane-proof construction, hurricane-resistant windows, and emergency generators that power most services within the apartments—coupled with a caring and dedicated staff, appear to minimize the fear associated with another big storm and to motivate potential consumers to become residents at McKeen Towers.

The Sisters are currently involved in updating the older building with new hurricane-resistant windows and improvements to the mechanical systems. Under consideration is relocation of the main chapel, which is often filled to capacity because it also serves neighborhood parishioners from adjoining apartment buildings. The original entry to the nursing home, which is not in use, features an extensive covered drop-off area with a patio deck surface above, at the second-floor level. This ambitious plan includes the enclosure of this drop-off space and extensive reconfiguration to accommodate a larger chapel for the entire community.

Environmental Therapy

Though much has been expressed about the water views and the project's convenient location with easy access to the West Palm Beach community, this ideal retirement lifestyle in Florida is complicated by the question of safety. Though McKeen struggled to increase occupancy in the early years, as a result of one-bedroom configurations, the past several years with active hurricane seasons promoted the concept of safety over the size of real estate. For many of these residents, going through another hurricane season alone was just too much. Because of its new construction materials and independent mechanical systems, the Towers can provide all the comforts of home, and adds the reassuring presence of support staff who spend much time in the building. The Towers as a home now provides safety and security even in the midst of the Florida hurricane season.

Outdoor Environment

Although the front of The Towers faces a city park, the amount of green space that is actually owned by the Sisters is severely restricted. As with any urban building,

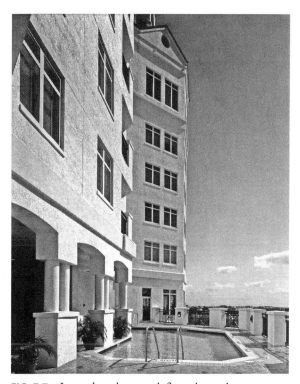

FIG. 7-7 Located on the seventh floor, the pool area provides residents with exercise, sun bathing, and dramatic views of the ocean *Courtesy of O'Keefe Architects Inc.*

ground-level space is at a premium. In this case, it is used to address parking requirements only and not garden or generous green spaces.

Covered walkways, balconies, and arcades are lovely features that enhance the regional flavor of the architecture and offer residents a choice of outdoor environments. French doors open to all of these areas and also bring the light inside. However, these multiple access points come with the expense of increased security oversight. It should be noted that balconies off the apartments are prized amenities and are limited in number, so that outdoor space for a majority of the residents is available only through these arcades and walkways.

The seventh-floor deck area features a swimming pool for the residents and spectacular views of the ocean. The exterior therapy deck on the second-floor level is a prime piece of real estate with plenty of potential, considering its proximity to the many medical services, including physical therapy, speech therapy, and activities. However, it suffers from lack of programming and is disappointingly unused and uninviting.

Quality of Workplace and the Physical Plant

Many beautiful common spaces are present in McKeen Towers, including the grand entrance and lobby, five dining rooms in skilled nursing, two dining rooms in assisted living, and the main dining room and breakfast café in independent living, as well as the entire seventh floor of the Tower, which is dedicated to a ballroom, chapel, fitness center, and pool. Wide hallways and tall ceilings set the tone, and all spaces are immaculately maintained.

In contrast, the existing 25-year-old nursing facility structure is clearly showing its age, and the community as a whole is visually divided by the new and old environments: the tired and dated versus the new and fresh approach to design, amenities, and workplace environments.

Universal workers perform laundry and housekeeping duties in assisted living and nursing assistants float between the assisted and skilled nursing areas of the building. Though distances may be at a minimum for residents, walking distances for staff are increased. With

FIG. 7-8 Typical independent living floor *Courtesy of O'Keefe Architects Inc.*

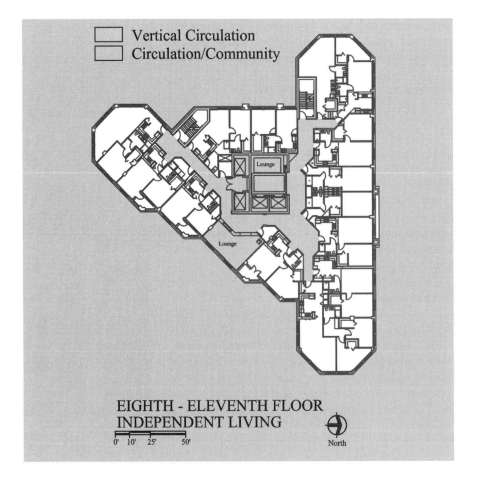

Vertical Circulation
Circulation/Community

Lounge

Lounge

EIGHTH - ELEVENTH FLOOR
INDEPENDENT LIVING

0' 10' 25'   50'

North

levels of care also split between floors, stairwells would seem to be the fastest method of traveling vertically. However, use of stairwells is restricted by code access and who among staff had the access code was not entirely clear.

Loading-dock access and kitchen designs seem to be the areas most criticized. Kitchen layouts require the wait staff to travel considerable distances to serve the residents in the Tower dining rooms.

Housekeeping also has its challenges, as service in the Tower is personalized and customized to the requirements and desires of each resident. Residents do not want a stereotypical hospitality approach to housekeeping and have confidence in their housekeepers' ability to know and meet individual preferences.

Operator Perspectives

The inclusion of both independent living and assisted living residents within the Tower was intended to act as a "feeder" of private-pay nursing care into the skilled nursing facility. However, not all of these residents come in as private-pay residents, and with the lack of restriction on the number of Medicaid patients, the operator may need to reevaluate its policies. In addition, the 12 rental penthouse units have been under consideration for conversion to life-care contract status, a change that would significantly increase cash flow.

Operational efficiency is challenged by the high-rise configuration and vastness of the common areas that must be maintained and staffed. A great deal of time and effort are required to maintain residential finishes, as well as the extensive common areas that help sell this retirement lifestyle. Included in the design mix are three separate kitchens, each with its own chefs and staff, and nine dining areas for a community population of only 230 residents. Approximately 203 full-time employees are maintained, so the ratio of residents to staff seems high.

McKeen Towers, however, offers a unique level of service to the more affluent residents of West Palm Beach. The extremely popular Caledonia Café serves only breakfast, with a made-to-order menu. The evening meal for a population of about 75 is served at two seatings in gracious and separate surroundings. The full-time concierge promotes resident well-being and knows more about individual lifestyles and preferences than any other staff person at the facility.

To the management's credit, although there are obstacles inherent in the high-rise design that add to the cost of staffing and operating the community, they manage extremely well around these perceived obstacles and "cannot imagine it in any other way."

General Project Information

PROJECT ADDRESS
McKeen Towers
311 South Flagler Drive
West Palm Beach, FL 33401

PROJECT DESIGN TEAM
Architect: O'Keefe Architects, Inc.
Interior Designer: Wellesley Design Consultants
Landscape Architect: Land Design South
Structural Engineer: McCarthy & Associates, Inc.
Mechanical Engineer: Tilden, Lobnitz & Cooper, Inc.
Electrical Engineer: M.P. Spychala & Associates, Inc.
Civil Engineer: Michael B. Schorah & Associates, Inc.
Dining Consultant: Professional Kitchens, Inc.

Gerontologist: N/A
Management/Development: N/A
Contractor: The Weitz Company

PROJECT STATUS
Completion date: January 1998

OCCUPANCY LEVELS
At facility opening date: 25%
At date of evaluation: 95%

RESIDENT AGE (YRS)
At facility opening date: 82
At date of evaluation: 82

PROJECT AREAS

INDEPENDENT LIVING RETIREMENT APARTMENTS

Project Element	Apartments		
	No.	Typical Size (GSF)	Size Range (GSF)
Studio units	14	450	450–624
One-bedroom units	49	650	560–1,024
Two-bedroom units	6	1,358	1,358–1,652
Total (all units)	69	69,075 GSF	
Residents' social areas (lounges, dining, and recreation spaces):		15,872 GSF	
Medical/health/fitness and activities areas:		6,848 GSF	
Administrative, public, and ancillary support service areas:		7,508 GSF	
Service, maintenance, and mechanical areas:		4,782 GSF	
Total gross area:		97,327 GSF	
Total net usable area (per space program):		76,037 NSF	
Overall gross/net factor (ratio of gross area/net usable area):		1.28	

ASSISTED LIVING

Project Element	New Construction	
	No. Units	Typical Size
Studio units	18	450 GSF
One bedroom units	16	700 GSF
Total (all units)	34	19,694 GSF
Residents' social areas (lounges, dining, and recreation spaces):		3,152 GSF
Medical, health care, therapy, and activities spaces:		1,096 GSF
Administrative, public, and ancillary support services:		7,897 GSF
Service, maintenance, and mechanical areas:		2,160 GSF
Total gross area:		33,999 GSF
Total net usable area (per space program):		25,757 NSF
Overall gross/net factor (ratio of gross area/net usable area):		1.32

SKILLED NURSING

Project Element	New Construction	
	No.	Typical Room Size
Residents in one-bed/single rooms	38	300 GSF
Residents in two-bed/double rooms	4	544 GSF
Totals	42	24,544 GSF
Social areas (lounges, dining, and recreation spaces):		2,552 GSF
Medical, health care, therapy, and activities spaces:		816 GSF
Administrative, public, and ancillary support services:		4,786 GSF
Service, maintenance, and mechanical areas:		2,160 GSF
Total gross area:		34,858 GSF
Total net usable area (per space program):		25,097 NSF
Overall gross/net factor (ratio of gross area/net usable area):		1.38

SITE AND PARKING

SITE LOCATION
Urban

SITE SIZE
Acres: 2.128
Square feet: 92,723

PARKING

Type of Parking	For This Facility			
	Residents	Staff	Visitors	Totals
Open surface lot(s)	27	0	3	30
Underground garage	26	0	0	26
Totals	53	0	3	56

CONSTRUCTION COSTS

SOURCE OF COST DATA
Final construction cost as of January 1998

SOFT COSTS
Total soft costs: $3,500,000

BUILDING COSTS

New construction except FF&E, special finishes, floor and window coverings, HVAC, and electrical:	$20,000,000
Renovations except FF&E, special finishes, floor and window coverings, HVAC, and electrical:	Included in above
FF&E and small wares:	Included in above
Floor coverings:	Included in above
Window coverings:	Included in above
HVAC:	Included in above
Electrical:	Included in above
Medical equipment costs:	Included in above
Total building costs:	$20,000,000

SITE COSTS

New on-site:	$1,500,000
New off-site:	N/A
Renovation on-site:	N/A
Renovation off-site:	N/A
Landscape:	Included in above
Special site features or amenities:	N/A
Total site costs:	$1,500,000

TOTAL PROJECT COSTS
Total project costs: $25,000,000

FINANCING SOURCES
Nontaxable bond offering through private sales

CARE COMPARISON

Source: www.medicare.gov—January 30, 2006
SNF staffing: 4.33 care hours/resident/day
SNF occupancy: 130 of 132 = 98.4%

Hours per Resident per Day	McKeen	FL Average	National Average
Not-for-profit	Yes		
Multifacility	No		
Levels of care	SNF		
Medicare	Yes		
Medicaid	Yes		
Licensed #	132		
# residents	130	110.3	95.3
% occ this day	98%		
RNs	0.35	0.50	0.50
LPNs	1.03	1.00	0.70
RN + LPN	1.38	1.50	1.20
CNA	2.95	2.80	2.30
RN + LPN + CNA	4.33	4.30	3.50

Part III

Assisted Living

> *"When I was young there was no respect for the young, and now that I am old there is no respect for the old. I missed out coming and going."*
>
> **J. B. PRIESTLY, 1894–1984**

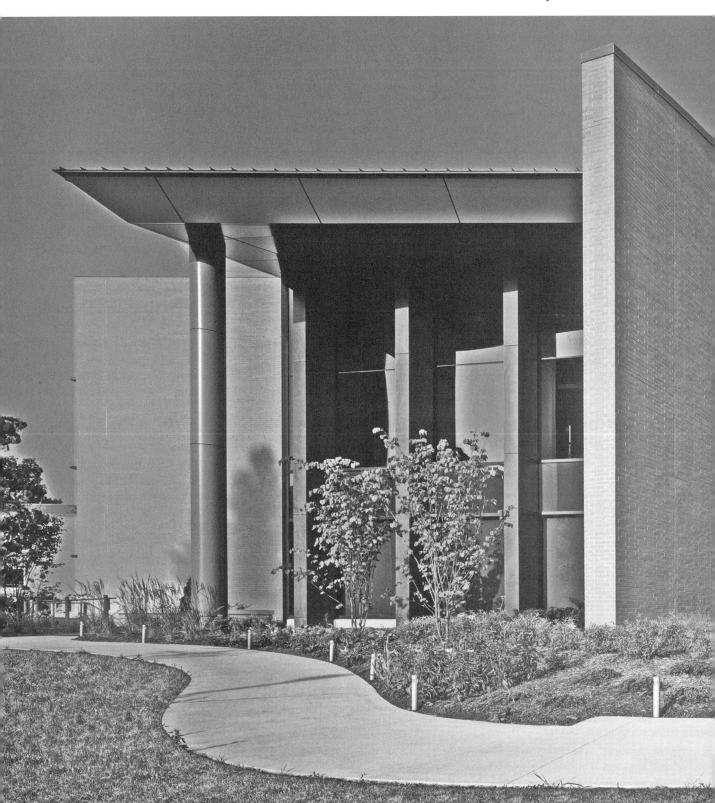

Chapter 8

Dominican Center at Marywood

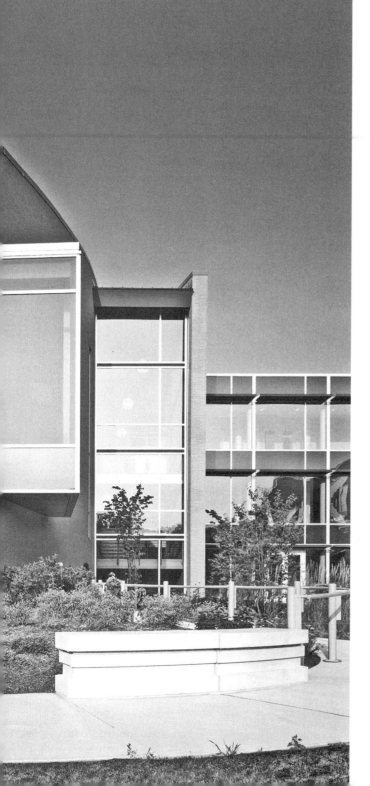

EVALUATION SITE: Dominican Center at Marywood

COMMUNITY TYPE: Assisted Living
- 31 assisted living apartments
- 10 nursing care apartments
- 10 dementia care apartments
- Exempt from state licensure for care

REGION: Midwest

ARCHITECT: Perkins Eastman Architects, P.C.

OWNER: Sisters of the Order of St. Dominic of Grand Rapids

DATA POINTS: Resident Room: 390 gsf (assisted living)
375 gsf (nursing and dementia)

Total Area:	1,572 gsf/resident
Total Area:	80,190 gsf
Project Cost:	$200.77/gsf
Total Project Cost:	$16,100,000
Investment/resident:	$315,686.27

Staffing: 1.2 care hours/resident/day (assisted living)
2.4 care hours/resident/day (nursing and dementia care)
Occupancy: 98% as of March 2006

FIRST OCCUPANCY: July 2005

DATE OF EVALUATION: March 2006

EVALUATION TEAM: John Shoesmith, AIA; Jane Rohde, AIA, FIIDA; Patricia Sprigg; Jeremy Vickers

FIG. 8-1 A contemporary approach to architecture for the elderly is evident in this exterior view of the chapel
Photograph: Hedrich Blessing/Christopher Barrett

Introduction

"How do we want to live together, pray together, socialize together, and come together as a community?" The answers to Sister Darlene Sikorski's questions are the formative forces behind the Dominican Sisters' vision for the ideal assisted living facility: a facility that would not only leave a lasting legacy for the Dominicans, but would also firmly state that the congregation is as vibrant and alive as ever.

Marywood was designed as a replacement home for the Dominican Sisters living in Aquinata Hall, an antiquated, 38-year-old traditional care facility with small resident rooms, small common areas, and double-loaded corridors. The Sisters designed a new building, with four households offering three distinct care levels, that would allow them to improve and expand the level of care they could offer. They decided early on that they did not want regulations to "overwhelm" the building and, as a religious order exempted from state regulation, were able to develop a facility free from licensing requirements. Although not licensed as such, the three levels of care offered to Sisters within the building are assisted living, dementia care, and nursing care.

In the planning stage, the Sisters asked that the building be "simple but elegant, functional and cost effective." The resulting environment certainly meets this call. Its forms are dynamic but simple. The detailing is refined, yet restrained. The building does not look anything like senior living projects of the past; instead, it offers a glimpse of what the future may hold. Despite the Sisters' exemption, the building was designed and constructed so that it could easily meet regulations with only slight modifications. The capacity for the building

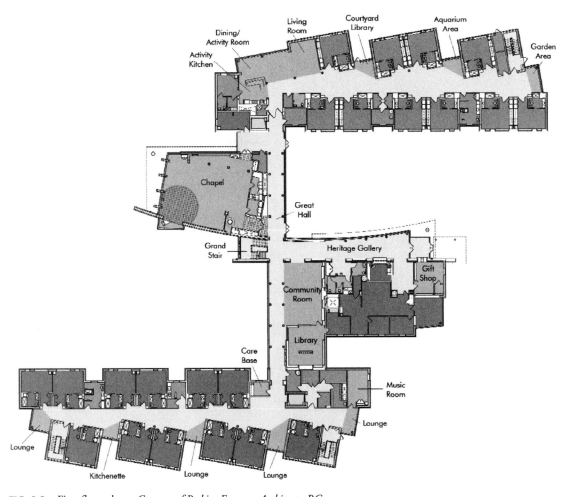

FIG. 8-2   First-floor plan   *Courtesy of Perkins Eastman Architects, P.C.*

to meet regulations in the future not only met the Sisters' desire to perhaps sell the assisted living portion eventually, but also put the facility on equal ground with other assisted living buildings.

This is an exceptional building that accomplishes most of what it set out to do. It expands the traditional definition of assisted living and senior living design and does so in a dynamic and successful way—for this alone, the project is commendable.

Designers' and Owners' Stated Objectives and Responses

OBJECTIVE: Respect and promote the Order's mission and vision by creating a "sense of place" and a visual landmark to celebrate their lives and communicate their presence to the public.

DESIGN INTENT: The Sisters' mission and vision are celebrated with a centrally located chapel and thoughtful placement of the building on a sacred site. The residence is situated prominently in the front of the site, which the Sisters consider the most sacred part of their campus. This careful positioning offers the approaching public a view of the building from every direction and places the chapel in the heart of the campus, a perfect location for the symbol of the Order's faith. Its visual presence is projected to the public and the campus through surrounding glass walls and a glass-enclosed tabernacle.

OBJECTIVE: Ensure the facility's future marketability to nonreligious entities.

DESIGN INTENT: To attract future developers, the assisted living wing could be sold floor-by-floor or in its entirety, and alcove studio units were designed to be easily converted to one-bedroom kitchenette apartments by the removal of walls between adjacent units and the conversion of closets to kitchenettes. Each apartment is prewired for cable television, high-speed Internet access, and future technologies. These amenities address the Sisters' current needs and are attractive to future lay residents. Outdoor courtyards are easily transformed into private enclaves for the Sisters or areas for public interaction.

OBJECTIVE: Create a fresh senior living design that departs from traditional typologies and addresses the simplicity of the Sisters' lifestyle.

DESIGN INTENT: An innovative design vernacular is expressed with clean volumetric forms, simple architec-

tural materials, a unique building layout, and the deconstruction of a typical double-loaded corridor. Careful site positioning resulted in a building that offers views for all resident rooms, the perception of a "building without walls," and wayfinding assistance via view corridors to sacred landmarks.

OBJECTIVE: Use green building practices wherever possible to protect the land and preserve the environment for future generations.

DESIGN INTENT: Green principles included design of the building to meet LEED Silver criteria, minimal site disturbance, and natural progressive water management.

OBJECTIVE: Design a building that promotes the provision of a higher level of care than previously available, and do so in an operationally efficient manner.

DESIGN INTENT: Grouping Sisters requiring similar levels of care into household clusters accommodates their needs more effectively than the previous scattered arrangement. The household cluster design supports a low staff-to-resident ratio of 1:10 in skilled care and 1:12 in assisted living. Support spaces are decentralized throughout the corridor.

Field Observations: Meeting the Objectives

OBJECTIVE: Respect and promote the Order's mission and vision by creating a "sense of place" and a visual landmark to celebrate their life and communicate their presence to the public.

FIELD OBSERVATIONS: Despite resistance from the neighborhood, the building was situated on the front of the property in a very prominent location. It stands clearly forward and separate from the Motherhouse, and is the first building apparent on the site when approached by car. The architect's attention to integrating the building into the natural slope of the site is commendable. The site integration allows the massing of a three-story building to complement its single-family neighbors across Lakeside Drive by appearing to be two stories as it faces them. It opens to three full stories on the west to take advantage of views of the existing wetlands and greenbelt.

The separate location of the new building forward and away from the Motherhouse is accentuated by brick that contrasts with the exterior of the existing building. The site, massing, and form of the new building set it apart so successfully that evaluators wondered if the color of the brick could have taken more of a cue from the Motherhouse without diminishing the desired distinction between the two buildings. Although it reportedly is not popular with its neighbors, the Sisters are happy with the new building and feel that it achieves their desired effect.

The simple volumes, geometries, and material used in the assisted living and nursing wings contrast with the more dynamic form, materials, and detailing of the building's entry and chapel. Curvilinear walls in both wings not only create visual interest, but also control views from within the chapel and accentuate the tabernacle inside and out.

OBJECTIVE: Ensure the facility's future marketability to nonreligious entities.

FIELD OBSERVATIONS: The created environment is certainly aesthetically appealing. The use of materials and attention to detailing are such that the building in itself is not overtly denominational. Instead, it provides a sophisticated canvas for the management and residents to include décor and objects that make a space feel more like home and to identify its use in a particular way. This is true even in the chapel area. The architecture allows the space to be nondenominational. It is the iconography brought to the chapel, rather than the space itself, that makes it belong to the Dominicans.

Common spaces included in the building address the Sisters' current needs and would be attractive to future lay residents as well. Each space is well designed, highly functional, and detailed and finished appropriately for the elderly. The quality and quantity of lighting levels in all spaces is outstanding and the lighting controls provide excellent flexibility. The inclusion of a wellness/fitness area with pool and holistic/massage therapy area are attractive assets for non-Sisters, and their location makes it easy to separate these facilities from the Sisters' area if the building were to be divided.

Resident rooms are generously sized. None of the studio units were joined to create a one-bedroom unit at the time of the POE, although it was not hard to imagine how they could be joined to create ample space. Wiring the rooms for Internet access is one amenity that is attractive to both the Sisters and future members of the lay public. More coordination could have occurred with room wiring, however, because the outlets are located in the bedroom portion of the rooms and not in the visiting area or built-in desk area adjacent the entries. Whereas the location of the outlet may not be problematic if the studios are joined to make a one-bedroom unit, the poor placement poses a challenge for the Sisters now and a potential problem for any units not combined

FIG. 8-3 The swimming pool at the wellness center where holistic therapy is administered *Photograph by John Shoesmith, AIA*

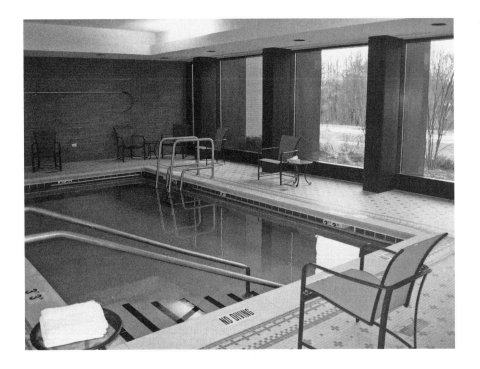

in the future. Currently, the Sisters who have computers keep them on the exterior wall adjacent to the bed, because of proximity to the outlet.

OBJECTIVE: Create a fresh senior living design that departs from traditional typologies and addresses the simplicity of the Sisters' lifestyle.

FIELD OBSERVATIONS: The created environment sheds many of our preconceptions of senior living while still being true to the sense of home for the Sisters who live there. (See Figure 7 in the color insert.)

The volumetric forms of the Marywood building are simply expressed and reinforced with material selection and detailing. Materials are used seamlessly from exterior to interior, reinforcing the concept of bringing the outdoors inside and the idea of a "building without walls." The brick volumes of the paired resident units contrast to the service spaces, which feature corrugated metal siding and punched window openings. Alcove spaces are expressed through floor-to-ceiling glass detailing. To tie the building together, the punched openings and storefront styles are repeated in the unit window openings for the bedroom and living room.

In an effort to reduce the perceived length of the corridor, units are paired and their orientation is skewed along one side of the corridor. This creates alcoves between each pair of rooms and increases opportunities for views to the outside by creating openings to the exterior at each of these points. Pairing the units in this way also allows service space to be located unobtrusively across from each alcove, as the eye is drawn to the alcove and its indoor/outdoor connection instead of the service space. The layout successfully minimizes the corridor length and the number and location of service spaces. The effect is greatest when moving from resident rooms toward core common spaces. Unfortunately, the effect is not equally strong in the opposite direction, as the positioning of the resident room limits the visibility of the alcoves. Even so, natural light enters the corridor at these points and helps to break up the corridor.

Activity lounges are sized to easily accommodate activity by small groups of residents. Unfortunately, activity in the alcoves is not programmed; as a result, the spaces are not being used as the Sisters had envisioned and furnished them. Some Sisters are using the alcove adjacent their units merely as an extension of their living rooms. The Sisters are in their first year of occupation and are still getting their feet underneath them operationally. It will be interesting to see if and how alcove use changes over time.

The commitment the design team made to incorporate natural light, connect the building to the outdoors, and provide views of established site landmarks to assist in wayfinding are definite highlights of the building.

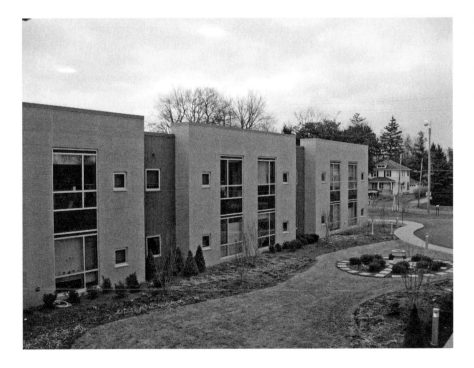

FIG. 8-4 A residential wing with volumes defined by use of differing materials *Photograph courtesy of Jane Rohde, AIA, FIIDA, JSR Associates, Inc.*

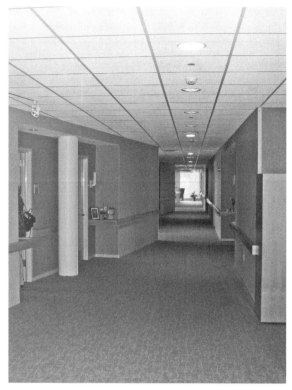

FIG. 8-5 A residential corridor with alcoves and inset entry doors *Photograph by John Shoesmith, AIA*

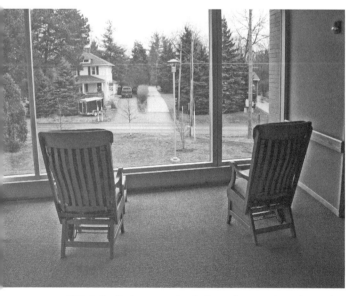

FIG. 8-6 By incorporating intimate lounges along the corridor length, natural light is introduced into the building *Photograph courtesy of Jane Rohde, AIA, FIIDA, JSR Associates, Inc.*

OBJECTIVE: Use green building practices wherever possible to protect the land and preserve the environment for future generations.

FIELD OBSERVATIONS: Marywood was designed to meet LEED Silver criteria, although there was and is no intention of certifying the building as such. The Sisters felt that some of the LEED requirements, such as providing a double-pipe system for recycling gray water, were cost prohibitive.

Low-E glass use and the indoor and outdoor shading systems have been effective. Many Sisters remarked that they like the Mecho shades because the multidirectional operation allows them to control both sunlight and views into their rooms.

Although the two-pipe heating system operates efficiently and is centrally monitored by the head of maintenance, the system has caused some issues. The location of air diffusers in resident rooms, difficulty in regulating thermostats, and lack of acoustical insulation at the units are all drawbacks the Sisters cite in reference to the system. The air diffuser blows air directly on the bed, and the Sisters think the units are noisy, although the review team did not find them noisier than average. It could simply be that they are noisier than the hot-water radiant system in the previous residence.

Furnishing costs were decreased by recycling and incorporating some of the Sisters' heirlooms into the new building. Where appropriate, pieces were reupholstered in more modern finishes to blend with the new interior color palette. Pieces selected for reuse are all appropriate for the elderly and appear to be easy for the Sisters to use (e.g., chairs are stable and have arms that allow Sisters to get in and out of them easily). Reuse of this furniture provides wonderful accent pieces and suitable seating that is very attractive and meaningful to the Sisters.

OBJECTIVE: Design a building that promotes the provision of a higher level of care than previously available, and do so in an operationally efficient manner.

FIELD OBSERVATIONS: Aquinata Hall, the Sisters' former residence, had a compact, double-loaded corridor design with narrow, small rooms that made for very short travel distances for staff. Sisters' needs were addressed in whatever room they happened to reside in at the time, and no Sisters were segregated to certain parts of the building based on health needs.

The households in the new Marywood building are designed so that Sisters with similar needs live together. The building includes two households of assisted living care, one of nursing care, and one of dementia care. Although none is currently licensed, they are designed so

92

Part III   Assisted Living

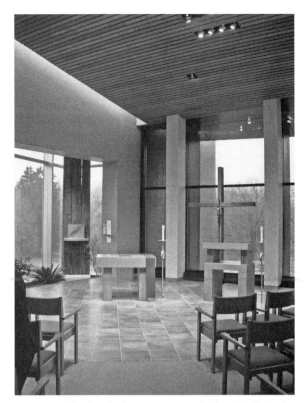

FIG. 8-7 The chapel where services are held and individuals can meditate *Photograph courtesy of Jane Rohde, AIA, FIIDA, JSR Associates, Inc.*

that licensing is possible for the future. The only exception made to the codes was the distance from resident rooms to the nurses' area.

The assisted living households are in the south end of the building and the dementia care household is in the north, with common spaces and the chapel between them. Staff who work with both groups of residents must travel great distances between the assisted living and dementia care households.

Staff cited many design elements that they felt detracted from operational efficiency of the building, including the length of corridors within each household and the perceived distance between staff and residents. Additionally, the distance of the stairs (versus elevators) from each nursing unit prevents staff from getting from one floor to another in a timely manner; the distance of the food-preparation kitchen in the Motherhouse from the serving kitchen in the building is also problematic. The staff feel that any operational efficiency gained by the staffing ratios in the households is undermined by the distance between each household.

It was interesting to observe that staff have transferred their traffic and work patterns from the old building to the

new one. Cleaning, linen, dining service, and medication carts are parked throughout the hallways, detracting from the intended residential feel, despite the numerous decentralized support spaces in each household.

Field Observations: Themes and Hypotheses

Creating Community

The Sisters have all known each other for many years, and this extended knowledge and relationship with one another mean they truly live together as a family. Such a well-developed sense of community makes special demands of the Marywood building, especially in light of the newly segregated care levels.

Marywood seems a sprawling campus to many of the Sisters, although they do consider the building and its amenities an improvement over the previous environment. Some Sisters have not actually traveled through the entire building, because the distances are too far for them. Some of the comments made by Sisters interviewed conveyed that they have not seen or are not aware of several common spaces available to them that are not adjacent to their households. Although most references to room size and configuration were positive, a Sister occupying a room at the end of one household reported that the pairing of the rooms and the distance to the common space make her feel somewhat isolated. She also worries that staff could not reach her quickly during an emergency.

Some of the Sisters feel that several community spaces are too large and located in too public an area to foster the type of community or household gatherings that they would like to participate in. One Sister mentioned that "social feeling was missing" because of the large, public spaces. Interestingly, the neglected alcoves provide abundant community space between each room pair to foster the social element in each household. Perhaps the space is overlooked for social interaction because it is too open to the corridor and not fully enclosed.

Making a Home

Resident bedrooms are one of the biggest positives of the Marywood center for the Sisters. Although all rooms are studios, the Sisters found them to be quite ample, and one Sister remarked that she felt her studio actually had four separate rooms: an entry, a visiting or parlor area, a bedroom, and a bathroom. The same studio unit type is replicated throughout the assisted living, dementia care, and nursing portions of the building, the only change in the room being the amount of built-ins provided in lieu of furniture as one moves from assisted living to nursing. The rooms were universally designed and seemed to suit each population effectively.

Designers obtained a code variance to provide a split door in the resident room between the sleeping area and the bath. Although not a problem for some Sisters to operate, these have not been as successful as expected. The weight of the doors is unmanageable for the frailer Sisters. The door hardware on the resident room entries and in common spaces is also problematic. Standard door closers were installed on these doors, but the resistance of the standard door closer combined with the weight of the door makes it extremely difficult for most Sisters to open the doors. Electronic free-arm closers, in which the closer is activated only when an alarm is sounded in the building, may have eliminated this problem.

Pairing the units to reduce the size of the corridors and hide service spaces is an effective way of diminishing what could have been two very noticeable institutional elements within the building.

The décor in the building also makes the Sisters feel at home. Incorporating heirloom furniture, using artwork that speaks to the Sisters' religious affiliation, and leaving the building as a canvas for the resident and staff décor is a brilliant way to allow the Sisters to adapt the building to their needs and vision, while leaving the fundamental design free from religious iconography to encourage future sale of the facility.

The Sisters would like a guest room where friends and family can stay in the building. Further, one Sister feels that eventually there may be a need for hospice rooms in the future where family, friends, or caregivers could visit and perhaps stay with a Sister needing hospice care. She did not feel that the 100% studio design lends itself well to this type of need.

Environmental Therapy

Administration and the Sisters both report that the abundance of windows and the resulting views, natural light, and feeling of connection to the outdoors have positive effects on the Sisters. Many Sisters commented on how wonderful it is to have a strong orientation to the outdoors, not only in the views afforded them from their rooms, but from the corridors and common spaces as well. The views to the Motherhouse act as a wayfinding landmark for some of the Sisters. The connection to the outdoors and natural light have resulted in less depression and improved general attitudes among the Sisters, according to the administration.

The outdoor feel and the abundance of natural light encourage the Sisters to do even more in an effort to save natural resources. During our review, we saw many of the Sisters opting to use natural light rather than the

FIG. 8-8 Dining room with serving and activity kitchen beyond, opening to residential corridor
Photograph: Hedrich Blessing/Christopher Barrett

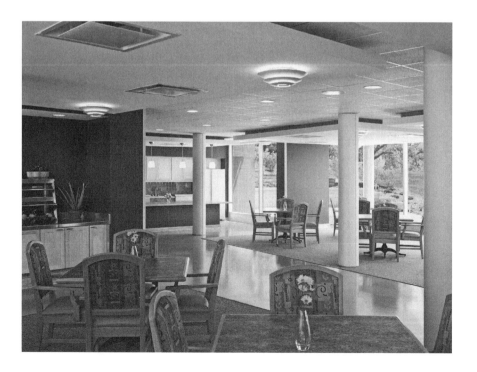

fixtures. Many corridor light fixtures were switched to the minimum required for ambulation, and lights were switched off completely in many common spaces, even areas in use.

Further, the connection to the outdoors and layout of the building are reportedly encouraging some Sisters to take walks in the winter months when they would not have done so previously.

Quality of Workplace and the Physical Plant

Long walking distances to the stairs versus elevators, to the main kitchen, and between staff and residents, and the distance between households all hinder efficiency and eliminate the benefits of higher-than-average staffing ratios, according to staff. Spaces designed for decentralized services have apparently not been totally or successfully embraced by the staff, as there were med carts and cleaning and dining carts throughout the hallways.

The Sisters and staff are pleased with the low-E glass and the shading systems installed inside and out. Maintenance monitors the two-pipe heating system and, despite some complaints from the Sisters about the thermostats, noise, and location of the system, maintenance says the system is efficient and easy to manage.

Interior materials were selected for their environmentally friendly and sustainable characteristics. Unfortunately, the composite rubber-and-cork flooring product has not worn well in its first year. It translates imperfec-

tions from the concrete underneath, looks dated, and is a constant concern for maintenance and administration.

Operator Perspectives

The Dominican Sisters are very pleased with the Marywood project and offered the following perspectives on the first seven months of operation.

The Sisters are happy with their decision not to license the building to prevent regulations from overwhelming the home-like environment. They recognize the practicality of eventually licensing the facility and are proud of their forward-thinking design. The facility was executed in a way that did not compromise their goals and will serve them well if they decide to sell or lease a portion of the building to a private, outside provider.

Despite the usual details and problems that crop up when adjusting to new surroundings, the Marywood project has exceeded the Dominican Sisters' expectations and is an enduring landmark that communicates the mission of the Sisters to the community and will continue to do so well into the future. The Sisters are proud of their new home and of the image it portrays to the community. One Sister delighted in telling us that she heard a visitor to the Motherhouse look out the window at Marywood and say, "If that is retirement then I'll be willing to retire tomorrow."

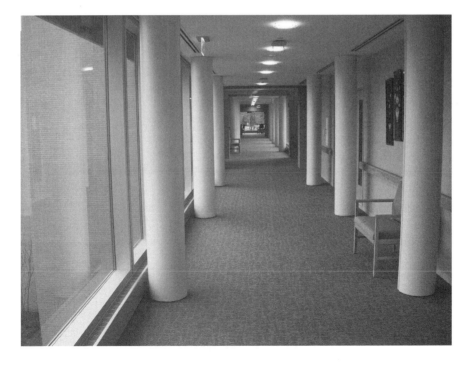

FIG. 8-9 The single-loaded corridor, with natural light penetrating the building and community spaces on the opposite side of the corridor *Photograph courtesy of Jane Rohde, AIA, FIIDA, JSR Associates, Inc.*

General Project Information

PROJECT ADDRESS
Grand Rapids Dominicans
Dominican Center at Marywood
2023 Fulton Street East
Grand Rapids, MI 49503

PROJECT DESIGN TEAM
Architect: Perkins Eastman Architects P.C.
Interior Designer: Perkins Eastman Architects P.C.
Landscape Architect: Wolff Clements & Associates, Ltd.
Structural Engineer: Graef, Anhalt, Scloemer & Associates, Inc.
Mechanical Engineer: OWP/P
Electrical Engineer: OWP/P
Civil Engineer: Moore & Bruggink, Inc.
Food Service: Baker Group

Liturgical Design: INAI Studio
Chapel Lighting: Gary Steffy Lighting Design, Inc.
Acoustical Engineer: Acoustics by Design
Pool Design: Innovative Aquatic Design, LLC
Contractor: Erhardt Construction

PROJECT STATUS
Completion date: July 2005

OCCUPANCY LEVELS
At facility opening date: 100%
At date of evaluation: 98%

RESIDENT AGE (YRS)
At facility opening date: 89
At date of evaluation: 89

PROJECT AREAS

Project Element	Units, Beds, or Clients	New GSF	Total Gross Area	Total on Site or Served by Project
		Included in This Project		
Assisted living (units)	31	390	12,090	31
Special care for persons with dementia	10	375	3,750	10
Skilled nursing care (beds)	10	375	3,750	10
Common social areas (people)	51	11,358	11,358	51
Kitchen (daily meals served)	200	1,427	1,427	200
Retail space (shops/restaurants, etc.)	1	366	366	1
Fitness/rehabilitation/wellness (daily visits)	30	963	963	30
Pool(s) and related areas (users)	100	1,163	1,163	100
Other (please describe): Chapel (users)	80	2,921	2,921	80

ASSISTED LIVING AND NURSING

Project Element	No. Units	Typical Size
	New Construction	
Single bedroom units (studio)	51	384 GSF
Total (all units)	51	19,590 GSF
Residents' social areas (lounges, dining, and recreation spaces):		11,358 GSF
Medical, healthcare, therapies, and activities spaces:		5,726 GSF
Administrative, public and ancillary support services:		3,738 GSF
Service, maintenance, and mechanical areas:		12,327 GSF
Total gross area:		80,190 GSF
Total net usable area (per space program):		52,739 NSF
Overall gross/net factor (ratio of gross area/net usable area):		1.5

SITE AND PARKING

SITE LOCATION
Suburban

SITE SIZE
Acres: 10.5
Square feet: 461,027
Area of entire campus: 33 acres

PARKING

Type of Parking	For This Facility			
	Residents	Staff	Visitors	Totals
Open surface lot(s)	0	26	24	50
Carports or garages	0	2	0	2
Totals	0	28	24	52

CONSTRUCTION COSTS

SOURCE OF COST DATA
Final construction cost as of June 30, 2005

SOFT COSTS

Land cost or value:	N/A
All permit and other entitlement fees:	$60,000
Legal:	N/A
Appraisals:	N/A
Marketing and preopening:	N/A
Other:	N/A
Total soft costs:	$1,600,000

BUILDING COSTS

New construction except FF&E, special finishes, floor and window coverings, HVAC, and electrical:	$7,730,000
Renovations except FF&E, special finishes, floor and window coverings, HVAC, and electrical:	$50,000
FF&E and small wares:	$500,000
Floor coverings:	$350,000
Window coverings:	$135,000
HVAC:	$2,438,000
Electrical:	$2,353,000
Medical equipment costs:	N/A
Total building costs:	$13,556,000

SITE COSTS

New on-site:	$606,000
New off-site:	$75,000
Renovation on-site:	N/A
Renovation off-site:	N/A
Landscape:	$263,000
Special site features or amenities:	N/A
Total site costs:	$944,000

TOTAL PROJECT COSTS
(include all fees and costs, except financing)
Total project costs: $16,100,000

FINANCING SOURCES
Conventional (private) financing

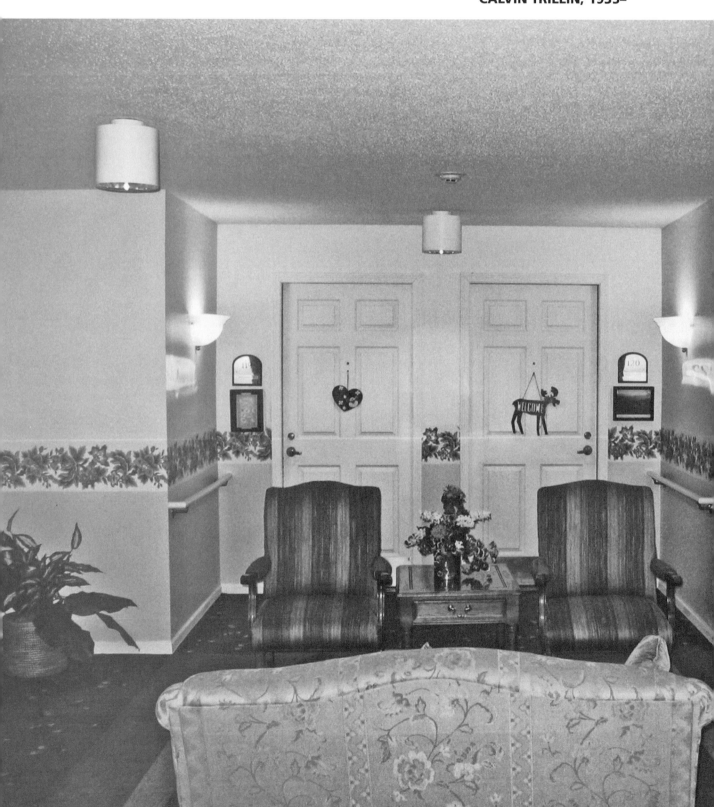

"The most remarkable thing about my mother is that for thirty years she served the family nothing but leftovers. The original meal has never been found."

CALVIN TRILLIN, 1935–

Chapter 9

Rosewood Estate of Roseville

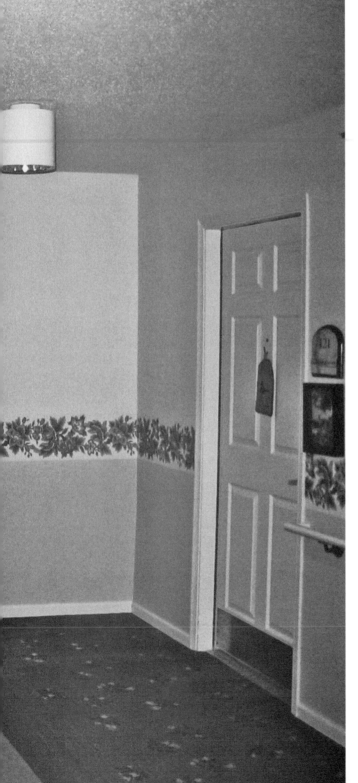

EVALUATION SITE: Rosewood Estate of Roseville

COMMUNITY TYPE: Assisted Living Facility
- 68 assisted living apartments

REGION: Northern Midwest

ARCHITECT: Arvid Elness Architects, Inc.

OWNER: Care Institute, Inc. (original owner was Liberty Rosewood Limited Partnership)

MANAGER: Sunrise® Senior Living

DATA POINTS:

Apartment Size:	363–630 gsf
Average Apartment Size:	550 gsf
Total Area:	892 gsf/resident
Total Project Area:	60,663 gsf
Total Project Cost:	$5,000,000
Investment/resident:	$73,529.41
Staffing:	1.74 care hours/resident/day
Occupancy:	98% as of October 2005

FIRST OCCUPANCY: July 1989

DATE OF EVALUATION: October 2005

EVALUATION TEAM: Mina Adsit, AIA; Terri Zborowsky, Ph.D. candidate; David Reimer; David Slack; Jeffrey Anderzhon, AIA

FIG. 9-1 A resident lounge surrounded by resident apartment entries *Photograph by Jeffrey Anderzhon*

Introduction

Snuggled into a suburban residential neighborhood adjacent to one of Minnesota's 10,000 lakes, the colonial architectural style of Rosewood Estate appears both completely at home and out of place in its northern plains surroundings. (See Figure 8 in the color insert.) To the layperson, however, the colonial-style building's location and visual approach convey a residential feeling and create a sense of home that is intuitively felt the moment the building comes into view. Designed and built at a time when assisted living facilities were still searching for both physical and care provision identity, Rosewood Estate, designed by Arvid Elness, provides a guiding example that nearly 20 years later is still considered a success. Completed and opened in 1989, Rosewood Estate was designed with 68 apartments varying in size from a 363-square-foot studio to a 521-square-foot one-bedroom apartment. Each living space, except the smallest studios, has a distinctive living area separate from the sleeping area and a full kitchen and bathroom.

Rosewood Estate was conceived as a congregate independent apartment facility that includes meals and housekeeping. In addition, residents could contract with an on-site, independent home health care agency for care provision services. As early manifestations of assisted living began to take on distinctive care provision characteristics, the facility quickly and easily adapted to the new concept and was very successful in its marketing efforts.

In 1993, a short four years after opening, Rosewood Estate added 40 more assisted living apartment units. The addition to Rosewood Estate does not have the same sensitivity to residents or staff as the original. Designed by a firm of Mr. Elness's contemporaries, it falls short in almost all respects, implicit or explicit, of the original residence. In fact, this addition detracts from the original and its only successes are from a marketing standpoint.

Set on a suburban lot in St. Paul, Minnesota, wedged between a fairly busy street and a lake, the facility takes advantage of the small area and of the topography of the lawn sloping from the street to the lake. The building is three stories with two above the street-level grade and a third, walk-out floor on the lake side. Each floor has resident apartments. The lower-level street side that is below grade is devoted to mechanical, support, and activity spaces that do not require windows.

The site is crowded with the original building, the 1993 addition, and parking for staff and visitors. The only space devoted to exterior resident activities is a short walking path around the parking lot to a small sitting area and dock overlooking the lake. Topography and the size of the lot prevent the facility from adding more outdoor spaces for residents. There are, however, very pleasing views from the lakeside apartments and public spaces. There is a well-used but crowded deck on the lake side of the building.

The building plan's apartment arrangement is arguably one of the first to recognize decentralization of building functions. Apartments are arranged around small social spaces that soften the public corridors and provide transitional space between public and private living areas. This arrangement gives the fairly large facility a more intimate feel and provides residents respite on their journeys to and from the central living and dining spaces. An added benefit is that the arrangement of the rooms decreases the distance between any apartment entry door and the main social spaces at the center of the building.

A conscious effort on the part of the design team has created an environment that is the antithesis of institutional—Rosewood truly displays the elements necessary to achieve a residential feel. As one approaches the building, one sees a colonial style that is compatible with the neighboring single-family homes, and its symmetry provides an intuitive welcome at the entrance. Understanding the entry sequence and the general arrangement of space within the building is second nature. No time need be wasted on orientation; one's attention can be immediately focused on the interior finishes and, more implicitly, on the care program housed within the surroundings.

Residential order of design and iconography abound throughout this facility, reinforcing the deinstitutionalization of the environment. The building features a secured main entry, controlled by the receptionist and flanked on one side by a covered porch complete with rocking chairs. Mirroring the covered porch, there is a dining room extension leading into a foyer with a high ceiling and the receptionist's area. This foyer features a decorative staircase to the second level and lies adjacent to a parlor with an eye-catching fireplace. The living room lies straight ahead as one enters the foyer. The resident apartments are located symmetrically on either side of the main social spaces. The arrangement of these spaces is residential in nature.

Placed in the context of the time of construction and the state of the care provision profession, Rosewood Estate provides a measuring stick against which many subsequent assisted living facilities were judged. This comparison succeeded in establishing fundamental criteria for "household" or "cluster" arrangements within a floor plate and established a definition of "residential"

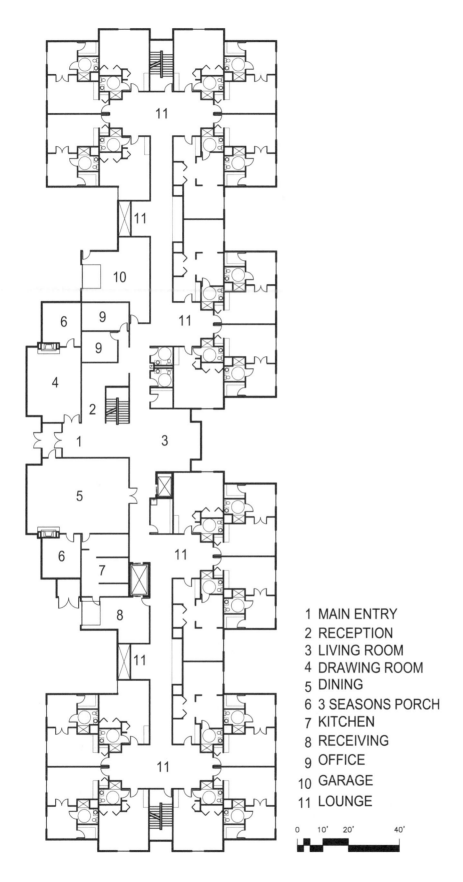

FIG. 9-2 Entry-level floor
plan *Graphic by Jason Reis*

1 MAIN ENTRY
2 RECEPTION
3 LIVING ROOM
4 DRAWING ROOM
5 DINING
6 3 SEASONS PORCH
7 KITCHEN
8 RECEIVING
9 OFFICE
10 GARAGE
11 LOUNGE

0   10'   20'   40'

and its expression, even in a large structure. Much has been learned over the years from the standards set by Rosewood Estate's design; much can still be taken from it as a lesson in providing a noninstitutional environment for increasingly institutional functions.

Designers' and Operators' Stated Objectives and Responses

AUTHOR'S NOTE: *Because of the age of this facility, there was no recoverable record of stated design objectives or design intents. Those indicated here have been gleaned from articles and publications regarding Rosewood Estate by the design architect and others.*

OBJECTIVE: Create a noninstitutional, home-like character.

DESIGN INTENT: Rosewood Estate utilizes residential, colonial-style architecture with simple detailing and symmetry. The site lends itself to a two-story street façade that is made more residential with high-sloped roofs, decorative dormers, accentuated masonry chimneys, and a distinctive entry porch. The floor plan distinguishes between the central portion of the structure and the two sides, thereby reducing the scale of the larger building and giving it the look of a smaller house added onto over the years. Residential construction methods, detailing, and finish materials throughout the construction provide both economy and a noninstitutional feel.

Organization of central common spaces is supported by features typical to an average home, such as the central monumental stair, drawing room, and opposing dining-room fireplaces. Furnishings enhance the noninstitutional ambiance. Long, unbroken, and repetitive corridors typical of nursing facilities are replaced by an arrangement of apartments around decentralized and more individualized lounges. The introduction of natural lighting, wherever possible, increases the feeling of spaciousness in both public and private spaces.

OBJECTIVE: Increase residents' social well-being through the architectural environment.

DESIGN INTENT: The use of a "cluster" design that provides social spaces surrounded by apartments enhances resident social interaction. The building provides opportunity and choice in resident activities and socialization, and the conscious emphasis on noninstitutional design lays the foundation for residents' social well-being.

OBJECTIVE: Emphasize independence and self-help.

DESIGN INTENT: Providing full apartments with fully accessible bathrooms for residents is the first step to independence. Residents can prepare their own meals in their kitchens or choose to dine in the congregate dining room. Laundry rooms on each floor are also provided for

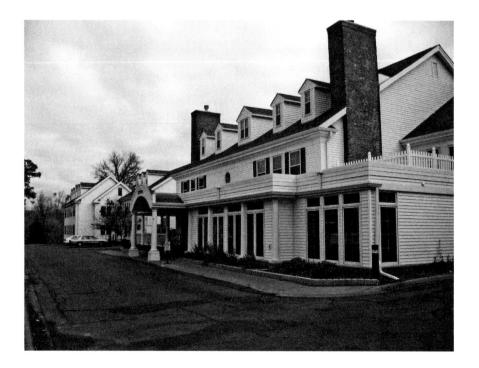

FIG. 9-3 Entry exterior with front porch just beyond main entry and 1993 addition in background *Photograph by Jeffrey Anderzhon*

resident use. As a nonlicensed facility, the Rosewood Estate care program includes only those services the residents chose to receive at the time the facility was opened. The residents can maintain their health programs independently of the facility and utilize Rosewood's services when necessary. The architecture lends itself to independence, because the cluster design decreases the length of the corridors leading to central common spaces and thus encourages participation in social activities and care provision.

OBJECTIVE: Dissolve the edges between the public or common areas of the building and the private living spaces in the facility.

DESIGN INTENT: The clusters provide a social area for apartment groupings of four to eight individual units. This feature is the initial step in designing an effective transition between public and private areas within the building. With this approach, the corridors disappear and become part of the living space for the residents. Residential interior finishes, the building layout, and a basic design that recalls residential architecture also work to meet this objective. Spaces familiar to each of our homes are fully defined and institutional finishes are removed. The entire building, beyond the individual apartments, becomes the residents' home.

OBJECTIVE: Deliver needed care to residents at a cost lower than traditional licensed nursing facilities.

DESIGN INTENT: The construction costs were lower for Rosewood Estate than for an institutional-model nursing facility because residential construction methods and materials were used. The savings are passed on to residents in the lower cost of housing and related services. Because residents can contract for as many or as few care services as needed or desired, the costs to residents are minimized. The combination of lower real estate costs and resident-controlled care costs provides an economical alternative to the traditional institutional nursing facility.

Field Observations: Meeting the Objectives

OBJECTIVE: Create a noninstitutional, home-like character.

FIELD OBSERVATIONS: The designers made a conscious effort to impart a residential feel to the facility. The colonial-style design immediately gives the structure an ambience that most people would associate with residential. The building massing, use of topography, and the addition of various architectural elements give the building the look of a large home, despite the fact that there are a substantial number of apartments within the structure. The gabled roof with its dormers and lapped siding, the formal and symmetrical massing, and the double-hung

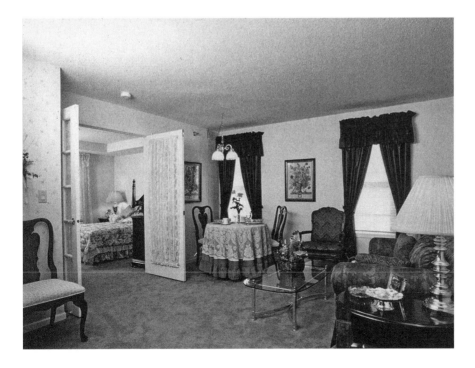

FIG. 9-4 Resident apartment with sleeping alcove
Image courtesy of ESG Architects, Inc.

operable windows reinforce the residential image of the building from the street.

The addition to the original facility sadly breaks the illusion that the structure is a house and not a congregate living facility. The addition also significantly detracts from the original architecture, even though it was intended to complement the original design. The lack of continuity is exacerbated by a huge electrical generator at the front of the building. Even to the most casual observer, the building addition is clearly a distraction from the original architecture and carries the entire structure significantly away from its home-like character.

Although the use of a colonial style in the design is not consistent with the building's northern plains location, it does feel comfortable on the wooded site adjacent to single-family residences. The larger parking lot is at a lower level than the street and is somewhat hidden by landscaping; additionally, the visitor parking near the building's entry is not overpowering enough to be objectionable.

The layout of the original building is well considered, follows a well ordered—if somewhat formal—residential design, and was one of the first designs to cluster apartments around social space. This contributes to a noninstitutional feeling and provides spaces where social interaction can take place on a variety of levels. It also reduces the visual presence of the corridor between centrally located common space and resident apartments.

Originally, the intervening lounges along the corridor received significant amounts of natural light, but these spaces were converted to offices as the need for staffing increased with the reduced acuity level of residents. Some of the lounges were reduced to small sitting areas with little natural light, which altered the function and ambience of those spaces. A preferable solution would have been to accommodate these offices within the 1993 addition and keep the original design in place to preserve the residential feel of the building.

Interior finishes and furnishings were selected in keeping with the residential theme. Carpet, warm wall colors, and detailing provide simple elegance, acoustical control, and durability. There is very little of the vinyl tile so prevalent in institutions for the elderly. The lighting, however, is very institutional. Most spaces are lit from ceiling-mounted fluorescent fixtures or recessed can lights, which provide light levels that may suit younger eyes but are substandard for older adults.

The apartments in the original design are one-bedroom, studio, or alcove units with full bathrooms and kitchens. The original intent was for residents to be fully independent and to have them contract for care assistance only when necessary. This approach amounted to nothing more than an age-restricted apartment building, albeit with congregate social spaces and a home health care agency. The layout of the apartments is definitively residential because the apartments were initially designed to be homes. The most popular unit

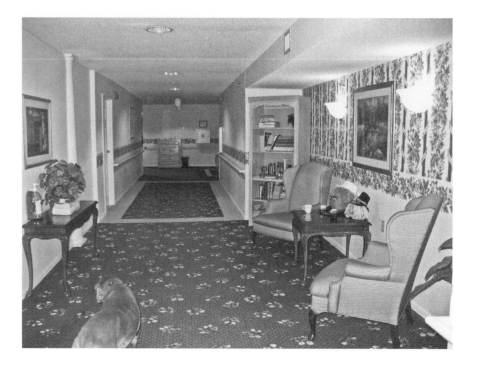

FIG. 9-5 The former corridor lounge was converted to offices, blocking the natural light that once flowed into this space *Photograph by Jeffrey Anderzhon*

is a 520-square-foot one-bedroom with a walk-in closet. According to staff, the most difficult apartments to market are those at the ends of the corridors, with longer walking distances to the dining room and central community spaces.

Although couples are welcome, room dimensions do not easily accommodate double or larger-sized beds. The only practical option for a couple interested in Rosewood Estate would be single beds placed some distance apart. These few downsides to the apartments do not appear to be significant barriers to high occupancy: the marketing department reports receiving some 400 inquiries per year for approximately 35 annual apartment turnovers.

OBJECTIVE: Increase residents' social well-being through the architectural environment.

FIELD OBSERVATIONS: Upon entering Rosewood Estate, the comfortable common areas, a dining room, and an attractive stairway greet the eye and impart a positive impression of the facility. On the day of the evaluation, 10 residents were seated near the entry. With the exception of one male and one female resident, they were not speaking to one another or even sitting near each other. One woman watched the birds in the aviary; others were situated in a living room area observing the receptionist and those entering and leaving the building. Six residents were seated in the dining room for either a late breakfast or early lunch; they each sat at their own table.

The airlock entry is equipped with two automatic doors, the purpose of which is largely defeated as the first and second entry doors open nearly simultaneously. Residents sitting near the front door certainly feel bursts of humidity and heat in the summer and cold in the winter. The foyer is too small to accommodate visitors as well as provide a sitting area for residents. Despite this fact, residents seem to congregate in this high-traffic area. It seems to be "the place to be."

Most staff members know each resident by name and greet residents as they pass in the hall. Residents seem pleased when staff take a moment to visit and seem to gather in areas where staff members are present. Fifteen-year-old furnishings in areas without staff do not show any signs of wear, but furniture of the same vintage in common areas near staff appear to be worn with frequent use. The areas seeing the least amount of use were the smaller, decentralized lounges in the cluster design.

The architectural environment's residential nature increases the social well-being of residents but falls just short of a true success. The diverse and ever-changing resident population and the design approach are partly to blame for the environment's few inadequacies. Because the original designers were forced to develop new ideas and approaches, given the lack of design precedents, the project has become a compilation of the design changes that followed its conception in the intervening years. It is easier to assess the various improvements to the building in this context. Our perspective

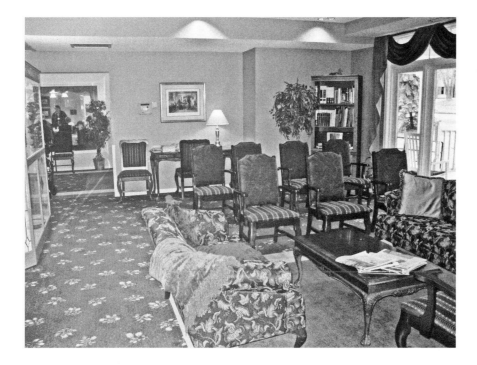

FIG. 9-6 The drawing room set up for resident activities *Photograph by Jeffrey Anderzhon*

would have been significantly different had Rosewood Estate not been forced to set its own precedents.

OBJECTIVE: Emphasize independence and self-help.

FIELD OBSERVATIONS: Because of Rosewood's pioneering new care provision model, independence and self-help were paramount to both the architectural design and the structure of the care program. The design emphasis on independence starts in the resident apartments. Private rooms with full kitchens and fully accessible bathrooms allow residents to move around their own rooms independently, regardless of their physical ailments. This same design allows residents to remain in their apartment homes as their health deteriorates and they need higher levels of care. The opportunity for residents to move about the interior of the building and participate in social activities was also well considered. Each floor level is fully accessible by either of the two elevators in the original design.

Unfortunately, the site does not allow complete independence, as there is no bus service or convenient stores and services within walking distance. This mandates reliance on friends, family members, or the facility van when residents engage in community shopping or cultural events. Additionally, the topography makes it very difficult for residents with ambulatory impairment to navigate around the site. This is particularly disappointing because the site is adjacent to a medium-sized lake resplendent with wildlife and natural beauty during all seasons.

OBJECTIVE: Dissolve the edges between the public or common areas of the building and the private living spaces in the facility.

FIELD OBSERVATIONS: Of all the objectives within the designer's scope, the issue of public versus private space was addressed most successfully. Rosewood Estate moved the design of elderly facilities toward a noninstitutional, nonmedical model by blurring the distinction between public and private spaces. The significance of the design as an industry benchmark should not be underestimated. Within this design there is a merging of congregate social spaces and private rooms. Many spaces are not clearly owned either by residents or by staff, which makes the spaces available to everyone in a manner that accommodates the moment or the individual.

To some extent, the concept of shared space is difficult for residents and staff to fully embrace. Thus, the purpose of the various spaces in Rosewood tends to be defined not by the intent of the original design but by residents' actual usage. This is not a failure of the architecture, but a failure of the population to understand the architecture and take full advantage of the environment.

OBJECTIVE: Deliver needed care to residents at a cost lower than traditional licensed nursing facilities.

FIELD OBSERVATIONS: When developing its new concept of environment and care provision, one of the facility's main objectives was to provide a more cost-effective alternative to institutionalized nursing care. There is really no question that the facility achieved this through a number of innovative approaches, including:

- Establishing the community within a nonlicensed facility.
- Using less expensive residential construction methods and materials.
- Providing only the care an individual requires, through an on-site home health agency.
- Promoting independence and self-help so that residents theoretically maintain their health longer and thereby reduce care costs.
- Avoiding regulated reimbursement costs, which allows more accurate and fairer compensation to the facility for care provision expenses.

Field Observations: Themes and Hypotheses

Creating Community

A sense of community is present within the Rosewood Estate facility and is in part created through the design of the facility. However, the community identity has boundaries that are present not as a result of the design, but from the personality that has emerged from the facility.

During the visit, about 30 residents gathered for a morning exercise activity held in the drawing room. Residents sat in very close proximity to each other, but spoke only to the staff member leading the activity. They seemed enthusiastic about the exercise, but did not use the activity as an opportunity to interact with other residents. Following exercises, the residents assembled in the lobby to enjoy refreshments before hearing a staff member read articles from the local newspaper aloud. Except for one male and one female resident holding hands and visiting, residents spoke only to the staff member.

Senior living communities often cater to older adults who are part of a specific affinity group. Rosewood Estate does not serve any such affinity group, and

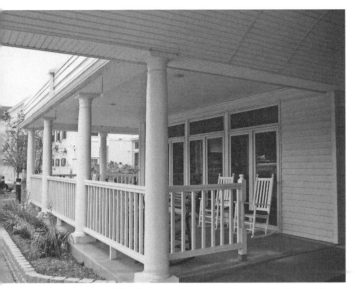

FIG. 9-7 The front porch at the main entry invites residents and visitors to linger *Photograph by Jeffrey Anderzhon*

as a result it struggles to encourage resident-to-resident interaction and nurture a significant sense of community. Because residents prefer spaces with a continual staff presence, underutilized rooms such as the chapel are vulnerable to remodeling for other purposes.

Making a Home

The deinstitutionalization of Rosewood begins before one even enters the facility: the colonial-style building truly looks like a home, and its location amongst other single-family homes in a residential neighborhood furthers the home-like design.

The planning stages for Rosewood occurred at the dawn of assisted living and certainly before there were licensure requirements for assisted living facilities. To that end, the apartment layouts do contribute to a home-like atmosphere because they are, in fact, homes for the residents. Ample closets for storage are designed into each unit. The proportions and dimensions of the rooms provide for both economy of space and flexibility in furniture arrangements. The selection and arrangement of windows in the units provide very good natural lighting; however, the artificial lighting again falls below standards acceptable for the elderly.

The full kitchens, bathrooms, and separate living areas in each living space encourage resident independence and also help to develop a homey feel. Residents can prepare their own meals and use the laundry rooms

on each floor to remain independent and really feel at home at Rosewood. The building layout makes it easy for residents to get around, and the cluster design definitely enhances the facility.

Regional/Cultural Design

Although the colonial design style selected for Rosewood Estate is not familiar to the facility's northern plains location, it was a suitable design choice. The style immediately brings a residential feel to the facility and is faithfully followed in both building massing and detailing.

Environmental Therapy

It appears that the quality of life for residents of Rosewood Estate is enhanced by the environment. The average age of residents is continually increasing, intimating that their length of stay is also increasing. When one compares Rosewood Estate and the stereotypical institutional nursing facility, there is no question that the environment of Rosewood Estate provides a therapeutic benefit. The comparison glows even brighter when one considers the fact that Rosewood Estate was conceived and constructed at a time when there were few or no alternatives to medical-model nursing facilities for elder care.

Outdoor Environment

The site on which Rosewood Estate is constructed is small and restrictive, and the topography, though providing a benefit to the building itself with its walk-out lower level, discourages resident usage. There is a lovely but small deck overlooking the lake that is a favorite spot for many residents.

Although the lake and wooded environs are attractive in any season, residents are generally able to enjoy the surroundings only from within the building. Aside from providing deer and bird feeders, little has been done to the exterior to promote resident participation in the outdoors.

Quality of Workplace and the Physical Plant

For the most part, staff seem pleased with Rosewood Estate as a workplace and the longevity of the tenure of most staff is indicative of this. As with many care facilities, Rosewood Estate has some difficulty in attracting professional staff, not so much as a result of the

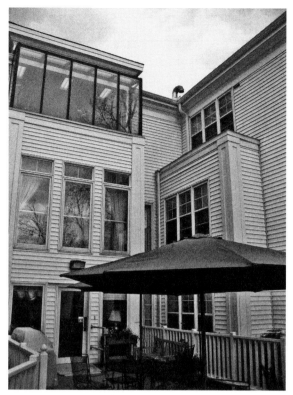

FIG. 9-8 The crowded and confined rear deck overlooks the adjacent lake *Photograph by Jeffrey Anderzhon*

workplace environment but because of the limited local workforce.

This environment has now been in use for some 15 years and has been adapted to meet the changing needs of the staff and of operations. The adaptations that have been made, for the most part, aid in providing a more efficient workplace, even if they have altered the original intent of the design. With an increased care program, and with additional burden placed particularly on the kitchen by the apartments added in 1993, the environment has been tested and the staff have adapted and innovated well.

Operator Perspectives

The operations of Rosewood Estate have evolved over the years, but always with the philosophy that the real estate and the operations should be separated for the benefit of both. Following private ownership and operations, the facility has come under the umbrella of Sunrise Senior Living, a large national organization that both owns and operates assisted living facilities. The current operators have not had the benefit of interaction with the designer regarding the original concept; thus, they have accepted the environment at face value and have successfully provided care to the residents within that environment.

Undoubtedly the current operators would have taken a different approach to the environment had they been the original operators. This is not to say that during the interview process they had criticisms of the environment on any major issue. However, the operator perspective on design in this case is one of adaptation rather than input. Additionally, the current operator provides a care program different from the original vision. Remarkably, the new care program has successfully adapted to the environment with considerably little environmental modification.

General Project Information

PROJECT ADDRESS
Rosewood Estate of Roseville
2750 North Victoria Street
Roseville, MN 55113

PROJECT DESIGN TEAM
Architect: Arvid Elness Architects, Inc.
Interior Designer: Arthur Shuster, Inc.
Landscape Architect: Damon Farber
Structural Engineer: Unknown
Mechanical Engineer: Unknown
Electrical Engineer: Unknown
Civil Engineer: Unknown
Dining Consultant: Unknown
Gerontologist: Unknown

Management/Development: Unknown
Contractor: Unknown

PROJECT STATUS
Completion date: July 1989
(addition completed 1993)

OCCUPANCY LEVELS
At facility opening date: 95%
At date of evaluation: 98%

RESIDENT AGE (YRS)
At facility opening date: 82.5
October 2005 average: 83.5

PROJECT AREAS

ASSISTED LIVING

AUTHOR'S NOTE: *Project data included for original project only, not for addition of 36 assisted living units in 1993.*

	New Construction	
Project Element	No. Units	Typical Size
Studio units	32	400 GSF
One-bedroom units	36	520 GSF
Total (all units)	68	31,720 GSF
Residents' social areas (lounges, dining, and recreation spaces):		7,890 GSF
Medical, health care, therapy, and activities spaces:		1,800 GSF
Administrative, public, and ancillary support services:		800 GSF
Service, maintenance, and mechanical areas:		7,256 GSF
Total gross area:		60,663 GSF
Total net usable area (per space program):		49,210 NSF
Overall gross/net factor (ratio of gross area/net usable area):		1.23

SITE AND PARKING

SITE LOCATION
Suburban

SITE SIZE
Acres: 1.92
Square feet: 83,635

PARKING
Type of parking: Open surface lot, 39 spaces

CONSTRUCTION COSTS

AUTHOR'S NOTE: *At the time this project was submitted for the* Design for Aging Review *in 1992, detailed cost data was not required. The cost data presented here is from several sources, including the original designer successor firm and the operator.*

SOURCE OF COST DATA
Final construction cost as of 1989

SOFT COSTS

Land cost or value:	Unknown
All permit and other entitlement fees:	Unknown
Legal and professional fees:	Unknown
Appraisals:	Unknown
Marketing and preopening:	Unknown
Total soft costs:	Unknown

BUILDING COSTS

New construction except FF&E, special finishes, floor and window coverings, HVAC, and electrical:	Unknown
Renovations except FF&E, special finishes, floor and window coverings, HVAC, and electrical:	Unknown
FF&E and small wares:	Unknown
Floor coverings:	Unknown
Window coverings:	Unknown
HVAC:	Unknown
Electrical:	Unknown
Medical equipment costs:	Unknown
Total building costs:	$5,000,000

SITE COSTS

New on-site:	Unknown
New off-site:	Unknown
Renovation on-site:	Unknown
Renovation off-site:	Unknown
Landscape:	Unknown
Special site features or amenities:	Unknown
Total site costs:	Unknown

TOTAL PROJECT COSTS

Total project costs:	Unknown

FINANCING SOURCES
Private financing

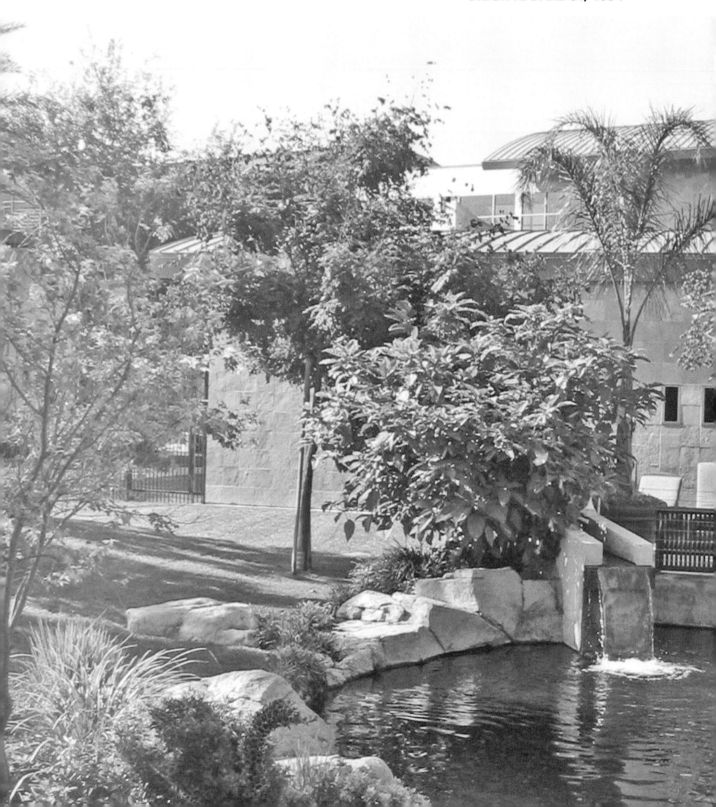

"It is sad to grow old but nice to ripen."

BRIGITTE BARDOT, 1934–

Chapter 10

The Fran and Ray Stark Villa

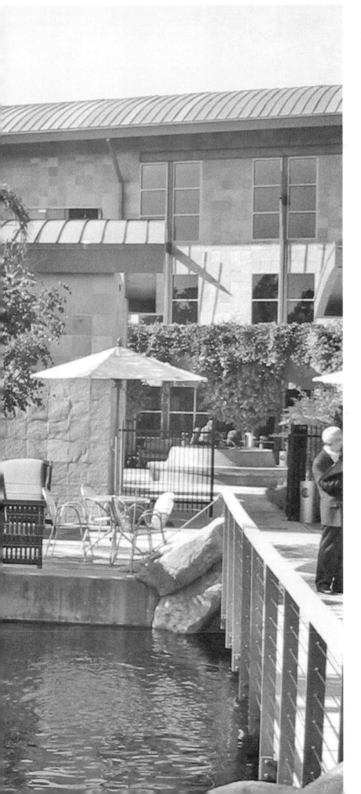

EVALUATION SITE: The Fran and Ray Stark Villa

COMMUNITY TYPE: Assisted Living Community, part of a CCRC

• 70 assisted living apartments

REGION: West Coast

ARCHITECT: SmithGroup

OWNER: Motion Picture and Television Fund

DATA POINTS:	
Apartment Size:	450–850 gsf
Average Apartment Size:	542 gsf
Total Area:	900 gsf/resident
Total Project Area:	63,000 gsf
Total Project Cost:	$16,000,000
Investment/resident:	$228,571.43/resident
Staffing:	1.6 care hours/resident/day
Average Age:	84.7 years
Occupancy:	95% as of October 2005

FIRST OCCUPANCY: October 2001

DATE OF EVALUATION: October 2005

EVALUATION TEAM: John Grace; Ryan Grace; Drue Ellen Lawlor, FASID; John Pace, AIA; Mitch Green, AIA; Jeffrey Anderzhon, AIA

FIG. 10-1 The Wasserman Koi Pond with Stark Villa beyond *Photograph by Jeffrey Anderzhon*

Introduction

The Fran and Ray Stark Villa sits near the east central portion of the Motion Picture and Television Fund (MPTF) Foundation's Woodland Hills campus. Founded in 1921, MPTF is a unique affinity group whose members share a professional interest in the entertainment business. Begun by Mary Pickford and Charlie Chaplin as a self-help support service for unemployed actors, MPTF has grown to embrace insurance, wellness, home health services, acute health care, and long-term care as parts of its mission.

The Woodland Hills campus has been a key part of MPTF since before World War II. Presently the campus includes 180 residential units and more than 250 health care beds. The hospital has seven levels of care, from intensive care to long-term and dementia care. Residential space includes 60 cottages, 50 "lodge rooms," and the subject of this evaluation, the 70-unit Fran and Ray Stark Villa assisted living residence.

Woodland Hills sits on the southern edge of the San Fernando Valley, west of Interstate 405 and inland from Malibu and the Pacific Ocean. When MPTF was established, Woodland Hills was a small, almost "country" community at the edge of large orchards. Over the next 30 years, the area filled with modest one-story bungalows of wood clapboard siding and cedar-shake roofs. Bougainvillea bursts into color below massive live oaks and cypress climbs into lower reaches of the canyons above Mulholland Drive. Woodland Hills is subject to the same marine layer that shrouds the Los Angeles basin many mornings a year, but its inland location and protective hills generally give it a sunny, dry, and hot climate.

Over the years, MPTF acquired about 80 acres, but has whittled the property down to the 40 acres that form today's campus; only half of the property is actually developed. The land slopes gently but consistently uphill from north to south, making the north end's hospital entry about three floors lower than the Villa entry to the south. Developed as needs became pressing and donations became available, the campus is an informal collection of mostly one-story buildings surrounded by mature, lovingly tended landscaping. The overall effect is relaxed and low-key, in many ways a good match for the bungalows in the surrounding neighborhoods.

By the mid-1990s, MPTF recognized that its existing campus might no longer meet the needs of current residents aging in place or respond to a consumer market in search of noninstitutional alternatives. San Francisco architect, the SmithGroup, was retained to produce a campus master plan, which called for:

- Phased development of the remaining land in clusters of buildings.
- A new north-south central pedestrian spine with parallel parking and service driveways at the edges.
- A new main-campus entry and center housing administrative and wellness functions.

FIG. 10-2 The Roddy McDowall Rose Garden at The Stark Villa is a richly landscaped retreat for residents *Photograph by Jeffrey Anderzhon*

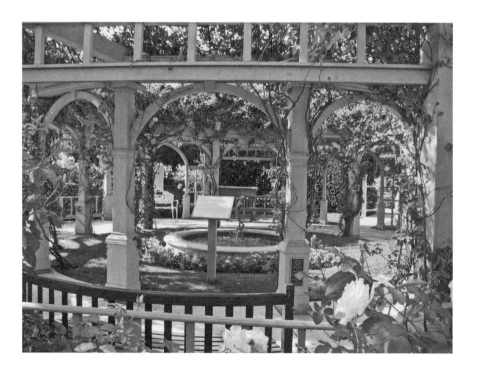

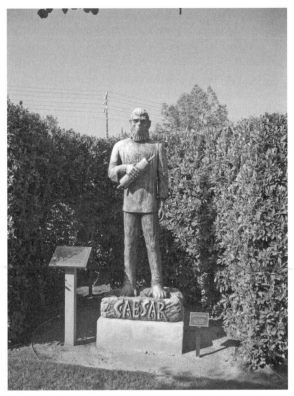

FIG. 10-3 Sculpture on the campus includes bronze tributes to John Wayne and Roddy McDowall and adds visual interest to the landscaped grounds *Photograph by Jeffrey Anderzhon*

SmithGroup was also hired to design the first of the new building clusters: an assisted living project. MPTF's intention was to offer older, frailer adults an alternative to the stand-alone cottages—which are better suited to more mobile, younger populations—and the institutional "lodge room" studios created in renovated hospital space.

MPTF built the existing campus through donations, and the assisted living project was no different. Once a major donor was identified during schematics—keeping in mind what had been termed an "8- to 10-year waiting list"—a significant decision was made to maximize the total number of living units within the already established development footprint and budget. The result, completed in October 2001, was a three-story, 63,000-gross-square-foot community with 70 apartment units, of which 70% are studios, 25% are one-bedroom units, and 5% are two-bedroom units.

The Villa is a distinctive piece of architecture that contrasts with both the existing campus environment and mainstream assisted living design. The barrel-vaulted roofs; nonhistoricized aesthetics; combination of stone, metal, and plaster exterior materials; and profusion of balconies and terraces give the project an unmistakably contemporary feeling. The massing and placement of lower and higher volumes that frame open spaces give the Villa an energy and dynamism

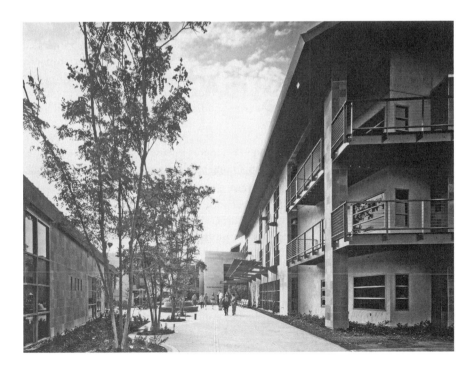

FIG. 10-4 The main entry courtyard is flanked by the distinctive assisted living building and separate meeting-room buildings *Photograph by John Edward Linden*

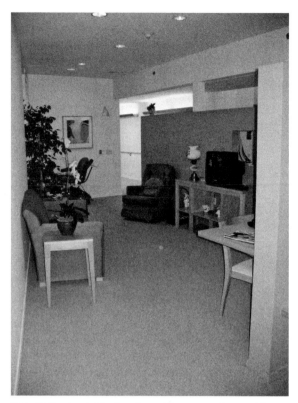

FIG. 10-5 A neighborhood transition space where resident socialization can take place in a casual setting *Photograph by Jeffrey Anderzhon*

that is a significant departure from the existing campus's predominately mid-century modern aesthetic.

The contemporary design approach continues inside with a double-height entry hall complete with a Hollywood staircase flowing from a second-floor balcony overlooking a portion of the dining room. (See Figure 9 in the color insert.) A second-level outdoor terrace makes the Villa seem almost cut in two by a stone wall that slices through the project from a koi pond on the east toward the shuttle-bus stop on the west. Furnishings have simple lines, accent walls have strong colors, and lighting eschews table lamps in favor of mid-century modern pendants, cove lighting, and wall-washers. Not your grandmother's assisted living residence, one is tempted to observe.

Designers' and Operators' Stated Objectives and Responses

OBJECTIVE: To exemplify aging in place by emphasizing dignity and independence for residents.

DESIGN INTENT: The Villa's layout employs several strategies to emphasize dignity and independence and to set the standard for aging-in-place models. The designers divided the building into six resident households, creating the potential for dining options on each floor and providing spaces and furnishings that support independent movement.

The Villa is Z-shaped, with roughly equal residential "arms" extending from the central entry and common areas on all three floors. Each arm has a social space at its interior corner, creating for each 12 to 15 residents a "family room" close to their apartments. The design further encourages ambulation by providing built-in benches along the hallway side of these social spaces, and wayfinding is aided by accent colors on prominent walls.

During the design stage, operations requested the ability to provide dining on each floor. The Villa design accommodates this with support kitchens and sub-dining rooms on the second and third floors in addition to the main dining room on the first floor.

OBJECTIVE: To provide a home-like atmosphere.

DESIGN INTENT: Single-loaded corridors with ample daylight and views, balconies for each unit, accessible upper-floor terraces, ground-level gardens, and patios all make the most of indoor-outdoor connections, reinforce the noninstitutional nature of the Villa, and firmly locate it in its southern California setting. The continuous sense of the outside is balanced by relatively simple, undecorated interiors intended by the design team to encourage residents to personalize both private and semi-public spaces.

The decentralized social spaces were also intended to help create a noninstitutional, home-like atmosphere. In theory, if residents of one wing frequented activities at a family room in another wing, then residents might feel that the entire building was part of their personal living space.

OBJECTIVE: To support a sense of community and social interaction among residents.

DESIGN INTENT: Decentralizing social and activity spaces created "attractions" throughout the Villa. Some spaces across the courtyard in an activity pavilion were placed specifically to promote resident mixing through movement. Game rooms, a spa, a business center, a potting room, an exercise room, an aviary, and a kitchen garden with raised planting beds are located with the intent to activate all floors of the Villa. A large second-floor dining terrace, the koi pond beyond the activity pavilion, and the rose garden across the entry drive pull residents

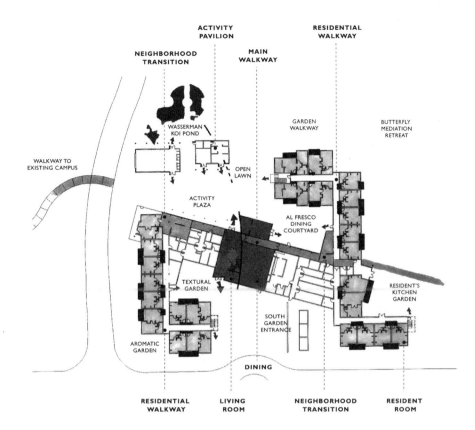

ACTIVITY PAVILION

RESIDENTIAL WALKWAY

NEIGHBORHOOD TRANSITION

MAIN WALKWAY

WALKWAY TO EXISTING CAMPUS

GARDEN WALKWAY

BUTTERFLY MEDIATION RETREAT

WASSERMAN KOI POND

OPEN LAWN

ACTIVITY PLAZA

AL FRESCO DINING COURTYARD

TEXTURAL GARDEN

RESIDENT'S KITCHEN GARDEN

SOUTH GARDEN ENTRANCE

AROMATIC GARDEN

DINING

RESIDENTIAL WALKWAY

LIVING ROOM

NEIGHBORHOOD TRANSITION

RESIDENT ROOM

FIG. 10-6 First-floor plan
Graphic by SmithGroup, Inc.

farther outside and enhance the possibility of interacting with residents from elsewhere on the campus.

OBJECTIVE: To address the particular interests of the motion picture and television industry.

DESIGN INTENT: Activity programming and some limited building features—such as cable television and Internet access in every apartment, first-run movies to be shown in the activity pavilion, barrel-vaulted roof shapes reminiscent of Hollywood soundstages, and a memorabilia gallery on the first floor—were all envisioned during the design stage to showcase the community's connection to the entertainment industry. Indicated on the plans but not initially outfitted or staffed was a radio production room, intended to allow residents to continue their avocation by producing programs to be broadcast throughout the Villa.

OBJECTIVE: To link to other buildings on campus.

DESIGN INTENT: Rather than acting as a single building block, the Villa embraces key aspects of the campus master plan. The plan's new north-south circulation spine runs through the heart of the Villa zone, widening into a courtyard fronted by the main Villa building and the activity pavilion. The circulation spine becomes a main organizing feature of the design, with the possibility of linking the kitchen garden to future development.

The main courtyard leads to the lovely Roddy McDowell Rose Garden and, beyond the garden, downhill to the existing campus. On the far side of the entry hall, a smaller courtyard leads to resident parking and the on-campus shuttle stop.

Field Observations: Meeting the Objectives

OBJECTIVE: To exemplify aging in place by emphasizing dignity and independence for residents.

FIELD OBSERVATIONS: The Villa works well for a population that is on average about two years older than designers anticipated during planning. The average age has increased from 83 years to almost 85 years campus-wide since 2002. According to staff, there is more demand for nonambulatory accommodation and new residents are now more frail at move-in than in the past.

Because the Villa was designed for aging in place,

changes in resident profile and code restrictions have resulted in less diversity than originally imagined. Licensed as a "Residential Care Facility for the Elderly," the Villa is not allowed to accommodate anyone who requires tube feeding, is bedridden, or requires 24-hour nursing supervision. This limitation makes accommodating nonambulatory residents on the three floors more difficult. License restrictions and slower-than-anticipated increases in occupancy have eliminated the use of the upper-floor dining areas for special populations. Approximately 40% of the residents use walkers and wheelchairs, and care staff provide approximately 1.6 hours of direct care per resident per day.

Residents and staff noted that the family rooms at the residential arms of the building layout are well used, particularly in the mornings. Some of the rooms are more popular than others, and the built-in benches near these areas are not as much appreciated as some of the rooms, because the detailing makes them uncomfortable to sit in, according to staff.

OBJECTIVE: To provide a home-like atmosphere.

FIELD OBSERVATIONS: The opportunity to personalize hallway spaces adjacent to apartments and motion picture memorabilia displayed throughout give the Villa a strong personality and sense of its residents. The "undecorated" hallway finishes create a gallery-like background for movie posters, awards, photos, and other mementos. Small niches at the first-floor lounge are filled with rotating collections of artifacts or crafts drawn from resident travels or hobbies. The stone wall in the dining room is used for resident portraits; many of these photos were taken at high points in residents' careers on stage and screen. As a result, the Villa projects a clear identity as the home to an unusual and colorful affinity group.

Prospective residents are not uniform in their appreciation of the modern interiors, contrasting them with the more relaxed, residential scale and style of the cottages. Marketing staff say that this difference gives them sales options: "Long Island vs. Manhattan," as one put it. Most campus prospects quickly look past these differences to more practical concerns, such as proximity to services or the potential need to move out of a cottage at a later date, add marketing staff.

OBJECTIVE: To support a sense of community and social interaction among residents.

FIELD OBSERVATIONS: Activity staff noted that although residents did not use the family rooms at first, their current use exceeds expectations. In fact, some areas are so popular—spots for checking e-mail and reading the newspaper are particularly busy in the morning—that staff said combining the activity corners and living rooms into one bigger room would better accommodate the residents who use the spaces. The staff also mentioned that the exercise room, a part of the activity pavilion, is too small given the current demand.

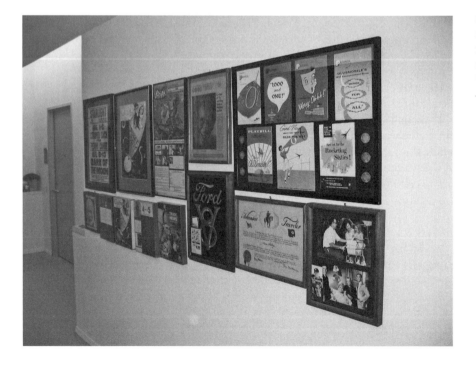

FIG. 10-7 Walls outside resident apartments display residents' accomplishments and what is important to them   *Photograph by Jeffrey Anderzhon*

Four activity staff are assigned to the 180 campus residents, including the cottages, lodge rooms, and the Villa. Villa residents walk to on-campus activities, such as entertainment industry events or a new improvisation class that has proven to be extremely popular. Residents from elsewhere on campus, primarily from the cottages, come to Villa happy hours and poetry readings.

Villa residents are quick to mention the strong sense of belonging they feel on campus. One resident noted, "There's a common language here. From the first day I walked on campus I knew nobody, but I knew everyone." In fact, Villa residents were the driving force behind the writing, photographing, editing, and producing of a book about MPTF: *Behind the Silver Screen.* The book chronicles the lives of more than 70 campus residents and is a source of pride for both residents and staff.

OBJECTIVE: To address the particular interests of the motion picture and television industry.

FIELD OBSERVATIONS: The most interesting development has occurred in the third-floor area originally assigned to the Radio Production Room. This has evolved into the MPTF Television Station and Studio, which develops, produces, edits, and broadcasts programming for on-site residents. Although residents are older and frailer, and thus able to do less than originally expected, the Studio has attracted younger volunteers, from recently retired 75-year-olds to local film-school students. This intergenerational mix has created its own community by emphasizing lifelong learning and taking advantage of the high levels of creativity inherent in this affinity group.

The head of the MPTF Foundation notes that the success of the Studio has "caused a sea change in our philosophy." The plan is now to "create a senior studio within the community, creating programming of interest to seniors across the globe." The director notes that "nobody ever retires from the entertainment industry," and that the Fund sees the Studio as "a chance to engage our population now and to keep young seniors engaged to the benefit of the entire campus."

OBJECTIVE: To link to other buildings on campus.

FIELD OBSERVATIONS: Villa residents have had to cope with a somewhat isolated setting since completion of the project because construction of the campus center was delayed. The completion of the adjacent wellness center, which will include an indoor pool, a fitness center, conference space, and administrative offices, will draw the community closer to the Villa. The wellness center will be open to all MPTF members, even nonresidents, and is expected to strengthen the link between the Villa and the rest of the campus.

Although the design objectives mentioned the koi pond and rose garden as important links between Villa and campus, use of both spaces might have been improved by more direct connections to the Villa entry courtyard. It does rain, even in southern California, and lack of covered access to the west courtyard's bus stop makes travel to the rest of the campus problematic during inclement weather.

Field Observations: Themes and Hypotheses

Creating Community

The Villa succeeds better than other campus buildings in creating a strong sense of community among this unique affinity group. The project's horizontal organization and indoor-outdoor connections give residents ample opportunity to find their own preferred places, and the communal setting and semi-public spaces give residents a chance to display their connections to the larger group.

Of credit to management is the sense that Villa residents consider themselves first and foremost to be a part of MPTF, and only secondarily a part of the Villa. Similarly, although the decentralized family rooms are well used, the evaluation team did not hear from either residents or staff about any strong connections to a particular household within the building. The casual placement of the family rooms and the strength of the single, straight main corridor may reduce the sense of household identity. In a larger project or one with specialized care settings, the sense of household might be more essential, but in the case of the Villa the lack of this connection does not seem crucial.

Making a Home

Dining on each floor, household-based floor plans, and family rooms encourage independent movement and choice and help to make the Villa more like a home than an institution. The built-in benches encourage residents to wander freely and explore other areas of the building with the security of pleasant rest stops along the way. Residents can claim the public areas throughout the Villa as their own—which is a critical part of feeling at home in one's surroundings.

Memorabilia and personal photos, pictures, and artwork adorn the walls of the Villa. Giving residents the authority to decorate their own space—private and public—is probably the best strategy for deinstitutionalizing the facility. Just as in the homes the residents left, they can leave their mark on the wall, not only for personalization but as a record and validation of their accomplishments, hobbies, and knowledge. The photos and cinema memorabilia are conversation starters and ways for residents to identify common interests among their neighbors.

The commonality among the group at the Villa is also a key part of feeling at home. The residents can relate to one another and participate in activities such as radio production and acting classes that take them back to their entertainment-industry days. They remain active, productive, and creative and can continue to feel useful. Carrying over activities they enjoyed before joining the Villa community helps residents settle in and continue their lifestyles in their new home.

Regional/Cultural Design

The Villa makes a strong architectural statement that anchors the project in its southern California setting and references the large-scale, dynamic sound stages that were the workplace for many residents. As a welcome departure from typical assisted living products, the Villa reinforces the value of regional design responses in senior living.

By contrast, some residents say the Villa does not fit into the existing campus setting as well as it might, and that it lacks the warmer, small-scale, residential feel typical of Woodland Hills. Designed in a style similar to the Villa, the new wellness center will likely make the Villa seem more at home at MPTF. Like the valley below the campus, which long ago lost its orchards to shopping centers and office complexes, the two new buildings may suggest a higher density and a more animated future for the campus.

Environmental Therapy

The Villa is a dramatic improvement in the options for communal living on campus, and its internal organization and site plan encourage residents to engage each other and the campus as a whole. The MPTF Studio on the third floor, the first-floor potting shed, and the kitchen garden are examples of the Villa's ability to evolve with resident needs. Another example is the new deli, recently opened in the second-floor dining space. Serving a lighter menu, the deli relieves the main dining room, which was sometimes crowded during mealtime.

Specific design or operational responses to early-stage dementia seem in need of reinforcement. Senior staff acknowledge that the need for dementia care is greater than before and believe that sensor technology and software can fill that gap. Similar assisted living projects elsewhere have created specialized dementia units within the assisted living setting, but perhaps the Villa's small, 70-unit size makes this difficult.

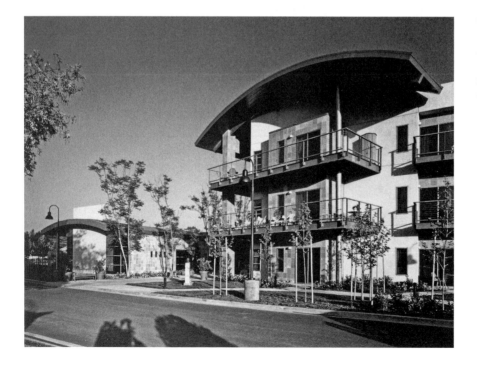

FIG. 10-8 The barreled roof design is reminiscent of a movie studio sound stage building. The building has generous resident balconies and luxurious landscaping © *John Edward Linden*

Outdoor Environment

Indoor-outdoor connections are one of the strongest parts of the design: corridors are single loaded, every unit has a balcony or patio, terraces give residents on every floor the chance to go outside without taking an elevator, and the dining room opens to the hardscaped spine courtyard on the east and the more landscaped bus-stop courtyard to the west. Constant views of trees, lawn areas, and outdoor plazas eliminate any institutional character.

Residents and staff, however, commented that use of the outdoors was less than expected, as spaces were "too hot" or "too cold" and that shade was "insufficient." The easterly and westerly orientation of both these spaces may be the problem, as low sun angles may create alternatively deep shade or glare and heat. Although orientation may not be easily changed, staff may be able to add furnishings, umbrellas, screens, portable heaters, or other devices to make exterior areas more pleasant to occupy.

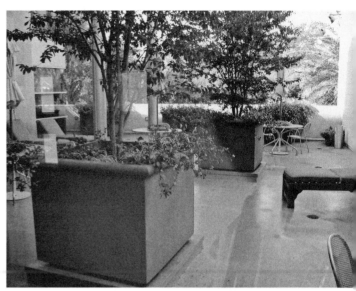

FIG. 10-9   A roof deck allows residents to enjoy the Southern California climate from several building locations
Photograph by Jeffrey Anderzhon

Quality of Workplace and the Physical Plant

Staff noted that the prevalence of outdoor views and natural light made the Villa a pleasant place in which to work, but that staff-support areas could use considerable improvement. Medicine rooms on both the second and third floors were lacking some of the equipment that would help them function correctly, they said. More janitor closets, big enough to easily accommodate large items such as carpet cleaning machines, are needed throughout the building. Storage rooms have been drafted to hold cleaning carts and linen, leaving staff with insufficient space.

Only one clean linen room per floor makes for longer walks for supplies and tends to keep linen carts in the halls for longer periods. Lack of storage shelving or closets at the decentralized activity rooms makes it more difficult for staff and residents to use these areas effectively. Staff meetings are made somewhat difficult by the lack of an enclosed conference room in the main building, and staff spaces on the whole were deemed too small.

Although the facility management director described the Villa's physical plant as largely "trouble-free," floor finishes, hall lighting, and the unit HVAC systems have caused some difficulties. Public-area carpets could have benefited from more pattern and coloration to better hide dirt and wear, particularly in the dining room. Corridor lighting was originally specified with some lamp types not locally available, and although lighting levels were good, energy costs were higher than expected. Management has responded by switching some fixtures and carefully monitoring lighting usage and energy. The split-system unit HVAC units manage resident room conditioning well, but in-the-wall piping was quite noisy at the outset and required considerable attention to reduce the noise.

Lack of communication between the kitchen consultant and management during the planning process resulted in an inappropriate main kitchen layout. Designed for cook-chill, the management decided during construction to use traditional cooking methods and to change a self-service cafeteria line to full wait service from a dish-up station. As it was too late to make significant changes in either layout or equipment, the space is cramped and makes meal preparation and service difficult. Dining tables and four-caster chairs function well for residents, and table linens were a feature from the start. The corridor that leads to first-floor resident rooms poses some guest relations difficulties for the hostess, but does not prevent the dining room from functioning as a unit.

Operator Perspectives

Senior management at MPTF is enthusiastic about both the Villa and its architect, noting that the SmithGroup's key staff are "great architects and a pleasure to work with." Given the chance to do it again, management might opt for fewer studios, more one-bedroom units, full kitchens for some units, walk-in closets in all units, and a second bathroom or two sinks in the bathrooms of larger units. Overall lighting in resident rooms would be increased and mini-kitchens redesigned to raise the refrigerator and lower the microwave. Closet doors, as well as locked valuables drawers, would be provided in all resident rooms.

Characterizing MPTF as a whole, several management staff emphasized that the organization "takes care of its own." With 500,000 members in southern California, MPTF has the advantage of developing long-term relationships with its clients. "We have a unique opportunity to know what our cohorts need," noted the executive director. In particular, senior staff acknowledge the traditional industry difference between those "above the line" and those "below the line." This knowledge translates to about 40% of all campus residents on some form of "scholarship," including about 10% of Villa residents. Looking forward, senior management hopes to activate the campus for the newly retired, creating "from old friends, new neighbors."

General Project Information

PROJECT ADDRESS
The Fran and Ray Stark Villa
23388 Mulholland Drive
Woodland Hills, CA 91364

PROJECT DESIGN TEAM
Architect: SmithGroup
Interior Designer: SmithGroup
Landscape Architect: Sitescapes
Structural Engineer: Taylor & Gaines
Mechanical Engineer: Stone Matakovitch & Wolfberg
Electrical Engineer: Stone Matakovitch & Wolfberg
Civil Engineer: RBA Partners
Dining Consultant: Cini Little

Gerontologist: N/A
Management/Development: N/A
Contractor: Millie & Severson

PROJECT STATUS
Completion date: October 2001

OCCUPANCY LEVELS
At facility opening date: Unknown
At time of evaluation: 95%

RESIDENT AGE (YRS)
At facility opening date: 79
At time of evaluation: 84.7

PROJECT AREAS

ASSISTED LIVING

Project Element	New Construction	
	No. Units	Typical Size
Studio units	48	450 GSF
One-bedroom units	18	650 GSF
Two-bedroom units	4	850 GSF
Total (all units)	70	38,000 GSF
Residents' social areas (lounges, dining, and recreation spaces):		9,000 GSF
Medical, health care, therapy, and activities spaces:		4,000 GSF
Administrative, public, and ancillary support services:		4,000 GSF
Service, maintenance, and mechanical areas:		8,000 GSF
Total gross area:		63,000 GSF
Total net usable area (per space program):		49,000 NSF
Overall gross/net factor (ratio of gross area/net usable area):		1.28

SITE AND PARKING

SITE LOCATION
Suburban

SITE SIZE
Acres: 2
Square feet: 87,120
Area of entire campus: 40 acres

PARKING

Type of parking	For This Facility			
	Residents	Staff	Visitors	Totals
Open surface lot(s)	10	10	4	24

CONSTRUCTION COSTS

SOURCE OF COST DATA
Final construction cost as of October 2001

SOFT COSTS
Land cost or value:	Leased
All permit and other entitlement fees:	Unknown
Legal and professional fees:	Unknown
Appraisals:	N/A
Marketing and preopening:	N/A
Other fees:	N/A
Total soft costs:	Unknown

BUILDING COSTS
New construction except FF&E, special finishes, floor and window coverings, HVAC, and electrical:	$10,000,000
Renovations except FF&E, special finishes, floor and window coverings, HVAC, and electrical:	N/A
FF&E and small wares:	Included in above
Floor coverings:	Included in above
Window coverings:	Included in above
HVAC:	Included in above
Electrical:	Included in above
Medical equipment costs:	Included in above
Total building costs:	$10,000,000

SITE COSTS
New on-site:	$2,000,000
New off-site:	N/A
Renovation on-site:	N/A
Renovation off-site:	N/A
Landscape:	N/A
Special site features or amenities:	N/A
Total site costs:	$2,000,000

TOTAL PROJECT COSTS
Total project costs: $16,000,000

FINANCING SOURCES
Project construction costs were funded through contributions

"If you live to the age of a hundred, you have it made, because very few people die past the age of a hundred."

GEORGE BURNS, 1896–1996

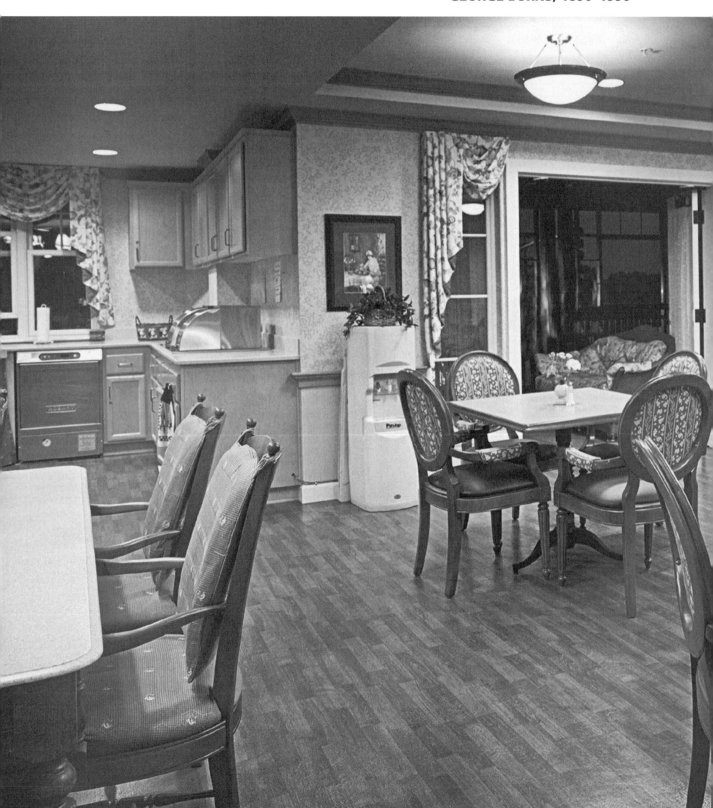

Chapter 11   Sunrise of La Jolla

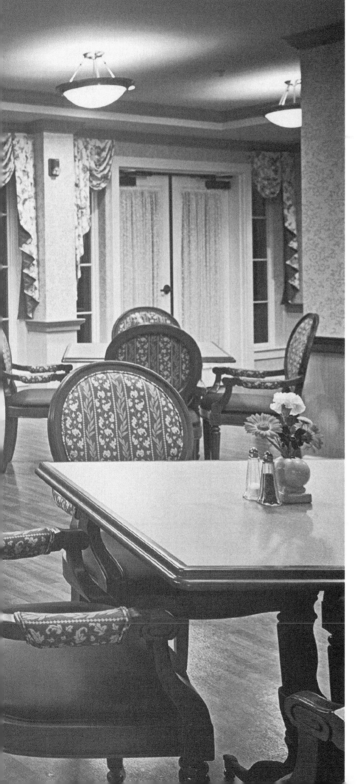

EVALUATION SITE: Sunrise of La Jolla

COMMUNITY TYPE: Assisted Living
- 31 assisted living apartments for 35 residents
- 19 assisted living apartments for 29 residents with Dementia

REGION: West Coast

ARCHITECT: Mithun

OWNER: Sunrise® Senior Living

DATA POINTS: Assisted Living

Resident Room:	300 to 650 gsf
Assisted Living for Dementia	
Resident Room:	300 to 650 gsf
Assisted Living Total Area:	747.17 gsf/resident
Assisted Living Total Area:	26,151 gsf
Assisted Living for Dementia	
Total Area:	470.44 gsf/resident
Assisted Living for Dementia Total Area:	13,643 gsf
Total Building Area:	39,794 gsf
Project Cost:	$201.74/gsf
Total Project Cost:	$8,028,000
Investment/resident:	$125,437.50
(hard costs only; soft costs not provided)	
ALF Staffing:	1.16 care hours/resident/day
ALF Occupancy:	92% as of April 2006

PROJECT COMPLETED: May 2003

DATE OF EVALUATION: April 2006

EVALUATION TEAM: Eleanor Alvarez; Terri Sherman; Mitch Green, AIA; Jeffrey Anderzhon, AIA

FIG. 11-1 Dining room for assisted living for those with dementia, with terrace beyond
www.architecturephotoinc.com

Introduction

In mid-morning, as the marine layer clears from the La Jolla sky and this populous San Diego suburb reaches a vibrant level of activity, one might drive past the structure housing Sunrise of La Jolla without thinking twice about the building. This is largely because it visually blends into the southern California colonial Spanish vernacular without missing a beat, and because this three-level, 50-unit assisted living facility (which houses 64 residents) occupies the northeast corner of one of the busiest intersections in this community. Just three or four blocks to the west is the Pacific Ocean, but the intervening development is primarily commercial and oriented to the ubiquitous automobile and to residents of La Jolla who are beyond the immediate neighborhood.

The tight site on which Sunrise of La Jolla sits is jam-packed with the built environment, both building and created mini-courtyard. Set just a few feet from the two bordering streets, there is not even enough room for a vehicular pull-off lane to drop residents or visitors off at the front door. In fact, the facility has had to make arrangements to share a grocery-store parking lot across the street to accommodate staff and visitor parking. It is not difficult to imagine how worrisome this would be for those residents able to venture from outside the facility walls, who step immediately into a world of vehicular traffic zipping past the building.

Upon entering Sunrise of La Jolla, one sees many of the hallmark features of the organization that pioneered the assisted living industry, though not necessarily rendered in their usual or traditional fashion. Visitors and residents are greeted by the trademark grand staircase and smell of cookies baking in the Bistro oven. (See Figure 10 in the color insert.) Although many of the standard elements are present, Sunrise of La Jolla is different in many ways from the company prototype. This is a Sunrise building embellished with a distinctive Pacific flair and ambience, beginning with the Spanish colonial exterior and continuing with a "California comfortable" embellished interior. It is not difficult to feel at home surrounded by the furnishings, the accessories, and the interior detailing.

The hectic facility location, constricted site, and imposing exterior belie the comfortable and inviting interior. Perhaps this environmental dichotomy is the factor that seems to prevent residents from venturing into the neighborhood. Alternatively, it was perhaps a subconscious response by the design team to the perceived care need of an aging-in-place resident population with lower acuity levels, in an effort to protect them from the outside dangers. In either case, the environment seems to wrap itself around the residents, providing them with an enclosure that is protective but that does provide enough opportunity, with its mini-courtyards and balconies, to satisfy a craving for enviable California weather.

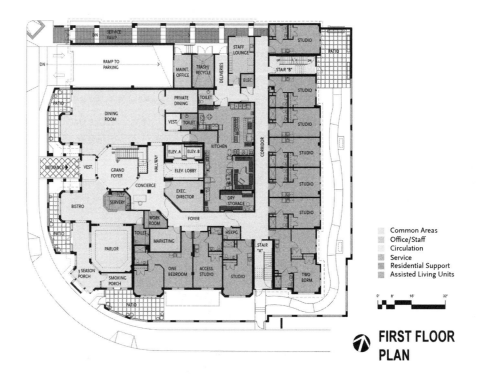

FIG. 11-2 First-floor plan, street level *Courtesy of Mithun*

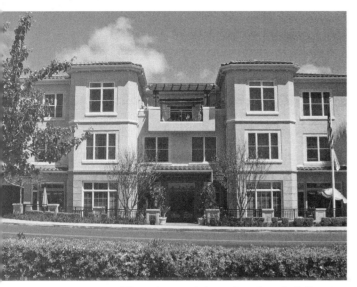

FIG. 11-3 The main entry is located at a busy La Jolla street intersection *Photograph by Jeffrey Anderzhon*

Architect's Statement

We were challenged with the task of designing a unique 50-unit assisted living community that enhances the quality of lifestyle available for seniors on the former site of a one-story branch bank. The goal was accomplished by creating an urban building solution, one where residents feel comfortable in close proximity to busy shops and restaurants, and abundant pedestrian and automobile traffic. From the upper floors, residents in west- and north-facing rooms enjoy views of the Pacific Ocean.

The aesthetic of the building embraces the California Mission style, with deep-set wood windows in thick stucco walls. The compact, three-story building with underground garage expresses a clear sense of arrival and an appropriate fit into the neighborhood.

Designers' and Owners' Stated Objectives and Responses

OBJECTIVE: Create a high-quality residential environment in an urban, mixed-use, oceanfront neighborhood.

DESIGN INTENT: This was accomplished by creating an urban solution where residents can feel comfortable in close proximity to busy shops and restaurants, and abundant pedestrian and automobile traffic. From the upper floors, views to the Pacific Ocean are available from every room facing west or north.

We used quality materials, including clad wood windows and doors, integral-colored stucco exterior, detailed roof eaves, and a barrel tile roof in the spirit of traditional building materials indicative of the regional Mission style. Ample glazing and porches encourage outdoor excursions by emphasizing the relationship between the indoor rooms and outdoor gardens.

OBJECTIVE: Maintain exterior and interior relationship.

DESIGN INTENT: To create a familiar residential atmosphere and carry through the consideration to detail, we paid special attention to the interior detailing, such as a wood staircase, crown moldings, base and chair rail trim, Mission-style furnishings, and a selection of warm colors.

OBJECTIVE: Transition from a commercial to a residential neighborhood.

DESIGN INTENT: During the planning stages, an assisted living project was considered appropriate by city planners for this commercial-zoned site. It would front the commercial context of the street, being comfortably close to the sidewalk, with common areas at the first floor that exhibit larger windows, furnishings, and lighting indicative of a small carriage hotel. Directly uphill from the site are several multifamily and single-family structures.

Field Observations: Meeting the Objectives

OBJECTIVE: Create a high-quality residential environment in an urban, mixed-use, oceanfront neighborhood.

FIELD OBSERVATIONS: The neighborhood in which Sunrise of La Jolla resides is but a neo-oceanfront neighborhood, requiring a significant walk to actually arrive at the ocean. As with many California communities, this one relies heavily on and caters more to the automobile than to pedestrian traffic. There is indeed considerable automobile traffic surrounding the facility, which in turn discourages pedestrian traffic. The retail shops in the neighborhood tend to expect automobile access over pedestrian access and their nature, as a result of real estate economics, tends to service a driving public. Little opportunity exists for residents of the facility to participate in outings involving these retailers, a lack exacerbated by the unfriendly mix of cars and people. Although the nature of the community is certainly beyond the control of the designer of an individual project, it does have implications for the design. Upon a very constricted site that, because of the costs of real estate, required a substantial yield, there is success here in balancing a quality environment for residents at a location that economically demanded as much building as possible.

In the case of Sunrise of La Jolla, small courtyards were created on the site that are well protected from direct sun and clearly distinct from public walks. Although these are small, they do provide resident access to green space in a location that makes it difficult to utilize park spaces elsewhere.

OBJECTIVE: Maintain exterior and interior relationship.

FIELD OBSERVATIONS: Though there is consistency in design both on the exterior and within the interior of the building, the relationship between the two is not seamless. The exterior is nicely done in a colonial Spanish style, complete with replicated arbors and stucco finishes. The interior is also nicely appointed, with rich furnishings and finishes that relate more to a Craftsman style of design.

A physical and visual relationship does exist between the two, although somewhat strained because of the tight site conditions. This is manifest in the small courtyards on the lower level and the arbored balconies on the upper levels. These tend to flow easily between interior and exterior spaces, to some extent blurring physical barriers.

OBJECTIVE: Transition from a commercial to a residential neighborhood.

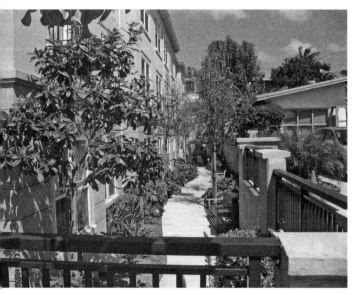

FIG. 11-4 A mini-courtyard separates the building from the busy street and provides a place for residents to enjoy the outdoors *Photograph by Jeffrey Anderzhon*

FIELD OBSERVATIONS: The transition from commercial to residential neighborhoods is somewhat beyond the control of the designer, although this project is certainly identifiable as residential. On the east side of this three-story building is a similarly sized apartment structure, but on the north are single-family, single-story residences. Thus, the transition is somewhat abrupt, at least on one side of the project.

The raised height of the first level, as well as the design treatment of the area between the public sidewalks and the building, does provide a softening edge to the building, which would logically assume a rather imposing stance on the busy street corner. In addition, because the site and surrounding environs slope from north to south and the adjacent properties sit at a higher grade, the building tends to feel less imposing than it might. Although the overall transition is not offensive, particularly to a commuter rushing through the intersection, the design does not overly exert itself to meet this objective.

Field Observations: Themes and Hypotheses

Creating Community

The building is located on a very busy corner, just south of the attractive La Jolla area. It appears that the neighborhood is in a transition that is beginning to produce a better aesthetic even as the La Jolla sprawl begins to encompass it. The neighborhood is noisy and commercial and has yet to transform into the charming, oceanfront lifestyle of La Jolla. The traffic buzzes by rapidly and is a concern for residents who want to venture outside. Designing a safe and easy entrance for residents and families was problematic in working with this site. When residents are getting on the facility van to go on an outing, the staff is required to stop passing traffic and to place orange traffic cones near the curb to ensure resident safety. As new residents move into the facility, the moving van must park nearly a block away, forcing the movers to roll all of the residents' belongings on a hand truck down the hill through the main entrance of the facility. All vendor deliveries also come through the front door, passing by both resident social areas and any visitors or residents who may be in these areas. This process creates an institutional feel, opens the doors to insects, and creates other maintenance issues.

As one approaches, the building feels very constricted on its small piece of land, surrounded by the

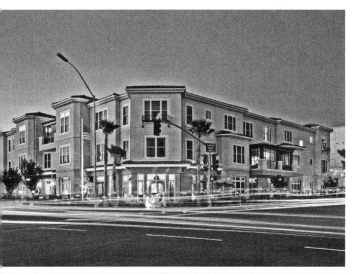

FIG. 11-5 Sunrise of La Jolla on a tight building site adjacent to a bustling vehicular intersection
www.architecturephotoinc.com

busy vehicular traffic. The outdoor space, though very limited, creates a partial barrier to the traffic, but blocks out the surrounding community as well, although the interior environment helps to compensate, through the ample use of light and visual accessibility to the exterior through beautiful balconies, terraces, and gardens. The upper-level living rooms and library have large, French doors that swing wide open and allow the ocean breezes to flow through the adjacent rooms. A safety railing and screen around the terrace on the memory care unit is nicely detailed and constructed for both security and beauty with an attractive, natural sun and wind screen.

Making a Home

The entry to Sunrise of La Jolla, the grand foyer, with its monumental staircase, is open and inviting and provides large, overstuffed chairs for guests as they wait for the resident they are visiting or for residents to relax in prior to an organized outing. Just off the foyer is the charming Bistro, with beverages and fresh cookies always available. Beyond the Bistro is a more formal parlor, complete with fireplace, comfortable seating, and décor that washes one with comfort and puts one immediately at ease. A three-season porch adjacent to the parlor allows residents to watch the busy street activity with the feeling of being outside.

The large dining room is on the opposite side of the foyer, and can comfortably accommodate all the assisted living residents in a single seating. In addition, there is a smaller, private dining room adjacent to the main room that is utilized by visiting families and for private events. The menus and food purchase selections are all centralized from the Sunrise home office, but adjusted to fit the regional differences of this location. Two menu options are offered residents at each meal.

The physical ambience is somewhat marred by a strong smell of deodorant and a subtle stale odor that permeates the first-floor areas. A definite absence of activity on the first floor in the late morning was observed, but later in the afternoon, a number of residents gathered in the Bistro area with their pets. The dogs and their owners were very relaxed and friendly and certainly gave a family-like feel to a setting that included considerable social interaction. The Bistro has become the favorite gathering spot and a very important social area for the residents, their families, and friends, although the cushions on many pieces of furniture were frayed, torn, and dirty.

On the resident floors, hallways are provided with enlarged areas for the flow of residents, staff, and equipment carts, and for use as intimate seating areas. The entrance of sunlight through large windows, as well as skylights on the upper level, adds a feeling of openness and spaciousness. The Sunrise principle of "This is the last place you will need to go to. We will take care of your needs, no matter what they are" is ingrained in the staff and further contributes to a feeling of family and

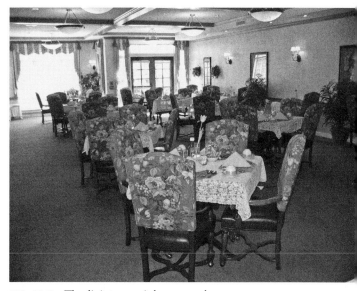

FIG. 11-6 The dining room is large enough to accommodate residents, guests, and wheelchairs *Photograph by Jeffrey Anderzhon*

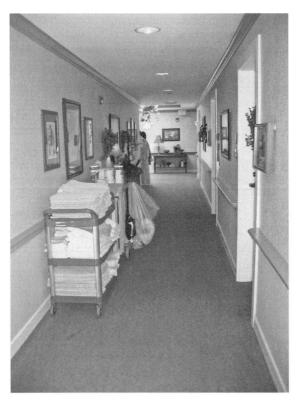

FIG. 11-7 Enlarged areas in corridors provide places for residents to rest or for cart storage, but these locations are not convenient for staff *Photograph by Jeffrey Anderzhon*

home. The apartments have small galley kitchens, but these are seldom used by residents, as they all take advantage of the provided meal program. The acuity level of residents suggests that they no longer are able or, at a minimum, care to perform cooking tasks. The apartment kitchens, however, are a nice feature for families visiting residents in the apartment or if a resident wants to make a snack.

As one leaves the elevator lobby on the third floor, the library provides a striking impression with its view of the distant ocean across the rooftops. The beautiful French doors open to allow abundant light, along with the breezes and smells of the Pacific, to fill the room. This level's apartments are very desirable and in demand because they provide the most attractive ocean views and are most remote from the street below.

Of the total of 50 apartments in the facility, seven are shared occupancy in either split-room studio or two-bedroom configurations. These apartments are certainly large enough to accommodate two residents, but the facility socioeconomic location and the detriment to personal privacy created by this arrangement are both distractions from the creation of a home-like feel.

Regional/Cultural Design

Sunrise Senior Living is one of the largest, if not the largest, providers of care for the elderly in the United States. They have achieved this by providing a quality and affordable service and product that is consistent throughout their system. In the past, these services have been housed in a recognizable built environment that emulates a large Victorian home, regardless of the facility location. Although this provides quick recognition for the provider and an intuitive understanding that a building is a home and not simply a facility, the built environment became formulaic and often ignored local or regional architectural vernacular and context. In addition, the approach to care provision necessarily tends to be stereotypical, with only marginal allowance for specific cultural diversity within the confines of the building.

At Sunrise of La Jolla, the large provider begins to wander from this path by accepting and perhaps embracing the culture, at least environmental culture, in which the structure is placed. This design fits so well into the surrounding environs that it is almost unnoticeable. This is not to say that it is either boring or without its own unique qualities, but these attributes tend to be revealed only after completion of the first, cursory examination. The building is a good design neighbor and, in fact, appears to be a leader in a design transformation of neighboring structures.

Once past the exterior and into the interior of the building, however, there is less local or regional design vernacular. Although the fit and finish of the interior is accommodating, there is more here that falls back on consistency with other Sunrise facilities, albeit with a somewhat updated feeling. This includes the monumental stair, which tends to immediately draw the eye to a grand and spacious foyer complete with receptionist desk.

It could be argued that because the overwhelming majority of residents of California are transplanted natives of somewhere else, the homogenous interior design is indeed culturally appropriate. Certainly, the interior is warm and welcoming, but it offers little in the way of either recognizing or celebrating the diversity of the residents, regardless of the extent of that diversity. This Sunrise interior could as easily be in any of the numerous other corporate locations without anyone being the wiser.

Environmental Therapy

Although Sunrise of La Jolla has nicely appointed community spaces on the first floor, they are minimized due to the limited site and building footprint. When used by only a few residents at a time they function well, but when larger gatherings occur, they become restrictive and a reflection of the site itself. Additionally, for residents to access these first-floor rooms, they must use the elevators and thus are faced with another barrier that lessens their desirability.

The activity and living room on the third level tend to be more frequently used. In particular, the activity room on this floor, though somewhat small, has become the community multipurpose room where current events are discussed and low-level resident exercises are performed.

On the second floor, where dementia assisted living residents are segregated, the living room is divided into living space and activity space. This area flows into the dining room and provides a fairly large area where a large mix of activities can occur. These spaces are more aptly sized for this floor's smaller population and more adequately organized to provide appropriate staff supervision and resident choice of either active or passive therapies.

Within the dementia area there is a "Snoezelen" room, another Sunrise trademark, that creates a peaceful environment for agitated memory care residents. Soothing sounds and serene videos of gentle streams and beautiful landscapes contribute to the calming milieu. Aromatherapy, fans, and subdued lighting are used to de-escalate agitated behaviors in a confused resident. The room is quite small, but seems adequate to meet residents' needs for a separate place where they can regain their composure. The room door has been removed to make it feel less cramped and confining, but this brings into question the integrity of a fire separation wall.

Outdoor Environment

The building and exterior gardens appear well maintained and designed to provide private space within a distinctively commercial area of the community. The patio located at the rear of the property is difficult to access and not used frequently by residents or their guests. It is definitely out of the mainstream of activity, although it does connect, by way of sidewalk, to the more attractive south courtyard. This mini-courtyard is well landscaped and nicely shaded, providing a buffer against the hard edges of the city street with the softness of a California planting area.

The front garden area adjacent to the main entrance provides an area visually and physically integrated with the entry and a comfortable place to sit while waiting for visitors or transportation, though there is little protective shade here.

The building's two balconies, one on the second level for dementia residents and one on the third level for

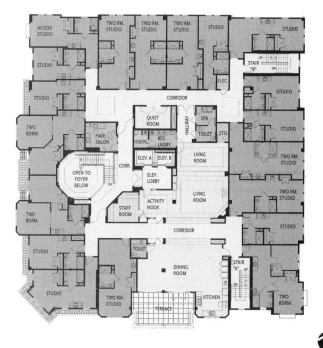

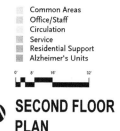

FIG. 11-8 Second-floor plan. This level is assisted living for those with dementia *Courtesy of Mithun*

Common Areas
Office/Staff
Circulation
Service
Residential Support
Alzheimer's Units

0'   8'   16'   32'

SECOND FLOOR PLAN

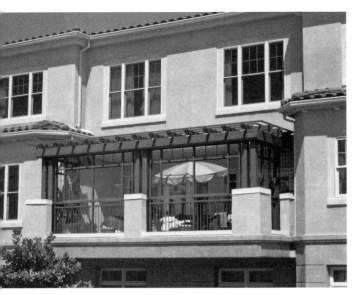

FIG. 11-9 The terrace for those with dementia blends with the architecture, is secured with safety vision panels, and provides adequate shade *Photograph by Jeffrey Anderzhon*

assisted living, are nicely proportioned and detailed. They provide comfortable outdoor seating areas that are inviting as well as secure, and the spaces flow easily and gently from the adjacent interior rooms.

The availability of parking is a major issue for this property. Parking on-site is limited to the area beneath the building. The grocery store across the street to the west provides complimentary shared parking for guests and staff, but crossing the busy street to reach this satellite parking area is less than ideal. There is no signage to direct visitors to these spaces, and the first-time visitor is faced with the chore of finding a parking place on one of the adjacent side streets and walking some distance to the building.

Quality of Workplace and the Physical Plant

The leadership team at Sunrise of La Jolla was experiencing some instability and turnover in the department manager positions. At the time of the evaluation, many of these key roles were filled with relatively new hires who were just beginning to learn how to work together as a team. Although management knew that the evaluation team would be present, the executive director was not available on the day of the visit to discuss impressions of the facility or the leadership team, leaving it unclear as to why this group of managers was experiencing turnover. Each department appears to operate independently, and there is little to no focus on overall integration or systemic functioning. It was clear, how-

ever, that the environment was not a contributing factor to this lack of cohesion.

When interviewed, the staff enthusiastically talked about the extensive training programs provided by Sunrise for staff at all levels. They described specific career tracks and felt support and the availability of good growth potential within the company. They believe that Sunrise encourages promotions from within and were pleased with the opportunities.

Resident care managers provide all of the needed services for residents, consistent within a universal worker model. Most of these care managers are certified nursing assistants (CNAs) or have some type of medical background. In this role, they provide laundry services and do light housekeeping and personal care assistance for residents. The work areas are discreetly blended into the resident living space and are efficient without being institutional. The floor plates are small enough to be naturally decentralized in storage and work areas that support the universal worker concept.

Staff in the memory care area is packed tightly into a room that functions as nurses' station, office, and reception area for the floor. Even though there is an effort to get away from institutional services, this area looked like a glorified medication room, with charts lining the walls and residents being checked for vital signs without benefit of privacy. The director was very enthusiastic about the Sunrise organization and very pleased with the systems and available support. She was very complimentary and stated that all of the details of the operation had been clearly thought through.

The memory care area has all of the predictable features of a Sunrise product: dress-up area, laundry folding station, baby dolls, tactile wall hangings, and the Snoezelen room. The staff commented that the storage space was adequate and well planned and remarked on the pleasing ambience of the facility as a workplace. Staff are clearly aware that they work with a fairly demanding clientele, generally in their mid-80s, and that they need to provide a high quality level of services.

Operator Perspectives

There are numerous competitive options in this geographic market for more upscale and expansive senior living accommodations and products. This contributes to the difficulty in filling this facility's smaller apartments and the several apartments designed to be shared occupancy. However, the assisted living apartments are generally occupied, indicating that this community caters to residents who have various care needs. The memory care unit is the option most often requested for resident placement and appears to fill a high demand for dementia care in the area.

The department supervisors interviewed were generally well pleased with the environment and its functionality. Surprisingly, almost all of these individuals commented on the amount of storage available for their purposes. All were pleased with this amenity, as well as the sensible locations of that storage and its ease of use. A number of staff had served in other Sunrise locations and preferred Sunrise of La Jolla to their past experiences, citing the environment as a major reason for this.

General Project Information

PROJECT ADDRESS
Sunrise of La Jolla
810 Turquoise Street
San Diego, CA 92109

PROJECT DESIGN TEAM
Architect: Mithun
Interior Designer: Martha Child Interiors
Landscape Architect: IVY Landscape Architects, Inc.
Structural Engineer: Putnam Collins & Scott Associates
Mechanical Engineer: Westgate Engineering
Electrical Engineer: AWA Electrical Consultants
Civil Engineer: Dudek Associates
Dining Consultant: N/A

Gerontologist: N/A
Management/Development:
Contractor: Suffolk Construction Company, Inc.

PROJECT STATUS
Completion date: May 2003

OCCUPANCY LEVELS
At facility opening date: 30%
At date of evaluation: 92%

RESIDENT AGE (YRS)
At facility opening date: 85
At time of evaluation: 85

PROJECT AREAS

ASSISTED LIVING

Project Element	New Construction No. Units	New Construction Typical Size
Studio units	19	300–350 GSF
One-bedroom units	8	425–550 GSF
Two-bedroom units	4	515–650 GSF
Total (all units)	31	18,134 GSF
Residents' social areas (lounges, dining, and recreation spaces):		3,800 GSF
Medical, health care, therapy, and activities spaces:		0 GSF
Administrative, public, and ancillary support services:		2,586 GSF
Service, maintenance, and mechanical areas:		5,431 GSF
Total gross area:		26,151 GSF
Total net usable area (per space program):		20,720 NSF
Overall gross/net factor (ratio of gross area/net usable area):		1.26

DEMENTIA-SPECIFIC ASSISTED LIVING

	New Construction	
Project Element	No. Units	Typical Size
Studio units	9	300–350 GSF
One bedroom units	7	425–550 GSF
Two bedroom units	3	515–650 GSF
Total (all units)	19	10,619 GSF
Residents' social areas (lounges, dining, and recreation spaces):		2,046 GSF
Medical, health care, therapy, and activities spaces:		0 GSF
Administrative, public, and ancillary support services:		473 GSF
Service, maintenance, and mechanical areas:		505 GSF
Total gross area:		13,643 GSF
Total net usable area (per space program):		13,138 NSF
Overall gross/net factor (ratio of gross area/net usable area):		1.04

SITE AND PARKING

SITE LOCATION
Urban

SITE SIZE
Acres: 0.46
Square feet: 20,228

PARKING

Type of Parking	For This Facility			
	Residents	Staff	Visitors	Totals
Lot(s) under building(s)	N/A	26	0	26

CONSTRUCTION COSTS

SOURCE OF COST DATA
Final construction cost as of June 2003

SOFT COSTS
Soft costs not provided by owner or architect

BUILDING COSTS

New construction except FF&E, special finishes, floor and window coverings, HVAC, and electrical:	$6,497,400
Renovations except FF&E, special finishes, floor and window coverings, HVAC, and electrical:	$540,000
FF&E and small wares:	Included in above
Floor coverings:	Included in above
Window coverings:	Included in above
HVAC:	$285,000
Electrical:	$705,600
Medical equipment costs:	N/A
Total building costs:	$8,028,000

SITE COSTS

New on-site:	Included in building costs
New off-site:	N/A
Renovation on-site:	N/A
Renovation off-site:	N/A
Landscape:	Included in building costs
Special site features or amenities:	N/A
Total site costs:	Included in building costs

TOTAL PROJECT COSTS
Total project costs: $8,028,000

FINANCING SOURCES
Private financing

Part IV

Assisted Living for Those with Dementia

"Happiness is good health and a bad memory."

INGRID BERGMAN, 1915–1982

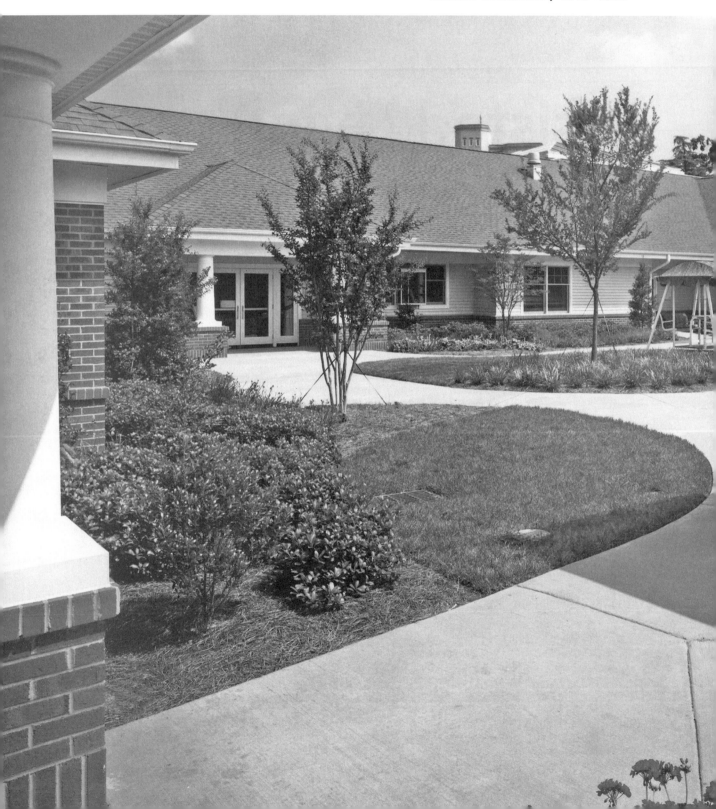

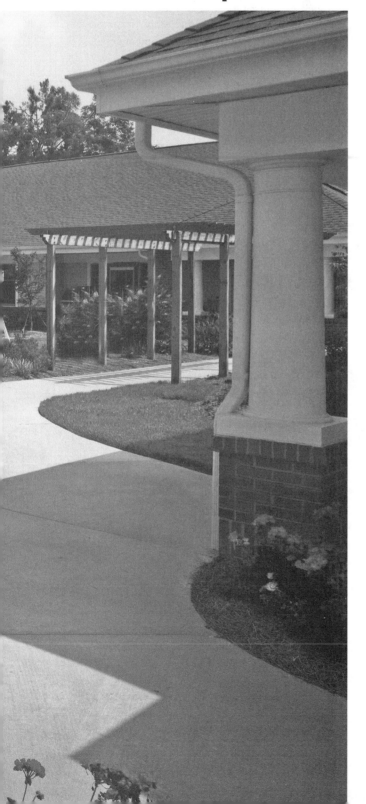

Chapter 12

Cuthbertson Village at Aldersgate

EVALUATION SITE: Cuthbertson Village at Aldersgate

COMMUNITY TYPE: Assisted Living for Those with Dementia, Part of a CCRC
• 45 assisted living apartments for those with dementia

REGION: Southeast

ARCHITECT: Freeman White, Inc.

OWNER: Aldersgate United Methodist Retirement, Inc.

DATA POINTS: Resident Room:	270 gsf
Total Area:	604 gsf/resident
Total Area:	34,000 gsf
Project Cost:	$118.00/gsf
Total Project Cost	$4,012,000
Investment/resident:	$89,155.55
Staffing:	3.02 care hours/resident/day
Occupancy:	98% as of August 2005

FIRST OCCUPANCY: June 2003

DATE OF EVALUATION: August 2005

EVALUATION TEAM: Ingrid Fraley, ASID; Thomas Hauer; David Slack; Mitch Green, AIA; Jeffrey Anderzhon, AIA

FIG. 12-1 The courtyard between households is where residents can enjoy the outdoors *Photograph by Tim Mueller*

Introduction

Aldersgate United Methodist Retirement Community, located on a 234-acre campus five miles from downtown Charlotte, North Carolina, is an ecumenical not-for-profit corporation dedicated to providing continuing care services to older adults.

Founded in 1948, the colonial-style architecture of the campus is surrounded by magnolia and pecan trees and is reminiscent of an age of southern hospitality and elegance. The campus opened with 132 apartments and 12 "infirmary beds" licensed by the state as intensive care. In 1960, another 242 beds were added in the new Wesley Care Center, and finally, in 1980, the Asbury Complex added another 100 intensive care beds. In subsequent restructuring, the Asbury building completely shifted to private-pay and all assisted-pay residents moved to the Wesley building. Assisted living was established at Parker Terrace. Independent living includes 300 apartments and cottages, with another 50 cottages planned or under construction.

As Aldersgate moved into the 21st century, a significant expansion and renovation program to enhance resident services and amenities was completed. One of the new residences is Cuthbertson Village, a licensed assisted living memory support center. The decision to build Cuthbertson Village was made in response to aging-in-place issues occurring within the campus. Cuthbertson strives to integrate a supportive environment designed to maintain each resident's functional independence by implementing personalized services and therapeutic activity programs.

Architect's Statement

Cuthbertson Village incorporates the "Eden Alternative" philosophy and "Main Street USA" concepts into a

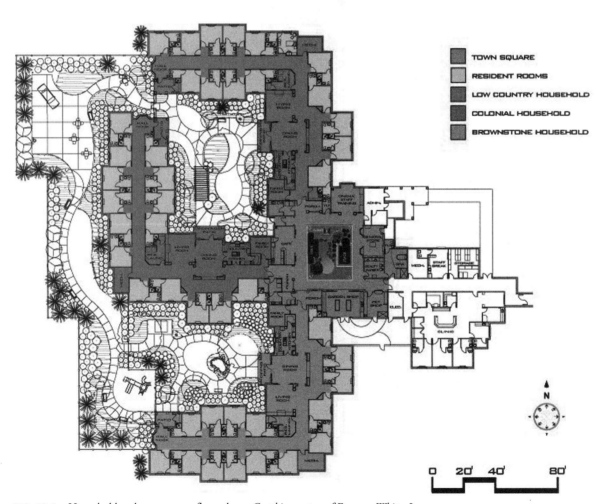

FIG. 12-2 Household and town square floor plan *Graphic courtesy of Freeman White, Inc.*

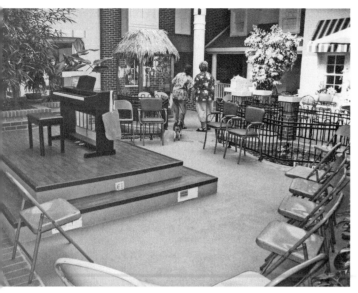

FIG. 12-3 Town-square events can cause congestion in many of the seating areas *Photograph by Jeffrey Anderzhon*

holistic environment for seniors with memory impairment, to promote positive interaction among residents, staff, families, and the community. (See Figure 11 in the color insert.)

The 45-bed village is divided into three households, each home to 15 residents who occupy private rooms and share a residential-scale living room, dining room, country kitchen, family room, and back porch. Each household connects to outdoor courtyards and to the central Town Square, which includes a general store, cinema, pet store, and café. There is also a garden shop surrounding a central garden with walking path, goldfish pond, stage, and aviary. Each area has expanded life-skill stations where residents are able to participate in or observe the activities, providing what the staff call "Purposeful Pathways" throughout the village. From morning until bedtime, residents are free to move throughout all areas of their household and village.

Designers' and Operators' Stated Objectives and Responses

OBJECTIVE: Provide a unique feature.

DESIGN INTENT: The Town Square space is the unique feature of the project. A tinted skylight gives views of the sky and allows soft light to enter the space throughout the day and evening. The space is big enough for special events in the cinema or on the bandstand, but small enough not to overwhelm residents. Decorative banners reflect the changing seasons, plantings vary with the holidays, and different activities are programmed to allow residents to reminisce about the traditions, holidays, and experiences of their lives.

OBJECTIVE: Create a holistic living environment for seniors with memory impairments to enhance their quality of life.

DESIGN INTENT: With the "Eden Alternative" as the project's guiding philosophy, residents live in an independent and caring environment that allows them to positively interact with and experience their surroundings. Fundamentally, the entire village creates strong visual, scent- and touch-connected experiences that create a holistic and caring living experience.

OBJECTIVE: Create an interactive community for residents, their families, staff, animals, and the larger Aldersgate community.

DESIGN INTENT: The village and households are filled with dogs, cats, birds, fish, and plants, to allow residents to continue having caring, purposeful experiences throughout their days. Family members and children visit regularly, providing the village with age diversity reminiscent of the communities residents lived in before moving to Cuthbertson. Planned activities for residents bring in different activity groups and children who enjoy the Town Square, play areas, and gardens as much as the residents do.

OBJECTIVE: Create an environment where residents are connected to the rhythms of nature and the changing seasons.

DESIGN INTENT: Different from some existing Alzheimer households, this community allows easy access to the outside from multiple locations, through French doors with sidelights that bring the outside in and cue residents to the garden areas. The skylight in the Town Square and the large windows throughout the households allow residents to experience the normal rhythms of the day and seasons, while the porches and gardens at the households allow residents to easily enjoy nature and the changing weather.

OBJECTIVE: Create stimulating wayfinding throughout the village for residents, to reduce agitation and unfocused wandering.

DESIGN INTENT: Throughout Cuthbertson Village, different visual icons and signage are used to strongly identify experiences for the resident. Each household has a distinctly different entry experience—from a brownstone

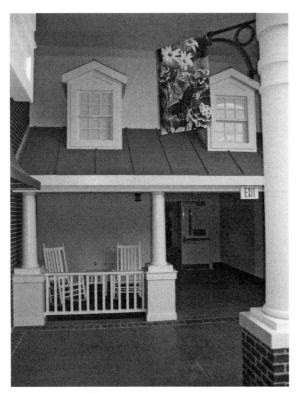

FIG. 12-4 Each household entry has its own front porch and design character *Photograph by Jeffrey Anderzhon*

stoop to low-country and colonial front porches—that strongly differentiates between residences. Bright, colorful signage at eye level is located at the activity centers and is reminiscent of signage the residents grew up with. In addition, as residents walk through the village, they pass through gates into multiple garden areas, enhancing a sense of freedom to move where they desire.

Field Observations: Meeting the Objectives

OBJECTIVE: Provide a unique feature.

FIELD OBSERVATIONS: Imagine a central square with a bandstand, sidewalks, and a perimeter of storefronts that are faithful replications of shops that would naturally spring up in any small town. Main Street has a definite "wow" factor and is certainly a visually appealing marketing tool for prospective residents and family members. The marketing value alone could be enough to justify the space, but even more noteworthy is that the space is actually used by residents, family, and staff. The various storefronts are well planned to maximize their visual appeal and memory enhancement. Although no

significant complaints were presented regarding the individual shops, it appeared that the general store and garden shop were too big and the theater and soda shop too small for the activities observed.

Staff comments focused on the center square, which is dominated by the bandstand stage and meandering water feature, which decrease the usable square footage during programs intended for the entire village. The functionality of group assembly is clearly challenged by the Main Street configuration. Activities planned on Main Street for all three households are difficult to accommodate. Folding chairs must be arranged in seating configurations forced into the spaces between planters, railings, water features, and the bandstand. As a result, the seating is often haphazardly placed and the tidy appearance of Main Street becomes cluttered.

Only one toilet room for residents and guests is available on Main Street, which presents a significant problem during large assemblies and even inconveniences smaller groups and family visitors.

The tinted glass atrium definitely enhances the outdoor atmosphere and did not appear to produce any significant glare. The space was quite pleasant with respect to light and temperature; however, acoustics suffered because of the use of hard finishes that were selected to enhance the outdoor theme. Some additional sound-deadening materials would be required to offset the effects of the concrete sidewalks, glass skylight, and storefront materials. Sitting in the soda shop, it was difficult to carry on a conversation, because our voices had

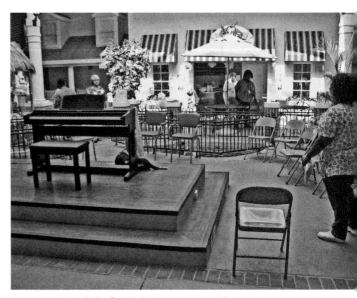

FIG. 12-5 Daylight floods the town square. The permanent stage can pose a tripping hazard *Photograph by Jeffrey Anderzhon*

to compete with the aviary and a musical program in the theater.

OBJECTIVE: Create a holistic living environment for seniors with memory impairments to enhance their quality of life.

FIELD OBSERVATIONS: The "Eden Alternative" was identified as a guiding philosophy because it would, ideally, allow residents to have broad and positive interactions with their surroundings. Main Street clearly takes to heart the interaction between the resident and the environment, providing strong sensory-based experiences. Opportunities for residents to participate in activities that suit their interests, habits, and abilities are clearly supported by the design of Main Street and the adjoining neighborhoods. Activity calendars are color-cued to identify the location and skill level of each activity scheduled. This was a particularly useful tool for the resident activity coordinators (RACs) to promote a more interactive and individualized agenda for each of the residents.

OBJECTIVE: Create an interactive community for residents, their families, staff, animals, and the larger Aldersgate community.

FIELD OBSERVATIONS: Main Street clearly acts as a gathering place, although frequency of visits by residents from the surrounding Aldersgate campus could not be documented. There seemed to be some perception that Cuthbertson was "the home" that more able campus residents should avoid. However, use by family members was clearly evident and Main Street is an important space for intergenerational visits. Although children are reportedly entertained by the water feature and pet shop, the addition of more interior space for their use, as well as a toy chest, were suggested by staff. Age-appropriate outdoor equipment and a basketball hoop were on the suggestion list as well.

OBJECTIVE: Create an environment where residents are connected to the rhythms of nature and the changing seasons.

FIELD OBSERVATIONS: The connection to the outdoor environment seemed to be the one area that clearly fell short of its mark. Main Street, with the exception of the view through the skylight, is an interior space. The only glass door accessing the courtyard from Main Street is in the garden shop. This door, as well as the dining room doors in each of the neighborhoods, displayed large, red "do not exit" warnings. Interviews with family members revealed that they use a circuitous route to the corridor ends in each neighborhood to gain access to the court-

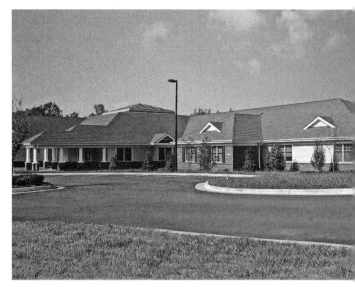

FIG. 12-6   The primary entrance lacks a strong presence. Proper identification would encourage visitors to use it without hesitation   *Photograph by Tim Mueller*

yards. Ironically, residents hesitate to use this door because they mistake it for a private apartment entry.

OBJECTIVE: Create stimulating wayfinding throughout the village, for residents to reduce agitation and unfocused wandering.

FIELD OBSERVATIONS: The storefronts and shop interiors of Main Street are well designed to encourage focused and meaningful activity. Each of the three neighborhoods has its own unique entrance feature from Main Street which plays off the image of a front porch, complete with a comfortable rocking chair. Two of the three porches were continuously occupied during the site evaluation. The third, a replication of a brownstone, is enclosed by a knee wall that limits visual access to Main Street and thus is seldom used. The dining, living, and kitchen components in each of the neighborhoods are visible to residents and easy to distinguish. Residents are easily drawn into these spaces.

The majority of the apartments are located down a double-loaded corridor and are somewhat disconnected from the social spaces. Each apartment entry is recessed by a short hallway. Visual connection to an apartment entry door is often obstructed, although this did not seem to be a problem for staff or residents. The door signage and pictures of the residents who occupy the adjacent rooms are placed in the main corridor and not at the apartment entry.

Ends of corridors feature an "oasis room" as a destination for residents. Though described by staff as having

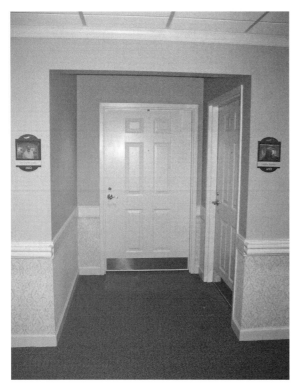

FIG. 12-7 Two apartment entrance doors share a private alcove, resulting in remote placement of interior signage on the corridor walls *Photograph by Jeffrey Anderzhon*

become a "personal sitting room" for the residents of that wing, use of this amenity was not observed during the evaluation.

Field Observations: Themes and Hypotheses

Creating Community

Overall, the design of Cuthbertson Village is aesthetically pleasing and supports both caregiver and resident. The staff seem to be highly motivated, well trained, and compassionate. There is a strong sense of community and a definite "family" within the facility.

The layout of the households could be improved. Although the co-location and visibility of the dining, living, and kitchen areas are well done, only four apartments are adjacent to this hub of activity. The remaining 11 apartments are distant from the core of the neighborhood, and the apartments at the extreme ends of the corridors are (understandably) the least popular. Residents of these rooms do not feel fully connected to the household social milieu.

Making a Home

The residents' rooms are quite small. Cabinet-wall HVAC units and doors that swing into the bathroom consume valuable square footage and eliminate options for resident furnishings. Built-in closets were passed over in favor of small wardrobes that eat up even more floor space. One family member told us that he was forced to change out his mother's clothing seasonally because of the lack of space.

Wood-look sheet vinyl covers the floor. This flooring is easy to maintain, and it was clear that residents' preferences for carpeting or area rugs would be problematic.

Lighting is poor and does not seem to meet minimum requirements for older adults. The ceiling-mounted fixture in the center of the room does not produce adequate illumination, and the wardrobe doors cut off the light required to access clothing. Floor and table lamps had been brought into several rooms to improve the lighting level, although they do take up yet more valuable floor space.

It was disappointing to see such small showers in the resident bathrooms. Although the showers may be large enough for a resident alone, they are too small for the staff to assist residents as needed. The square footage of the bathrooms is small, and there is very little storage space for resident linens or toiletries. Flooring coloration should provide more contrast with the toilet, to assist visual cueing. Lighting in the bathrooms consists of an overhead light and a vanity light over the mirror that are only marginally better than the resident room lighting.

Resident laundry and mechanical rooms occupy prime real estate in the heart of the household. Although the location makes the laundry visible and available to residents, the area is also used for linen storage and clean and dirty utilities, because of inadequate storage facilities. Locating these service areas in the heart of the household imparts an institutional feel.

The family rooms in each household seem to be underutilized. Staff, administration, and family members could not recall these rooms being used on a regular basis by residents and family members. Interactions that might happen in the family room seem to take place either in residents' apartments or on Main Street.

The spa, placed in an area that was "left over," feels noticeably like an afterthought that helped the facility comply with code requirements. Although the spa has a pleasant décor, it is isolated from the three neighborhoods on the opposite side of Main Street. A family member we questioned about bathing preferences was not even aware that the spa existed, or that it was an option for bathing. The remote location and the unfor-

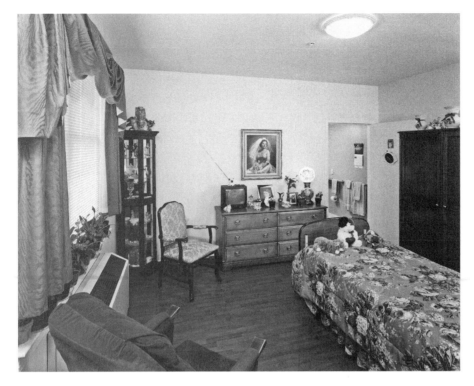

FIG. 12-8 Small wardrobes in each room do not provide adequate storage and complicate the placement of personal furnishings © *Tim Buchman 2006*

tunate need to cross Main Street in a bathrobe to reach the spa force many residents and staff to use the showers in the resident bathrooms by default.

Regional/Cultural Design

Although the aesthetic of Main Street is largely based upon a small North Carolina town, in reality its design and components reflect the general central-square identity of many American towns.

Environmental Therapy

Main Street is easily and safely used by residents on a continuous basis and thus must be deemed successful. The storefronts and shop interiors of Main Street

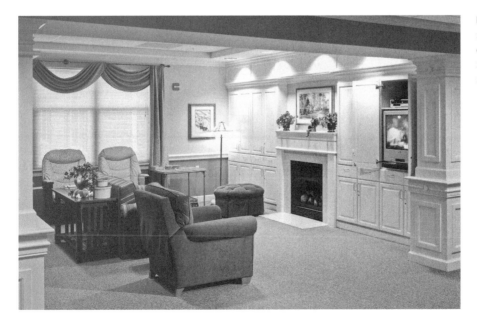

FIG. 12-9 The family room is residential in design but underutilized by residents © *Tim Buchman 2006*

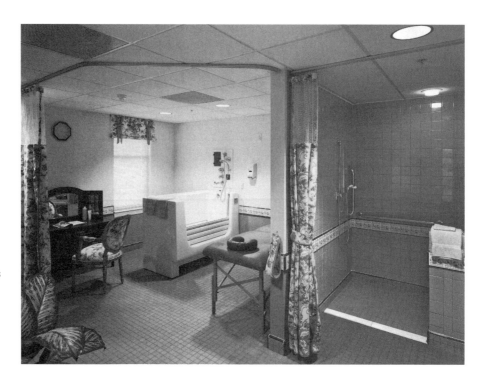

FIG. 12-10 Warm colors and residential inspired décor, including a vintage dressing table, result in a senior-friendly bathing room © *Tim Buchman 2006*

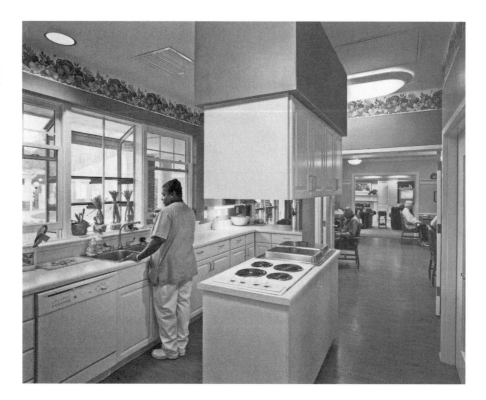

FIG. 12-11 Though visually pleasing, the kitchen islands lack counter space for cooking and serving, and the overhead cabinets become "head knockers" © *Tim Buchman 2006*

encourage resident use, and the front porches of each household are generally well designed and very popular. The dining, living, and kitchen components in each of the neighborhoods are visible to the residents and easy to distinguish. Residents are easily drawn into these spaces and make use of them as they were designed.

Outdoor Environment

It was disappointing that there is no direct and clearly understood access from Main Street to an exterior courtyard. The courtyards, though spacious, have little to offer in terms of amenities. The addition of shade-producing vegetation or furnishings, as well as raised planters for small activity gardens, would be beneficial to residents. Porch swings and gliders would provide passive activities for residents to enjoy.

The wandering sidewalks are confusing because the household entries from the courtyard side are not clearly delineated. A resident may leave one household, wander through the courtyard, unknowingly enter another household, and be completely confused as to the location. Residents who enter a household via the French doors into the dining room are reported to feel odd and hesitant about intruding into the dining space.

Quality of Workplace and the Physical Plant

Resident activity coordinators provide care in the individual neighborhoods and, with the exception of housekeeping and maintenance duties, are empowered to do anything and everything for residents. Caregivers receive specialized, ongoing training and are supported by Aldersgate's commitment to accommodate residents' changing needs.

The kitchen design should be reexamined with regard to function. It currently serves as the meal-serving kitchen, recreational kitchen, and a medication room. Drugs are administered at a workstation in the kitchen area. Not only did the space seem small, crowded, and totally inappropriate for the delivery of medications, but most states would prohibit this activity from taking place in the kitchen. This process is an operation most care providers would not want to associate with a kitchen.

Although staff did not complain, the "head-knocking" cabinets over the island contribute to the sense of confinement and block natural light from fully penetrating into the room. Bulky food delivery carts further tightened the space.

Food is prepared in a commercial kitchen at a remote location on campus and is delivered on a covered golf cart. The cart arrives at a delivery door and the food is carted through Main Street and the household corridors to the serving kitchen. This requires at least two trips for each meal to each household, one for hot foods and one for cold. The hot food is transferred to in-counter steam tables. Countertops on either side of the steam tables would assist in the plating of food.

Because the current kitchens do not have sanitizing dishwashers, dirty dishes have to be carted out of the households as well. Although new dishwashers have been requested in the upcoming capital budget, the issue of an ice machine remains unresolved. The household refrigerators are not large enough to handle the household ice needs.

Operator Perspectives

The environs of the campus are within a transitional neighborhood. Originally a blue-collar neighborhood, it has evolved into an ethnic neighborhood. This is advantageous for staffing but presents a marketing problem for the operator. There is concern about the future of the campus in this neighborhood, and the operator is currently in discussions with the University of North Carolina planning department, as well as the City of Charlotte, to gain a greater understanding of the future of the area and Aldersgate's involvement with and future within the immediate community. These discussions have a significant bearing on how Aldersgate approaches care provision and addresses future needs. However, the functionality of Cuthbertson Village and the population it serves has been pleasing to the operator, providing a necessary level of care in a pleasant environment.

General Project Information

PROJECT ADDRESS
Cuthbertson Village at Aldersgate
3800 Shamrock Drive
Charlotte, NC 28215

PROJECT DESIGN TEAM
Architect: Freeman White, Inc.
Interior Designer: Freeman White, Inc.
Landscape Architect: Site Solutions
Structural Engineer: King/Guinn Associates
Mechanical Engineer: Freeman White, Inc.
Electrical Engineer: Freeman White, Inc.
Civil Engineer: Site Solutions
Dining Consultant: N/A

Gerontologist: N/A
Management/Development: N/A
Contractor: Bovis Lend Lease

PROJECT STATUS
Completion date: June 2003

OCCUPANCY LEVELS
At facility opening date: 92%
At date of evaluation: 98%

RESIDENT AGE (YRS)
At facility opening date: 81
At date of evaluation: 88.9

PROJECT AREAS

DEMENTIA-SPECIFIC ASSISTED LIVING

Project Element	New Construction	
	No. Units	Typical Size
Studio units	45	270 GSF
Total (all units)	45	11,700 GSF
Residents' social areas (lounges, dining, and recreation spaces):		10,100 GSF
Medical, health care, therapy, and activities spaces:		750 GSF
Administrative, public, and ancillary support services:		300 GSF
Service, maintenance, and mechanical areas:		1,400 GSF
Total gross area:		34,000 GSF
Total net usable area (per space program):		24,250 NSF
Overall gross/net factor (ratio of gross area/net usable area):		1.40

SITE AND PARKING

SITE LOCATION
Small town

SITE SIZE
Acres: 3.4
Square feet: 148,104
Area of entire campus: 234 acres

PARKING

Type of Parking	For This Facility			For Other Facility			Totals
	Residents	Staff	Visitors	Residents	Staff	Visitors	
Open surface lot(s)	N/A	20	18	220	85	30	373

CONSTRUCTION COSTS

SOURCE OF COST DATA
Final construction cost as of May 2003

SOFT COSTS
Land cost or value:	N/A
Basic architectural and engineering:	$300,840
Expanded architectural and engineering:	N/A
All permit and other entitlement fees:	Unknown
Legal:	N/A
Appraisals:	N/A
Marketing and preopening:	$98,000
Total soft costs:	$398,840

BUILDING COSTS
New construction except FF&E, special finishes, floor and window coverings, HVAC, and electrical:	$2,107,810
Renovations except FF&E, special finishes, floor and window coverings, HVAC, and electrical:	N/A
FF&E and small wares:	$393,050
Floor coverings:	In above
Window coverings:	In above
HVAC:	$626,400
Electrical:	$383,400
Medical equipment costs:	N/A
Total building costs:	$3,510,660

SITE COSTS
New on-site:	$72,980
New off-site:	N/A
Renovation on-site:	N/A
Renovation off-site:	N/A
Landscape:	$29,520
Special site features or amenities:	N/A
Total site costs:	$102,500

TOTAL PROJECT COSTS
Total project costs: $4,012,000

FINANCING SOURCES
Nontaxable bond offering

"Old age is like a plane flying through a storm. Once you are aboard, there is nothing you can do."

GOLDA MEIR, 1898–1978

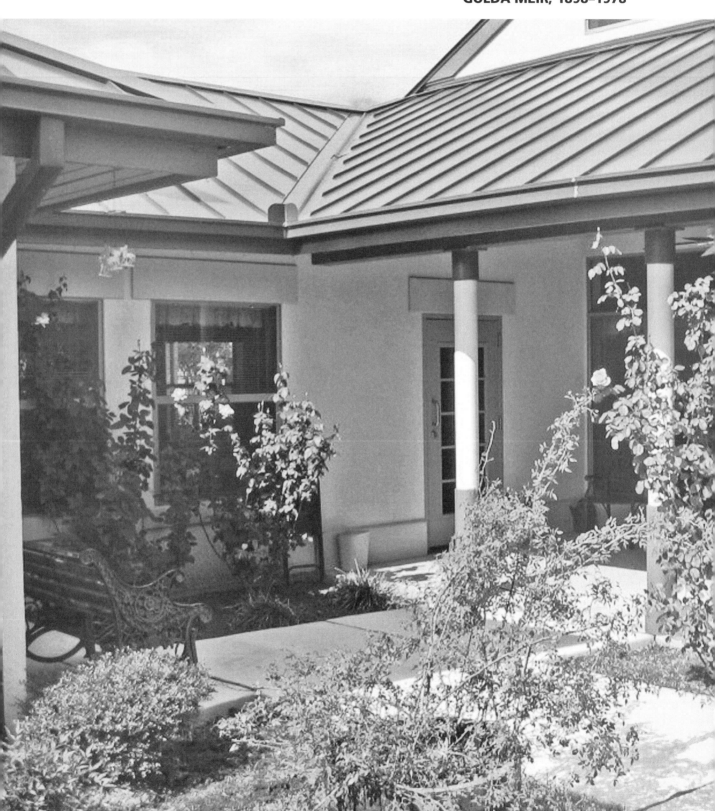

Chapter 13

Freedom House at Air Force Village

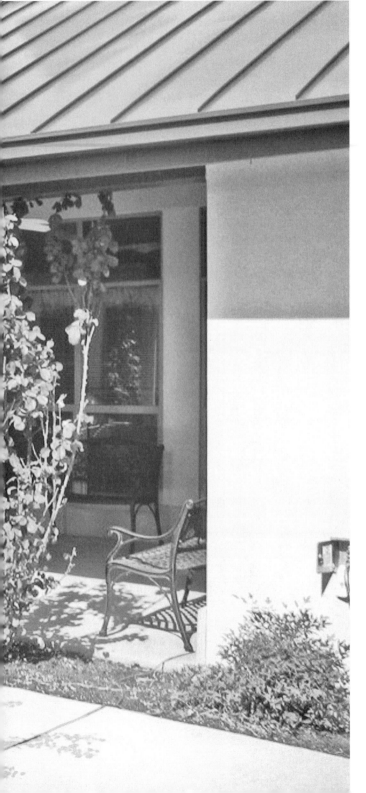

EVALUATION SITE: Freedom House at Air Force Village

COMMUNITY TYPE: Assisted Living for Those with Dementia
- 54 assisted living residents with dementia
- Day care for 22 children

REGION: Southwest

ARCHITECT: Rehler Vaughn & Koone, Inc.

OWNER: Air Force Village Alzheimer Care and Research Center

DATA POINTS:

Resident Room:	248 gsf
	(single-occupancy)
	396 gsf (shared-occupancy)
Total Area:	839 gsf/resident
Total Area:	45,312 gsf
Project Cost:	$175.76/gsf
Total Project Cost:	$7,963,932
Investment/resident:	$147,480.22
Staffing:	3.80 care hours/resident/day
Occupancy:	100% as of November 2005

FIRST OCCUPANCY: Phase I—July 1998, Phase II—June 2003

DATE OF EVALUATION: November 2005

EVALUATION TEAM: Mark Proffitt; Bill Bonn, AIA; Amy T. Carpenter, AIA; Margaret P. Calkins, Ph.D.; David Green; Andrew Alden; Russell McLaughlin; Robert Lagoyda; Mitch Green, AIA; this evaluation completed in conjunction with the Society for the Advancement of Gerontological Environments (SAGE)

FIG. 13-1 A household covered porch allows residents to enjoy the outdoors without exposure to direct sunlight *Photograph courtesy of SAGE/Society for the Advancement of Gerontological Environments*

Introduction

Since 1999, the Society for the Advancement of Gerontological Environments (SAGE) has conducted walk-through post-occupancy evaluations as part of the annual AAHSA fall meeting. Conference attendees have a unique opportunity to tour an innovative community and hear the results of a one-day post-occupancy evaluation from a diverse panel of experts in the field. In addition to the goals of the sponsor for the community, SAGE also benchmarks the environment against a set of key therapeutic goals that represent the SAGE philosophy: a philosophy that emphasizes person-centered concepts. Freedom House at Air Force Village was an ideal candidate for a SAGE post-occupancy evaluation because the vision of the project from the beginning was to create a place to understand the cause, care, and cure for people with Alzheimer's and related dementias. Moreover, the project, constructed in three phases, had a unique opportunity to make changes in the environment based upon experience or post-occupancy research.

Air Force Village is located 10 miles outside of San Antonio, near the Lackland Air Force Base in the arid Texas hill country. All residents have the distinction of being retired officers from branches of the uniformed services or their spouses. As officers in the military, many of the residents have lived throughout the country in communal settings, but are accustomed to a high level of service. In recognition that the existing nursing home was not supportive for people with memory loss, the Alzheimer's Care and Research Center Foundation was created in 1993 to raise the funds and awareness necessary to create an appropriate setting for residents with dementia and a place for ongoing associated research.

The Foundation opened the first phase of Freedom House for 27 residents in 1998. Designed to resemble a collection of houses in a Texas hill-country vernacular style, the building is broken into three households with nine residents each. The households are named after the first three Air Force Chiefs of Staff: Spaatz, Twining, and Vandenberg. With the building broken out into small households, residents have less information to process and familiar domestic patterns can be maintained. Each household has its own kitchen, dining room, living room, bathing spa, porch, and outdoor garden. Attention was paid to creating a hierarchy of zones from public to private.

Resident rooms are arranged around a central living room with a cathedral ceiling, instead of double-loaded corridors. The three households form a neighborhood that is connected by a central den and then glass walkways to the community building, which contains a social hall, chapel, and child day care as well as administrative and research offices. As funds were raised, the second phase of the project, also for 27 residents, opened in 2003 with an additional neighborhood of three more

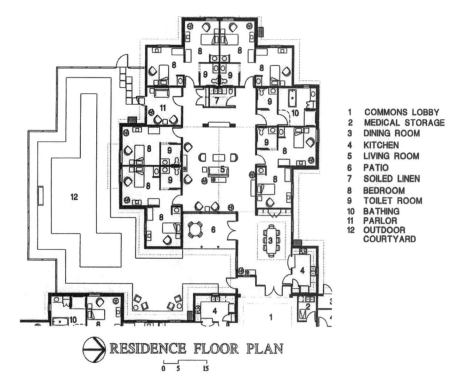

FIG. 13-2   A typical household floor plan with centered resident social space *Courtesy of Rehler Vaughn & Koone, Inc.*

1	COMMONS LOBBY
2	MEDICAL STORAGE
3	DINING ROOM
4	KITCHEN
5	LIVING ROOM
6	PATIO
7	SOILED LINEN
8	BEDROOM
9	TOILET ROOM
10	BATHING
11	PARLOR
12	OUTDOOR COURTYARD

RESIDENCE FLOOR PLAN

0   5   15

households of nine residents each, designed with slight modifications based on the lessons learned from operating the first phase. A larger courtyard garden with a gazebo was created between the two neighborhoods. The anticipated third phase of construction will include three additional households, each with nine residents who are in the end stages of dementia and need hospice care.

Freedom House demonstrates a commitment to innovative therapeutic design and innovative programming, along with research. The small nine-resident households create a calm, familiar setting where people with memory loss can thrive. The child day center for 22 children and the extensive gardens create opportunities for residents to engage in familiar, productive roles. The flexibility of the environment allows staff to treat each resident individually as a person and respond to that resident's unique needs. Family members feel very much at ease visiting and often participate in the daily activities of the households. One spouse of a resident declared her adoration to the evaluation group with this clear statement: "Once you make the decision to go to Freedom House, you never have to make another. You are so free!"

Architect's Statement

The project, along with its program of care, is based on the concept of a home. All functions and activities of daily living are an integral part of the therapeutic environment. The number of people with whom a resident must interact is limited to nine household members. Three such households form the total of 27 residents in each phase of the project. An activities center, day care, and research and education center round out the major uses. Project scale and image reflect the surrounding Texas hill-country vernacular.

Designers' and Operators' Stated Objectives and Responses

OBJECTIVE: To create a residential, home-like environment.

DESIGN INTENT: Reduce the scale and number of interactions among residents.

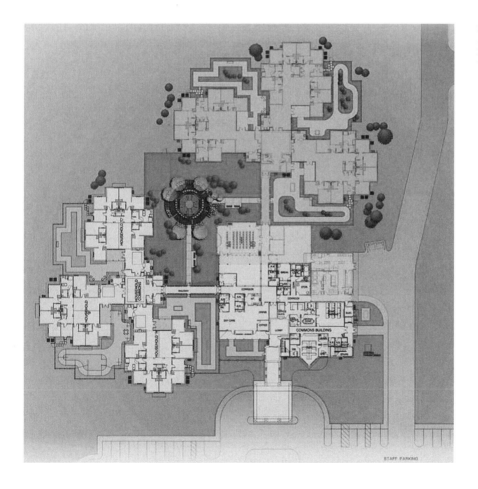

FIG. 13-3 Overall floor plan with Phase I and Phase II *Courtesy of Rehler Vaughn & Koone, Inc.*

OBJECTIVE: To promote movement and ambulation.

DESIGN INTENT: Provide visible and open, yet secure, yard spaces.

OBJECTIVE: To encourage participation in activities.

DESIGN INTENT: Provide familiar daily activities within a residential setting.

OBJECTIVE: Create a research and education center.

DESIGN INTENT: Provide a prominently located research office and classroom.

OBJECTIVE: To be compatible with the site context.

DESIGN INTENT: Use indigenous materials and vernacular building forms.

Field Observations: Meeting the Objectives

OBJECTIVE: To create a residential, home-like environment.

FIELD OBSERVATIONS: Dividing the building into households of nine residents has reduced the scale that residents with memory loss must comprehend, and offers opportunities to replicate the domestic patterns of a home. A clear theme that was emphasized when family members of residents were interviewed was the family atmosphere of the households. They also sensed that the households were quiet and noticed that staff did not wear uniforms. One family member said, "Immediately, my mom felt like she was home."

Each of the three households connects to a central area called the "den," although the evaluators felt that it did not live up to this name and felt more like a "hub." This hub has a faux fireplace and small seating area. All 27 residents have access to this space, and throughout the day several residents, as well as the household dog, were seen sitting in the area. While very little institutional clutter was found in the households, the hub contains staff desks, equipment, and carts. Laudable efforts were made to use residential-style desks and armoires for charting binders, but the area still has a mixed institutional appearance, which is in sharp contrast to the more residential atmosphere of the households. As this area is located at the front door to the households, it was felt that this space should project a stronger residential tone.

The three households are visible from the den area. As you step into the households, you immediately enter a dining room with an adjacent kitchen visible through a pass-through window. In Phase I, the dining room had a series of display shelves directly visible across from the doorway filled with small decorative items and books. In Phase II, the shelves were removed because staff thought they had a cluttered appearance. The evaluation team felt the dining room looked less residential without the shelves and that it was a missed opportunity to create an orientation point. Residents dine in smaller groups in a family style that encourages conversation. In fact, several family members as well as staff join residents for meals.

Beyond the dining room is an open living room adjacent to a porch. Rather than hallways, residents circulate through the living room to reach their rooms. Although the evaluators liked the use of the living room instead of corridors, some of the details of the space needed further study. This large space has a high ceiling with clerestory windows, but the space is dark, due mostly to the windows being located under a deep covered porch area and to the inefficient artificial lighting. The number and location of doors around the perimeter of the room do not promote the creation of a typical social furniture grouping found in a home. Most of the furniture floats in the middle of space, and the focus of the space is solely on the television set. This may be a concern for some residents with cognitive issues. The tall ceiling in the room resulted in a live acoustical space, making conversations difficult for residents to hear and comprehend.

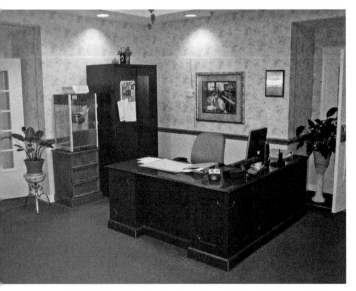

FIG. 13-4 Nursing desk and armoire for charts are a hub of activity but are often cluttered *Photograph courtesy of SAGE/Society for the Advancement of Gerontological Environments*

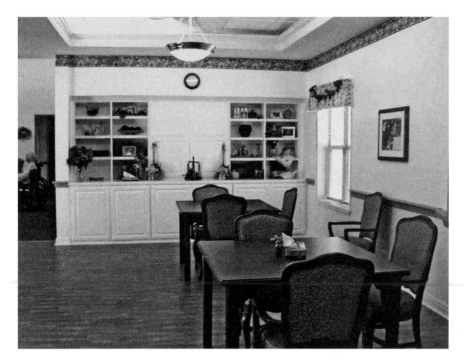

FIG. 13-5 The Phase I dining room incorporates display shelves. They were eliminated in Phase II *Photograph courtesy of SAGE/Society for the Advancement of Gerontological Environments*

OBJECTIVE: To promote movement and ambulation.

FIELD OBSERVATIONS: Freedom House has extensive outdoor gardens for residents to enjoy. Each household has a secure garden, and there is a large garden with a gazebo located between the two neighborhood phases, which is accessible via glass-enclosed walkways that lead to the community building. Some residents have participated in planting the gardens, and staff indicated many residents enjoy the spaces all year around. Raised planting beds and containers were seen in all of the garden areas.

The majority of the gardens are not visible from the public spaces of the households, which may discourage their use by some residents. Staff use cameras to view the garden areas, and a tone sounds to let them know when the door to the garden is opened. The large garden with a gazebo is located beyond the locked door of the households. It appears to be intended more for planned events, versus the more informal use of the patio gardens located within the households. The hot Texas climate and bright sun may also limit use of this space, because of comfort issues. Although porches provided shaded places near the doors for residents to sit, significant glare was visible reflecting from the metal roofs and white, untreated concrete.

Encouragement of ambulation and movement relies upon wayfinding. Outside, the household gardens are arranged in a circular loop, with one primary entry and exit at the front porch to encourage easy use. Wayfinding inside was somewhat less easy and hence less successful.

Because each of the households uses essentially the same architectural layout and is connected to the common spaces in the same manner, interior finishes, details, and exterior views are the only way to orient residents. In an effort to differentiate each of the households, the entries have distinctive architectural details over the doorways and different finish colors.

The evaluation team thought the architectural details were too subtle and located out of the view of most people with memory loss, who tend to look downward. The color differences within the pastel color schemes were very subtle and did not stand out enough to constitute a significant wayfinding cue. In Phase I, the large shelves in the dining room, located across from the entry door, served as the best orientation device for finding the household, but these were eliminated in the second phase. It was not clear that the items on the shelves were designed to be distinctly different, which the evaluation team thought was a missed opportunity. In Phase II, with no shelves, it was harder to differentiate the three households from each other.

In an effort to locate their rooms, some residents have placed landmarks outside their doorways on a provided shelf. One Air Force navigator chose to use small flags to identify his room. Memory boxes were used in the first phase of the project, but not included when the second phase was built because the staff did not believe them to be effective. Research has found that objects do aid residents with early-stage dementia to find their

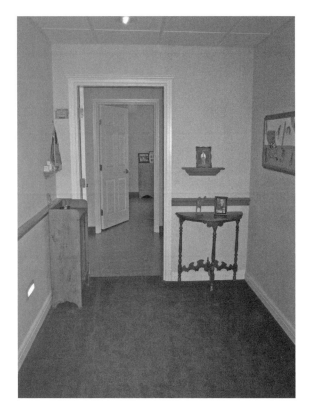

FIG. 13-6 A resident room entry, with display shelf and personal furnishings, helps to differentiate one room from another *Photograph courtesy of SAGE/Society for the Advancement of Gerontological Environments*

rooms, but the design of the shelves or boxes also plays a pivotal role in their success. The evaluation team believed that the memory boxes would have been more effective as an orientation device if they had been larger, deeper, and better lit.

OBJECTIVE: To encourage participation in activities.

FIELD OBSERVATIONS: During the visit, the evaluation did not see many planned activities in the households. Residents were often found watching the television in the living rooms or spending time in their own rooms. The kitchen provided on each unit offers the opportunity for participating in familiar domestic activities within a residential setting. However, the space is separated from the dining room by a doorway and a pass-through window with a counter. This arrangement does not make it conducive to group activity within the space, but one-on-one activities would be possible.

One area that family members and staff thought was missing was a den area for the men to play billiards or socialize in separate from the women. This type of space was being considered as part of the third-phase edition.

OBJECTIVE: Create a research and education center.

FIELD OBSERVATIONS: Freedom House is the only non-profit community in San Antonio that offers on-site research focusing on dementia. Freedom House research is conducted in collaboration with the University of Texas Health Science Center Medical School, under the directorship of Dr. Donald Royall. Current research focuses on early identification and measurement of Alzheimer's, medications that delay the onset of symptoms, and identifying genetics associated with Alzheimer's and related dementias. In addition, Freedom House serves as a model setting for research on the impact of the environment, caregiving, and program activities, though it is not clear how much environmental and behavioral research has been conducted. As part of the Alzheimer's Care and Research Center Foundation, Freedom House also has a resource library and caregiver education program to inform caregivers, provide support, and supply referral services.

OBJECTIVE: To be compatible with the site context.

FIELD OBSERVATIONS: Overall, the massing of buildings feels residential, with each of the households expressed

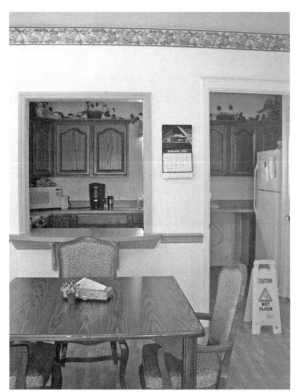

FIG. 13-7 The kitchen pass-through wall separates kitchen and dining room and discourages resident activity in kitchen *Photograph courtesy of SAGE/Society for the Advancement of Gerontological Environments*

individually through the architecture. The building has a hacienda compound appearance. The stucco façades and standing-seam metal roofs appear at home in the Texas hill country. (See Figure 12 in the color insert.) Creative touches, such as the use of stars as metal accents, emphasized the Texan location, as well as the military background of the residents. The evaluators found the large porte cochere to be out of scale in relationship to the rest of the project. A treatment that downplayed the size of an extended roofline to create a covered drop-off would have projected a more residential ambience.

Field Observations: Themes and Hypotheses

Creating Community

Freedom House is located remotely from the main community building on the Air Force Village campus. A pedestrian walkway is available as a connector, but it is apparent that most people drive to reach the building. This location does not help the Freedom House residents to be a part of the overall CCRC community.

Within the main section of the building, a chapel and activity space provide opportunities for all the residents to interact, but this area is used primarily for planned activities, as the two neighborhoods require a pass code to enter or exit. One of the lessons learned when implementing the second phase was to downplay the location of the doorway leading to the community building, so residents would not see people coming and going. However, staff indicated that some residents do move between the two neighborhoods.

Most of the emphasis has been placed on the small-scale households, which promote a family atmosphere that clearly resonated in interviews with the family members. One member stated that "you come to care for everybody . . . it's just a family." Another said, "I am a caregiver, but I need care too, and I get hugs . . . even now after several years since my wife has passed."

Making a Home

An essential concept of creating a home environment is promoting both privacy and autonomy of the residents. The majority of the rooms in each household are semi-private, but utilize an L-shaped design to provide each resident with his or her own space. Some of the rooms maintain privacy with a curtain, but a wall and doors separated others. One resident in a room separated by a curtain found this arrangement to be quite normal, and

she remarked to an evaluator, "I do not share a room; I share a bathroom with that person over there."

When other residents were asked their preference, most of the male officers clearly indicated that they would rather have a private room with a bathroom. Staff members felt that this was part of the background of military men who wish to "remain in control." Staff and family members supported the idea of shared rooms because it provided some residents with a caregiving role or comfort knowing someone is nearby.

The only time family members did not like a shared arrangement was during the very end stages of the disease, when family and friends would gather during the resident's final days. A private space for visiting with family members or staff was originally placed in each household, but removed in the second phase because it was rarely used. The evaluation team felt that this type of space was still needed, either adjacent to the household or within the household, as the majority of the rooms are shared. In the third phase of the community, which is intended for residents in the end stages of dementia and hospice care, staff and family members strongly believed—and evaluators concurred—that the

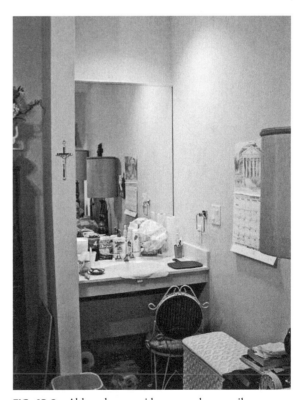

FIG. 13-8 Although two residents may share a toilet room, a separate sink for each resident is also provided in the sleeping space *Photograph courtesy of SAGE/Society for the Advancement of Gerontological Environments*

rooms should provide for privacy or have places for family members to spend time in private.

Regional/Cultural Design

Overall, the buildings appear residential, with each of the households expressed individually in the architecture. The building has a hacienda compound appearance. The stucco façades and standing-seam metal roofs are appropriate in the Texas hill country landscape. The use of stars as metal accents emphasized the culture of the state of Texas as well as the military background of the residents. The interior décor of the households maintains a residential appearance with the inclusion of residential-style furniture.

Environmental Therapy

The multiple-household design for nine residents each permitted staff to locate residents with similar needs close to one another. Efforts are made to group residents by cognitive and functional needs and allow them to age in place. Residents are rarely transferred to another household or to the nursing home unless it is absolutely necessary. Therefore, the programming for daily events can be easily customized for individual needs. Overall, the small-scale environment created a very calm environment with many of the sights, smells, and feel of a home. The air was filled with the smell of baking cookies in one household. As a result of the strong home ambience, institutional elements, although rare, were jarringly out of place. One such element was the use of vinyl flooring in some of the resident rooms.

The community respects the choices of the resident, which was reflected in one interviewed resident's statement that "no one dictates what you do." Accordingly, the environment has been designed to be enabling so residents can maintain their functional abilities and continue to make their own choices. For example, the wardrobe in each resident room is designed with two compartments: one for the bulk of the clothes and the other side where one or two choices can be placed for less effortful daily selection. This side can also be arranged so that clothing is visible in the order in which one normally dresses, to visually cue residents. Another example is the effective use of color. Continence for some residents with dementia often depends on situational issues, such as being unable to find a white toilet when it is placed against a white wall on a white floor. By using a contrasting color on the floor and walls, the toilet is made to visually stand out and provide a reinforcing visual cue.

Outdoor Environment

Extensive outdoor spaces were planned into the project. An outdoor courtyard that is available for the child day care also serves as a separate entrance. Each of the households has its own garden space, complete with a porch and circular path. The household gardens are enclosed by wooden fences that have a residential appearance. One of the lessons learned was that more outdoor space was needed for the households. Therefore, when Phase II was constructed, a large courtyard with a gazebo was created between the two neighborhoods. Raised planting areas and furniture were found throughout the gardens so residents can sit and enjoy gardening. Each of the households has a deep front porch—a welcome relief from the bright Texas sun. The outdoor space would have been enhanced by dyeing the white concrete, as it was found to be a source of glare. This was also true of the metal roofs. Some of the paths had inserts of brick pavers that had shifted and would be difficult to negotiate with walkers or canes.

Quality of Workplace and the Physical Plant

Staff at Freedom House are clearly integrated into the mission, management, and operational approach of the setting. A key qualification of a staff member, according to management, is being "caring and compassionate with a willingness to learn." It was evident that the staff had input when changes were made to the floor plans of the households in Phase II based on the operation of Phase I. Staff members are a critical part of the family atmosphere and take their meals with the residents.

The den/hub is the primary workspace for staff members in the neighborhoods. Much of the institutional clutter visible was in this area, and it would have improved the ambience to screen some of these elements from view in a back-office area. Staff felt that this area was too small and too open for necessary private communications, and would have preferred to have a small conference space adjacent to the area. With the movement in the industry toward cross-trained care team staffing, private meeting spaces will be seen in the future as being just as important as the nurse station was in the past.

Some of the storage and utility spaces were enlarged during the second phase of construction. Some features that were still found lacking included the need to have a dishwasher in the household kitchen to facilitate cleaning. Currently, staff have to do some dishes by hand. A

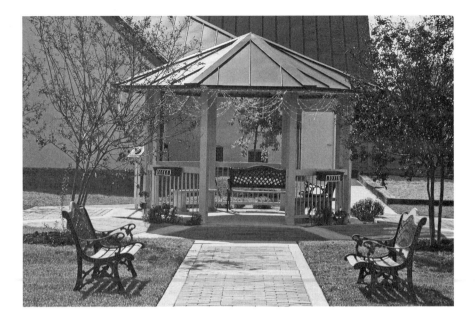

FIG. 13-9 A gazebo with benches provides a place to rest, but some brick pavers have shifted, creating difficulty for walking residents *Photograph courtesy of SAGE/Society for the Advancement of Gerontological Environments*

laundry room was provided in the first phase adjacent to the hub, but eliminated in the second phase. In Phase II, staff have to run back and forth to a central laundry location, which they find inconvenient.

Because Freedom House provides assisted living, a call system was not required by the Texas state code. Staff must rely upon either hearing a resident call for assistance or having a roommate call for assistance. Although the acoustically live living room helped with this issue by carrying voices, some staff were concerned about not being able to hear residents.

Operator Perspectives

AUTHOR'S NOTE: *As this project was constructed in two phases, there was an opportunity for the operator to evaluate the first phase and modify environmental issues in the second phase. This is a listing of those modifications:*

- The visual prominence of the entry/exit to the neighborhood was reduced to keep residents from shadowing staff and visitors when leaving.

- One fire separation was created at the entry to a neighborhood instead of one at each household, so that during a fire drill there is less disruption.
- The size of the patio space for the households was increased.
- The rarely used household parlors were converted into increased storage areas and a small private telephone niche.
- The size of the utility room and linen storage in each household was increased.
- Instead of privacy curtains, walls and a door are used to separate the semiprivate rooms.
- Equipment was switched from a tilting therapy tub to a therapy tub with a lift-up door. Some residents did not like the movement of the tilting tub.
- Instead of a small memory box, which staff did not find effective, a shelf was installed outside each door for residents to place orientation items.
- The display shelves were removed from the dining room to reduce the cluttered appearance.

General Project Information

PROJECT ADDRESS
Freedom House at Air Force Village
5100 John D. Ryan Blvd.
San Antonio, TX 78245

PROJECT DESIGN TEAM
Architect: Rehler Vaughn & Koone, Inc.
Associate Architect: Nelson-Tremain Partnership
Interior Designer: N/A

Landscape Architect: Rehler Vaughn & Koone, Inc.
Structural Engineer: Steve G. Persyn
Mechanical Engineer: Murray & Associates
Electrical Engineer: Murray & Associates
Civil Engineer: Brown Engineering
Dining Consultant: N/A
Gerontologist: N/A
Management/Development: N/A
Contractor: Phase I—Spaw Glass; Phase II—Concept
   Builders

PROJECT STATUS
Completion date: Phase I—July 1998, Phase II—June 2003

OCCUPANCY LEVELS
At facility opening date: 50%
At date of evaluation: 100%

RESIDENT AGE (YRS)
At facility opening date: Unknown
At date of evaluation: 85

PROJECT AREAS

DEMENTIA-SPECIFIC ASSISTED LIVING

Project Element	New Construction	
	No. Units	Typical Size
Private rooms	6	248 GSF
Shared occupancy rooms	24	369 GSF
Total (all units)	30	11,076 GSF
Residents' social areas (lounges, dining, and recreation spaces):		12,729 GSF
Medical, health care, therapy, and activities spaces:		832 GSF
Administrative, public, and ancillary support services (includes child day care):		3,712 GSF
Service, maintenance, and mechanical areas:		10,950 GSF
Total gross area:		45,312 GSF
Total net usable area (per space program):		34,362 NSF
Overall gross/net factor (ratio of gross area/net usable area):		1.32

SITE AND PARKING

SITE LOCATION
Suburban

SITE SIZE
Acres: 4.4
Square feet: 191,664

PARKING

Type of Parking	For This Facility			
	Residents	Staff	Visitors	Totals
Open surface lot(s)	0	27	57	84

CONSTRUCTION COSTS

SOURCE OF COST DATA
Final construction cost as of June 2003

SOFT COSTS
Land was donated
Total soft costs: $1,080,153

BUILDING COSTS
New construction except FF&E, special finishes,
   floor and window coverings, HVAC,
   and electrical: $6,142,368
Renovations except FF&E, special finishes, floor
   and window coverings, HVAC, and electrical: N/A

All FF&E, floor coverings, window coverings,
and small wares: $741,411
HVAC: Included in above
Electrical: Included in above
Medical equipment costs: N/A
Total building costs: $6,883,779

SITE COSTS
All site costs are included in building costs

TOTAL PROJECT COSTS
Total project costs: $7,963,932

FINANCING SOURCES
Entire project completed with donated funds

"Old age is the most unexpected of all the things that can happen to a man."

JAMES THURBER, 1894–1961

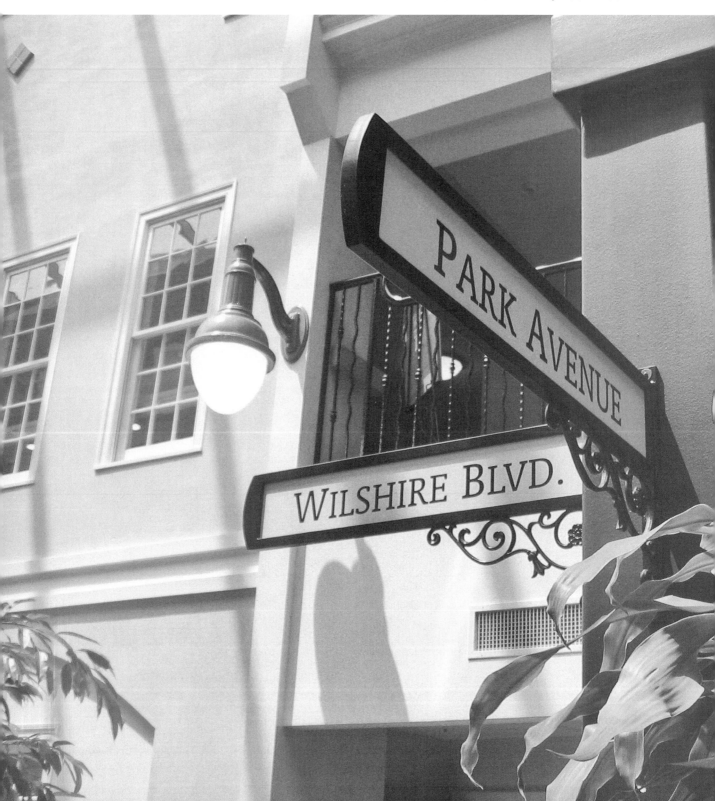

Chapter 14   The Forest at Duke

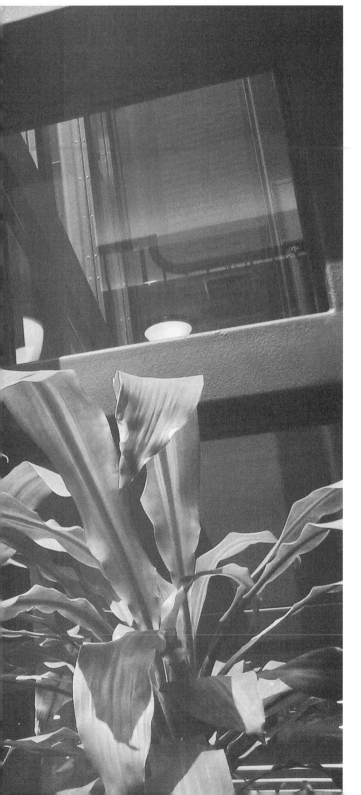

EVALUATION SITE: The Forest at Duke

COMMUNITY TYPE: Assisted Living for Those with Dementia
- 16 assisted living apartments
- 18 assisted living apartments for those with dementia
- 50 nursing care beds

REGION: Mid-Atlantic

ARCHITECT: Calloway Johnson Moore & West, P.A.

OWNER: The Forest at Duke, Inc.

DATA POINTS: Resident Room: 456–641 gsf
                                                        (assisted living)
Resident Room: 250 gsf (nursing care)
Total Area: 1,159.09 gsf/resident (assisted living)
Total Area: 39,409 gsf (assisted living)
Total Area: 612.80 gsf/resident (nursing care)
Total Area: 30,640 gsf (nursing care)
Total Area: 79,346 gsf
Project Cost: $181.44/gsf
Total Project Cost: $14,396,527
Investment/resident: $171,065.79
Staffing: 1.89 care hours/resident/day (assisted living)
                    4.00 care hours/resident/day (nursing care)
Occupancy: 99% as of August 2005

FIRST OCCUPANCY: February 2005

DATE OF EVALUATION: August 2005

EVALUATION TEAM: David Slack; Thomas Hauer;
Ingrid Fraley, ASID; Mitch Green, AIA; Jeffrey
Anderzhon, AIA

FIG. 14-1   Street signs tout upscale locations as part of the
resident orientation strategy   *Photograph by Jeffrey Anderzhon*

Introduction

The city of Durham, North Carolina, is recognized for its outstanding medical facilities and clinical services, as well as corporate centers for technology, research, and teaching. The success of this community can be largely attributed to the presence of Duke University, North Carolina Central University, the University of North Carolina–Chapel Hill, and North Carolina State University in nearby Raleigh. In addition to these institutions of higher learning, more than 300 medical and health-related companies are located in the Research Triangle.

Nestled in the heart of this area, The Forest at Duke, a continuing care retirement community, offers superior accommodation and a healthy lifestyle while promoting a distinct and visionary approach to caring for seniors. More than 400 people from 28 states reside at The Forest and enjoy the holistic philosophy and exceptional living experience. Programs ranging from exercise and aerobics classes to leisure and lap swimming are available through the activities department. At the clinic, good health and well-being are addressed through lectures on timely topics, support groups, screenings, personalized assistance, and access to the numerous programs and activities offered by the surrounding universities.

For more than a decade, a unique population comprised of "professors, gardeners, authors, CEOs, community volunteers, opera buffs, engineers, librarians, homemakers, and artists" has found comfort, security, and the freedom to live life to the fullest at The Forest.

The history of the campus spans about 20 years. Originally the Pickett Farm, the acreage evolved into a retirement campus in the mid-1980s, with the first buildings opening in 1992. The lobby of the main building sets the style for the campus with a signature stained-glass window, grand staircase, and interior water feature. Graceful and well-appointed interior spaces exemplify the spirit of southern hospitality with a cosmopolitan flair. Living and dining rooms, along with an exquisitely paneled pub, are reminiscent of the Grand Old South.

The adjoining health center moved away from this southern tradition and contrasts with the architectural theme and interior design throughout other areas of the campus. Based upon a series of best practices, research articles, and seminars, the health center has well-intentioned goals, including an emphasis on privacy and dignity issues, familiar items to distinguish resident rooms, outings for residents, a skylight to bring the outside in, and other small touches such as the elimination of medication carts.

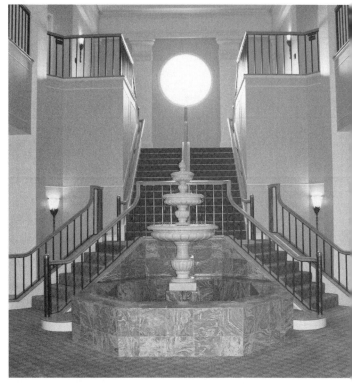

FIG. 14-2 The campus at The Forest at Duke has an upscale southern ambiance. This grand staircase is the focal point of the main building entry and lobby *Photograph by Jeffrey Anderzhon*

Our evaluation focused on the additions to the health center. However, its context and relationship to the remaining campus and resident lifestyle must not be ignored, and are discussed in later sections.

Architect's Statement

The continuing care retirement community, which opened in 1992, is building an addition to its health care center. Scheduled for completion in 2003, the project will create two distinctly different environments for assisted living. On the second floor there will be residential apartments with common areas and support services. On the ground floor there will be two special care "neighborhoods" with homes, streets, and gardens. A new village center will become the focal point of the entire health care building, providing amenities such as a chapel, town hall, fitness center, and spa. A unique cross-section allows the interior "street" in the village center to be a two-story skylit space. This addition is part of a larger project that will involve renovations to the existing health care unit and to the community center.

6 Neighborhoods

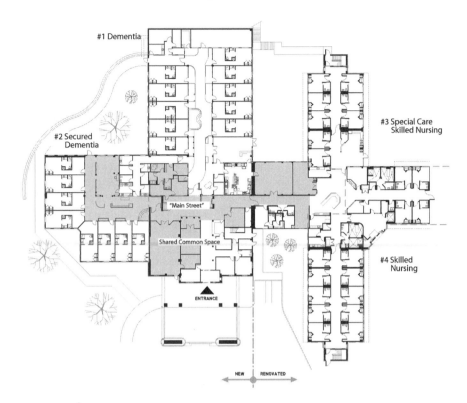

#1 Dementia

#2 Secured Dementia

"Main Street"

Shared Common Space

ENTRANCE

#3 Special Care Skilled Nursing

#4 Skilled Nursing

NEW   RENOVATED

FIG. 14-3 Lower-level floor plan indicates the relationship of the renovated skilled nursing wings to the new assisted living wings for dementia residents   *Courtesy of Calloway Johnson Moore & West, P.A.*

Designers' and Operators' Stated Objectives and Responses

OBJECTIVE: Accommodate two distinct populations of assisted living residents within a two-story building.

DESIGN INTENT: A unique building cross-section creates two types of apartment plans and a central two-story atrium. The ground level accommodates two special-care dementia units. The second floor provides apartments and support spaces for residents who are frail but without major cognitive impairment.

OBJECTIVE: Provide an environment that supports a high quality of life for cognitively impaired assisted living residents within a CCRC.

DESIGN INTENT: The village-like environment provides residents suffering from dementia with a familiar and interesting framework for their daily lives. Each resident has a home with a bedroom, a living room, garden space, and front door opening onto an interior street. The street leads to a village center with a chapel, beauty shop, town hall, fitness center, and general store.

OBJECTIVE: Provide an environment that supports a high quality of life for assisted living residents without significant cognitive impairment.

DESIGN INTENT: The second floor, which houses residents without significant dementia, is an environment that simulates the character of the independent living areas within the CCRC. Residents live in 640-square-foot apartments and have access to a living room/library and a dining room.

OBJECTIVE: Improve quality of life for residents of the existing health care center.

DESIGN INTENT: The existing health care center, now part skilled nursing and part medical/institutional assisted living, will be converted to skilled nursing care to meet the growing needs of the CCRC. The new village center will provide common space and a focal point for the entire health care population.

OBJECTIVE: Improve the circulation pattern between the existing community center and the health care center.

DESIGN INTENT: A new "skyway" provides a connection between the third floor of the addition and the commu-

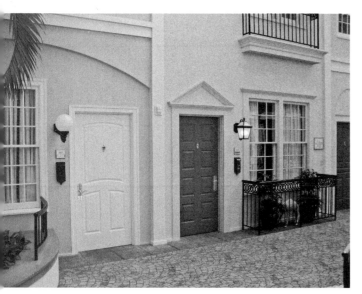

FIG. 14-4 One-of-a-kind details in millwork, lighting, design, and color identify dementia resident room entrances *Photograph by Jeffrey Anderzhon*

nity center of the CCRC, enabling residents and staff to walk between the community center and the health care center without passing through the private zones of the facility. The skyway also provides a direct route for CCRC residents to the new clinic on the third floor of the addition. The existing clinic in the community center will be demolished to provide space for an expanded arts studio and other amenities.

OBJECTIVE: Improve quality of food service and in turn improve health care.

DESIGN INTENT: The new addition contains a 600-square-foot pantry kitchen on each floor. These new pantries will serve the dining rooms for the new assisted living building as well as the renovated dining rooms for the existing skilled nursing population.

Field Observations: Meeting the Objectives

OBJECTIVE: Accommodate two distinct populations of assisted living residents within a two-story building.

FIELD OBSERVATIONS: Within the two-story structure, there are six households that provide support to assisted living and skilled nursing residents. The program mandated that the new construction as well as the remodeling of the existing nursing facility should feel like one building. Lines defining the old and new buildings were

eliminated; the finished product includes three adult care assisted living neighborhoods and three skilled nursing neighborhoods to meet six levels of care. This blurring of environmental design accommodates the facility's goal to induce less psychological resistance as residents are required to move into a more appropriate neighborhood to meet their evolving health care needs.

The Carlton neighborhood has 16 one-bedroom apartments with kitchens. It serves residents who need minimal assistance. The Gatsby, an Art Deco-themed "restaurant," provides meal service.

The Regency Square neighborhood has 12 apartments for those residents in early stages of Alzheimer's disease who do not require heavy medical care and are not at risk of elopement. Residents dine at Denali's, an Italian-themed "restaurant."

The Biltmore neighborhood is secured and has eight special-care units for those residents with behavioral problems, physical limitations, and end-stage dementia. Meals are served in an eat-in kitchen featuring a 1950s diner décor.

The Riviera neighborhood is also secured and has eight special-care units for residents at risk of elopement

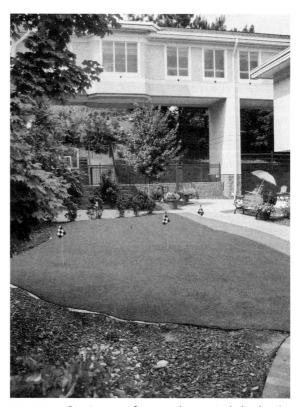

FIG. 14-5 Creative uses of courtyard spaces include a beach area complete with lounge chairs and beach umbrella, as well as a putting green *Photograph by Jeffrey Anderzhon*

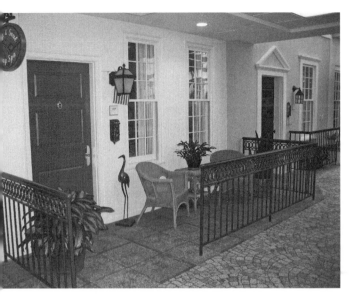

FIG. 14-6 Front porches at apartment entries are defined by metal railings that also serve as the code-required handrails for the corridor *Photograph by Jeffrey Anderzhon*

but with lighter medical needs than those in the Biltmore. A simulated outdoor café, Niko's Bistro, serves all meals.

The Holbrook is a remodeled neighborhood within the original health care structure, which has 30 intermediate-care beds grouped in three wings of 10 residents with intermediate physical and medical limitations. La Maison, a French-styled "restaurant," serves meals to residents.

The Olsen neighborhood, also remodeled within the original health care structure, has 20 skilled nursing beds, including respite care for residents with the most severe physical and medical limitations. Residents dine in "The Metro."

OBJECTIVE: Provide an environment that supports a high quality of life for cognitively impaired assisted living residents within a CCRC.

FIELD OBSERVATIONS: Regency Square incorporates a front-porch design that includes different materials and detailing within the porch and façades of each of the 10 apartments. The variation gives each residence its own character. Similar to a front porch on a small-town home, it provides a nice transition between private and public space and can accommodate two people sitting and conversing. A skylight over the common area adds natural lighting in a very unobtrusive manner.

This neighborhood, however, is located on a dead-end corridor, so "people watching" is limited to watching residents move from their apartments to another space in the neighborhood. The administration predetermined the furnishings and decoration, which makes it difficult for residents to personalize their own spaces.

The Riviera exploits the neighborhood theme, but enlarges it via the three-story atrium and imposes home fronts under an extensive skylit roof system. The atrium is clearly visible from the glass entrance elevator and windowed viewing areas on the second-floor hallways. Grand scale and visibility are the key environmental factors for this space. Questions regarding privacy, human scale, and the goal of minimum distractions for this special-needs population quickly come to mind.

The Biltmore is a smaller unit, closed off from the rest of the health center and without the distractions and commotion experienced in other neighborhoods. The residential atmosphere is very appealing, with an eat-in kitchen and living area in the same space. The only concern here is whether the residents would relate better to a Carolina mountain or beach-home motif than the kitchen's "1950s diner" theme.

OBJECTIVE: Provide an environment that supports a high quality of life for assisted living residents without significant cognitive impairment.

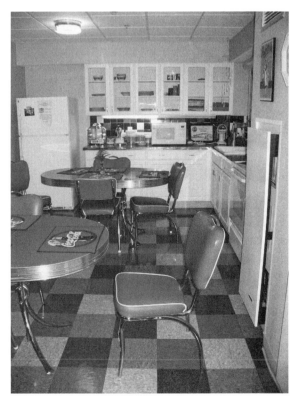

FIG. 14-7 Dementia residents in this neighborhood have all three meals at a 1950s diner. This space also serves as their activity kitchen *Photograph by Jeffrey Anderzhon*

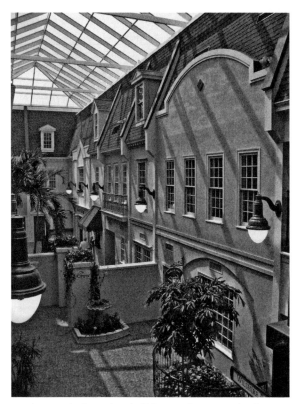

FIG. 14-8 An imposing skylight stretches across the dramatic three-story streetscape of the Riviera dementia neighborhood on the first level *Photograph by Jeffrey Anderzhon*

FIELD OBSERVATIONS: The second-floor Carlton neighborhood offers apartments the same size as the smallest units in the independent building and therefore may ease the transition for some residents as they move into the health care center.

Several apartments surround the large atrium overlooking the Riviera, whereas others overlook the smaller Regency Square atrium. They are all connected by largely unremarkable corridors, with little decoration or theme.

The Carlton lounge offers reading and coffee in an atmosphere described as a "grand hotel." Although some decorative motifs were successful, the small square footage and its location at the entry to the neighborhood do not promote neighborhood interaction.

OBJECTIVE: Improve quality of life for residents of the existing health care center.

FIELD OBSERVATIONS: The Olsen neighborhood within the original health center was refurbished with new carpet and paint. The large nurses' station was removed; its replacement is a work area disguised as a coffee bar.

The Holbrook neighborhood, again a part of the original health center, had a similar facelift, but it kept the more traditional nurses' station intact. The refurbished living room has a nice, comfortable family atmosphere with plenty of framed photographs of resident family members. An outdoor porch is also available to residents.

OBJECTIVE: Improve the circulation pattern between the existing community center and the health care center.

FIELD OBSERVATIONS: The fully enclosed, climate-controlled "bridge" offers good views into the garden spaces below and is an interesting feature. Due to site limitations, the skywalk begins at the community center and terminates at the top floor of the three-level health care center, where administrative offices, a conference room, a classroom, and community health clinic are located. The bridge is well executed in a transitional style, with appropriate seating areas along the way. The charm and appeal of this structure ease the transition from the community center to the health care center.

OBJECTIVE: Improve quality of food service and in turn improve health care.

FIELD OBSERVATIONS: Large pantry rooms secured for staff use only are carefully located and shared by two of the themed "restaurants." Food is prepared in a remote commercial kitchen; initially, batch cooking was done in units of 30, but has been reduced to units of 12. The food is delivered in insulated carts, one cold and one hot, to the pantry rooms.

Access into the health care center to deliver food occurs in two ways. Deliveries can come in through the rear of the Olsen and Holbrook nursing neighborhoods or by way of the connecting bridge from the community center, past the administrative offices and health clinic and down the signature glass elevator. The process is reversed at the end of mealtimes to accommodate the transfer of used materials, and can interfere with resident, staff, or visitor use of these prominent areas.

Meal service is at 8:00 a.m., noon, and 6:00 p.m. Residents may build their meals from a limited menu, and each course is served restaurant style. The serving staff is accommodating and polite, and staff supervisors take the time to stop by each table to inquire if the service is satisfactory. The dining experience is commendable and relaxing. Each of the dining rooms resembles a small, upscale restaurant and incorporates predining areas where residents can wait until meal service is ready to begin. Another outstanding feature is the flexibility of allowing capable residents to dine in any of the "restaurants" that they wish, breaking the monotony of daily routines and to some degree promoting social interaction. However, staff commented that "silverware and table settings on dining tables look pretty but are dangerous weapons when set out in a dementia unit."

Room service is available in the skilled neighborhoods only when the resident is incapable of using the dining room. In other areas, meals may be delivered for a period of three days when approved by the nursing staff to accommodate acute, short-term illnesses.

Nourishment carts with juices and snacks are provided twice daily and unfortunately take the place of a mini-pantry that residents could access on an as-desired basis. Coffee is served daily in the Olsen neighborhood coffee shop.

Field Observations: Themes and Hypotheses

Creating Community

Each neighborhood is uniquely identified by color, furnishings, and a decorative theme. Neighborhood streets on the first floor lead to Main Street where a chapel, beauty shop, town hall, fitness center, and general store are located. However, physically getting there is an issue. The second-floor neighborhoods are not physically a part of the Main Street theme, except that they have the view from above and are encouraged to use the unsecured first-floor area and its amenities. A number of vignettes appeared to have been staged designs or undertaken as photo opportunities rather than out of concern for resident comfort. Having said all of that, the general feeling is certainly not institutional. Decorative elements incorporated a variety of finishes, colors, and textures that are great eye candy.

Although the effort expended to create Main Street is evident, one may be tempted to wonder if the design envelope was pushed to the point of losing sight of the basic needs of older adults. In spite of the passion, dedication, and vision of the design team to eliminate everything that "smacks of nursing home," one could argue that it is not necessary to design an illusion that tries to avoid, at all costs, anything having to do with long-term care while providing long-term care services in a very conventional manner.

The evaluation team members have provided their insights regarding the design and construction of the health care center, but feel that further study of this unique environment and its impact on residents is warranted. Will it be a benchmark for 21st-century design? Will it stand with Woodside Place and Roseville Estate 20 years in the future as the design that challenged conventional care for older adults?

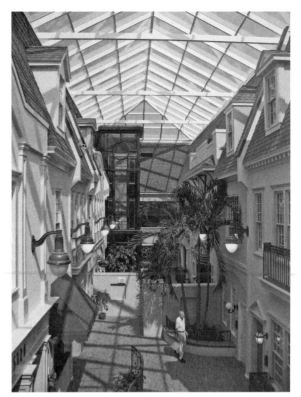

FIG. 14-9 A courtyard wall in the midst of the atrium space separates The Riviera dementia neighborhood from resident social functions such as the chapel, movie theater, and boutique *Photograph by Jeffrey Anderzhon*

Making a Home

The assisted living apartments in the Carlton neighborhood contain 641 square feet, the same amount of square footage as the smallest independent living unit elsewhere on this CCRC campus. A sitting area with kitchenette occupies the front portion of the apartment, with a bedroom and bathroom in the rear. The kitchenette, although providing additional cabinetry for personal storage and locked medications, seemed too large considering that three meals a day are served in the dining areas.

Throughout the remaining assisted living units, the square footage decreases to 456 square feet as a result of eliminating the kitchenette. Medication storage cabinets are located in each bedroom closet. The cabinet is low to the floor and difficult for staff to access. Staff reported that the "Riviera residents are very suspicious and even combative" when staff access their closets.

The closets are without light, compounding the difficulty in accessing medications, not to mention the correct clothes. In the Alzheimer's units, closet hardware was designed to provide a frontal view of clothing rather than the traditional side view.

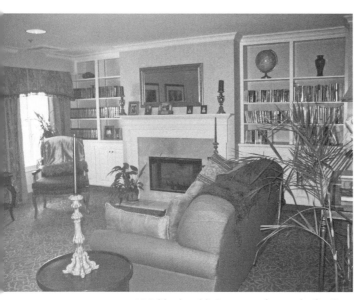

FIG. 14-10 Neighborhood living rooms feature the familiar fireplace and an abundance of decorative items that enhance the residential décor   *Photograph by Jeffrey Anderzhon*

Interior finishes were subject to change from room to room. Carpeting, cabinetry, and wall finishes varied, conceivably offering choice to residents as to which unit scheme they preferred. The result is an effective marketing tool, which one hopes makes the residents feel more at home, but comes at the expense of economy of scale and raises maintenance concerns for product repair and replacement.

Every unit has a private bathroom, the design of which seems to be adequate, and the sight line from the bathroom to the bedroom was achieved successfully. A curtain is used in lieu of a door. Some residents advised that the location of the towel bar directly above the grab bar was a poor location, as towels tended to hide the grab bar. An additional electrical outlet would have helped accommodate a variety of appliances.

Spa areas are available to those residents interested in bathing rather than showering. By appointment, residents can access their neighborhood spa or the Body and Soul Day Spa for bathing, hair care, and massage needs. Soft lighting, music, aromatherapy, plants, and interesting finishes there emulate day spas in upscale metropolitan cities.

Main Street is a remarkable creation of façades modeled after historic townhouses, accented by trees, benches, lampposts, and a fountain. (See Figure 13 in the color insert.) This space provides a truly striking common area for residents, although the actual impact on residents' well-being is uncertain. Real materials along with architectural detailing support the illusion of Main Street.

Although care has been taken to avoid synthetic materials and fake props, it is curious that the designers selected a carpet pattern that mimics a cobblestone street.

The enormous glass skylight, with its north-south orientation, allows direct sunlight to fall upon Main Street throughout the day. Depending upon the time of day and weather conditions, the direct light can cast some very confusing shadows or become bright enough to require sunglasses. The temperature was consistent and comfortable as a result of the radiant heating within the floor. It was reported that residents in the secured portion of Main Street (the Riviera) preferred to stay in their rooms because it "gets cold in the atrium."

The unsecured portion of Main Street is relatively small in comparison to the stunning glitz of the Riviera neighborhood. Destinations offered to residents include the Ritz Theater, an opulent and well-appointed space with comfortable seating and expensive electronic equipment and lighting. Although the movies only play on Wednesday nights, not much attention has been paid to wheelchair or walker storage in the theater.

The chapel façade was well conceived, but the interior configuration is small and limited to 12 persons. It therefore serves as a quiet meditation room rather than an area for interdenominational services, holiday services, or even the mourning of a passing resident.

Town Hall functions as a small community room. and Simone's, located on Wilshire Boulevard, displays well-dressed window mannequins and offers an upscale boutique atmosphere for imagined shopping trips.

The secured portion of Main Street is the most visible neighborhood in the facility, home to those residents with dementia and those at risk of elopement. It is the "wow" factor for visitors and family members, especially those entering via the glass elevator, and it creates a convincing illusion for marketing purposes. Residents, staff, and family enter the secured neighborhood through a small, decorative, wrought-iron door hidden within the walls that divide Main Street into its two components.

A charming walkway allows a short stroll past Niko's Bistro and eight resident rooms designed as full townhouse façades. Although the space is charming and attractive to prospective residents' families, the staff has mixed feelings about the neighborhood. Comments from interviews included "We shouldn't be parading people through Riviera or other places; it's upsetting." These "residents' homes should be private and quiet."

Although this portion of Main Street is competently executed with faithful replications and use of genuine materials, it does seem a bit overwhelming to be the common space for eight Alzheimer's residents at risk of elopement. There are small triumphs throughout the entire project, but unfortunately the secured portion of Main Street is not one of them.

Regional/Cultural Design

Although the detailing and finishes are indeed authentic, the concept can be construed as "fantasyland" in its approach. The Forest at Duke was conceived, detailed, and constructed as a high-end retirement community in the finest sense of gracious southern living. The residents are highly educated and affluent, and the campus reflects the expectations and tastes of its population through attractive and consistent design.

The addition, though highly publicized, is completely inconsistent with the existing campus and resident lifestyles. Regional and cultural influences have been eliminated in favor of metropolitan chic. Although the more sophisticated décor clearly avoids tried-and-true themes such as country cute or Williamsburg traditional, it may have little meaning to special-needs residents who spent their golden years in a campus lifestyle and surroundings that emulate the Old South.

Environmental Therapy

A therapeutic recreational program is provided by the health and wellness center on a daily basis. To develop activities that are meaningful, residents' interests and abilities are reviewed regularly. Individualized programs are created or modified to promote physical and mental health, as well as to meet cultural, social, and spiritual needs.

In this project, the built environment suggests that residents move within the complex to explore different neighborhoods and amenities. One of the original program goals was to provide residents with an "outing" experience. Although that experience is in part accomplished by the location and decorative detailing of destinations such as the Ritz Theater, the path to get to these spots is sometimes confusing. Although an expert in wayfinding was consulted and the design of interior signage was definitely modeled after the hospitality industry, the nomenclature and destinations that might have provided orientation seem intuitively unfamiliar. The names of the neighborhoods and dining rooms did not mean anything to the evaluation team and it was difficult to become acclimated without intensive study of the floor plan.

Outdoor Environment

Three outside areas are available for resident enjoyment: Central Park, the Wandering Garden, and Tranquility

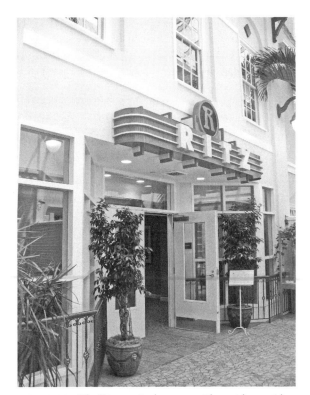

FIG. 14-11 The Ritz movie theater provides residents with occasional "outings" for socialization *Photograph by Jeffrey Anderzhon*

Terrace. In the tradition of North Carolina's outdoor amenities and interests, golf, basketball, and the beach can be found in Central Park. A putting green, small basketball court, and sandy beach complete with lounge chairs and sun umbrella await young and old alike. Unique sculptures, the soothing sounds of water, and an outstanding wall mural are positive contributions to the exterior environments.

However, it must be noted that each of these exterior spaces was carved out of the hillside, and as a result they are completely surrounded by building or retaining walls that eliminate any natural breeze and the natural sight line to the horizon. In one case, the courtyard is at least a story and a half below the surrounding grade and thus feels somewhat confining. This feeling is exacerbated by the presence of gunite concrete as the finishing material for the hillside, which is not compatible with the quality and finishes of the surrounding construction. In fact, it gave the odd feeling of being in a zoo with an observation platform high above.

Quality of Workplace and the Physical Plant

The unique design of the health center is appealing to employees because it is different from a normal work environment. It also seems that buying into the vision of management is necessary to be an effective employee.

The CNAs are responsible only for the direct care of residents. They are not involved in medication distribution, housekeeping, meal service, or any transportation to dining or activity programs. Due to the differing levels of resident care, CNAs cross-train in each of the neighborhoods and are rotated so that "no one has the hardest job all the time."

The size of the building—more than 60,000 square feet housing 92 residents—necessitates a lot of walking to reach all the residents. The Carlton was frequently mentioned in reference to this issue, not only for its size but also for the configuration of the apartments. To visit the 16 units, one has to navigate the corridors around all the skylights overlooking the Riviera neighborhood and Regency Square. "It's hard to walk those long distances," said one staff member.

Lighting levels in general are inadequate for the resident population. Carpet and wall colorations contributed to the absorption of artificial light. Because many of these units are located off a skylit area with

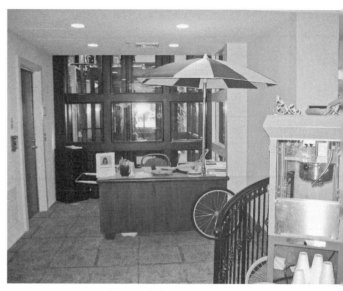

FIG. 14-13 Nursing desks and charting areas are disguised as pushcarts *Photograph by Jeffrey Anderzhon*

higher levels of illumination, temporary disorientation may be expected as residents with sensitive eyes traverse from very bright to very dark environments.

It appeared that several interior design choices revolve around visual effect rather than practicality or utility for the elderly. Product variation and color choices are used to personalize many of the resident neighborhoods. Part of the amazing amount of one-of-a-kind items included different mailboxes at every door, different door styles at every resident room entrance, different colors on every façade on Main Street, different light fixtures at the resident unit doors, and different decorative railings on the front porches. The efficiencies in price, quantity, and maintenance that would normally be expected are lost to the variations, and the commitment to senior-friendly products may have been sacrificed in the name of design as well. Reportedly, "it would be nice not to have the wrought iron for dementia wanderers and runners. It has contributed to skin tears."

Operator Perspectives

As stated by the operator, "This building is awesome, and makes it much, much easier for families to support moving Mom or Dad to assisted living or skilled nursing." For the operator, this reaction is welcome news and in reality must have credibility, as the addition continues to experience high occupancy levels.

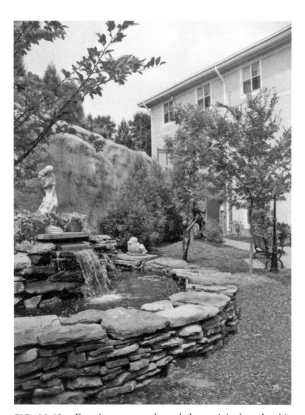

FIG. 14-12 Exterior courtyards are below original grade, this one features a retaining wall of faux stone *Photograph by Jeffrey Anderzhon*

General Project Information

PROJECT ADDRESS
The Forest at Duke
2701 Pickett Road
Durham, NC 27705

PROJECT DESIGN TEAM
Architect: Calloway Johnson Moore & West, P.A.
Associate Architect: Dishner Moore Architects
Interior Designer: Calloway Johnson Moore & West, P.A.
Charlotte Thompson & Associates
Landscape Architect: Charles E. Burkhead
Structural Engineer: Calloway Johnson Moore & West, P.A.
Mechanical Engineer: David Sims & Associates
Electrical Engineer: Calloway Johnson Moore & West, P.A.
Civil Engineer: The John R. McAdams Company

Dining Consultant: Culinary Design Service
Gerontologist: N/A
Management/Development: N/A
Contractor: Weaver Cooke Construction

PROJECT STATUS
Completion date: February 2005

OCCUPANCY LEVELS
At facility opening date: 72%
At date of evaluation: 99%

RESIDENT AGE (YRS)
At facility opening date: 88
At date of evaluation: 88

PROJECT AREAS

Project Element	Units, Beds, or Clients	Included in This Project New GSF	Renovated GSF	Total Gross Area	Total Served by Project
Senior living/assisted living/personal care (units)	16	22,657	—	22,657	—
Special care for persons with dementia	18	16,752	—	16,752	—
Skilled nursing care (beds) (includes dementia nursing beds)	50	—	30,640	30,640	50
Common social areas (people)	96	3,232	1,560	4,792	96
Kitchen (daily meals served)	273	1,200	—	1,200	645 (total CCRC)
Retail space (shops/restaurants, etc.) (Retail space in HealthCare addition will serve HealthCare population of 91. The community center has additional retail space.)	91	274	—	274	91
Fitness/rehabilitation/wellness (daily visits)	N/A				13
Pool(s) and related areas (users)	N/A				25
Other (please describe)	N/A				
Clinic/administrative space (average visits/day for clinic)	N/A	—	9,297	9,297	22

ASSISTED LIVING FACILITIES

Project Element	New Construction	
	No. Units	Typical Size
One-bedroom units	16	641 GSF
Total (all units)	16	10,256 GSF
Residents' social areas (lounges, dining, and recreation spaces):		975 GSF
Medical, health care, therapy, and activities spaces:		1,874 GSF
Administrative, public, and ancillary support services:		184 GSF
Service, maintenance, and mechanical areas:		1,809 GSF
Total gross area:		22,657 GSF
Total net usable area (per space program):		12,572 NSF
Overall gross/net factor (ratio of gross area/net usable area):		1.8

DEMENTIA-SPECIFIC ASSISTED LIVING

Project Element	New Construction	
	No. Units	Typical Size
One-bedroom units	18	456 GSF
Total (all units)	18	8,208 GSF
Residents' social areas (lounges, dining, and recreation spaces):		2,499 GSF
Medical, health care, therapy, and activities spaces:		1,913 GSF
Administrative, public, and ancillary support services:		0 GSF
Service, maintenance, and mechanical areas:		1,593 GSF
Total gross area:		16,752 GSF
Total net usable area (per space program):		11,103 NSF
Overall gross/net factor (ratio of gross area/net usable area):		1.51

SKILLED NURSING

Project Element	Renovations	
	No. Beds	Typical Room Size
Residents in one-bed/single rooms	50	250 GSF
Total	50	12,500 GSF
Social areas (lounges, dining, and recreation spaces):		3,804 GSF
Medical, health care, therapy, and activities spaces:		2,060 GSF
Administrative, public, and ancillary support services:		380 GSF
Service, maintenance, and mechanical areas:		400 GSF
Total gross area:		30,640 GSF
Total net usable area (per space program):		18,764 NSF
Overall gross/net factor (ratio of gross area/net usable area):		1.65

OTHER FACILITIES

Project Element	New Construction	
	No.	Size
Clinic	1	3,334 GSF
Connector to community center	1	2,068 GSF
Administrative, public, and ancillary support services		1,739 GSF
Service, maintenance, and mechanical areas		1,593 GSF
Total gross area		9,297 GSF
Total net usable area (per space program)		6,666 NSF
Overall gross/net factor (ratio of gross area/net usable area)		1.4

SITE AND PARKING

SITE LOCATION
Suburban

SITE SIZE
Acres: 1.34
Square feet: 58,650
Area of entire campus: 47 acres

PARKING

Type of Parking	For This Facility			For Other Facility			
	Residents	Staff	Visitors	Residents	Staff	Visitors	Totals
Open surface lot(s)	0	10	10	283*	40	27	370
Carports or garages	0	0	0	80	0	0	80
Totals	0	10	10	363	40	27	450

*Includes 80 spaces in cottage driveways

CONSTRUCTION COSTS

SOURCE OF COST DATA
Final construction cost as of February 2005

SOFT COSTS

Land cost or value:	N/A
All permit and other entitlement fees:	$32,485
Legal:	$15,082
Appraisals:	N/A
Marketing and preopening:	N/A
Other (miscellaneous):	$170,363
Total soft costs:	$1,908,098

BUILDING COSTS

New construction except FF&E, special finishes, floor and window coverings, HVAC, and electrical:	$6,032,689
Renovations except FF&E, special finishes, floor and window coverings, HVAC, and electrical:	$361,034
FF&E and small wares:	$1,043,861
Floor coverings:	$315,478
Window coverings:	Included in above
HVAC:	$1,189,357
Electrical:	$1,636,946
Medical equipment costs:	Included in FF&E
Total building costs:	$10,579,365

SITE COSTS

New on-site:	$1,640,778
New off-site:	N/A
Renovation on-site:	N/A
Renovation off-site:	N/A
Landscape:	$268,276
Special site features or amenities:	N/A
Total site costs:	$1,909,064

TOTAL PROJECT COSTS
(include all fees and costs, except financing)
Total project costs: $14,396,527

FINANCING SOURCES
Nontaxable bond offering

CARE COMPARISONS

AUTHOR'S NOTE: *The Forest at Duke does not participate in Medicare/Medicaid; thus, care comparison data is not available.*

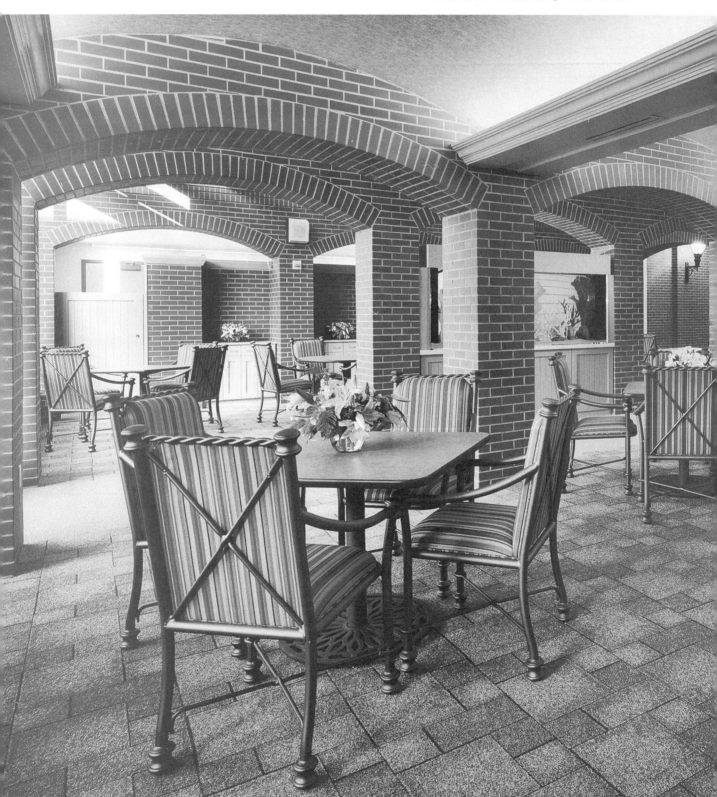

Chapter 15

The Village at Waveny Care Center

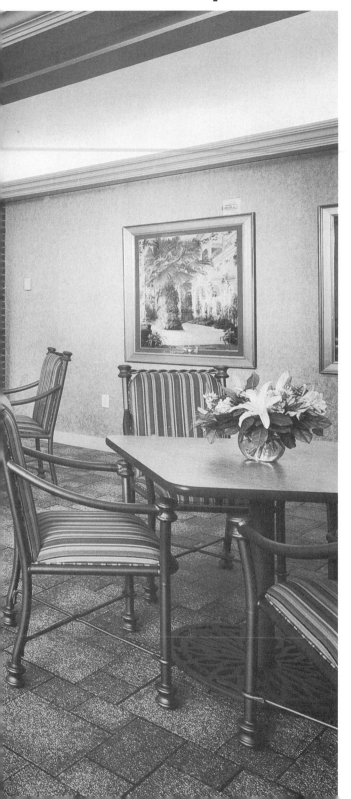

EVALUATION SITE: The Village at Waveny Care Center

COMMUNITY TYPE: Assisted Living for Dementia
- 52 assisted living apartments for those with dementia
- Adult day care for 40 clients

REGION: Northeast

ARCHITECT: Reese, Lower, Patrick & Scott, Ltd.

OWNER: Waveny Care Center Network, Inc.

DATA POINTS:

Resident Room:	300 gsf
Total Area:	1,242 gsf/assisted living resident
Total Area:	702 gsf/assisted living + adult day care resident
Total Project Area:	64,630 gsf
Project Cost:	$189.18/gsf
Total Project Cost:	$12,226,838
Investment/resident:	$235,131.50 (assisted living only)
Investment/resident:	$132,900.41 (assisted living + adult day care)
Staffing:	2.9 care hours/resident/day
Occupancy:	50% as of August 2004

FIRST OCCUPANCY: September 2001

DATE OF EVALUATION: August 2004

EVALUATION TEAM: Mitch Green, AIA, Jeffrey Anderzhon, AIA; James Mertz; Douglas Tweddale

FIG. 15-1 Residents can enjoy a meal in the community bistro and share in the activities of The Village's Main Street *Courtesy RLPS Architects/Larry Lefever Photography*

Introduction

New Canaan, Connecticut, is a community of tree-lined streets and colonial houses that conjure images of Norman Rockwell artwork. It is a community where residential iconography abounds within the built environment and where residential scale is a welcomed norm, particularly as compared to the urban environment of New York City just to the southwest. New Canaan provides respite from the societal issues that can accompany urban living and diminish quality of life for city dwellers.

It is fitting that The Village at Waveny Care Center began with direct inspiration from the New Canaan aesthetic and perhaps also from New Canaan's sense of community. It is also fitting that the word "village" is part of the community name. This assisted living facility was designed as the home for 52 Alzheimer's and memory-loss residents, who occupy four distinct households on two levels; there is also adult day care for up to 40 memory-loss clients. Located on a constricted site and designed as an addition to an existing 76-resident nursing facility of 1970s vintage, the exterior of the Village building conforms to the 1970s institutional aesthetic and appears consistent with previous construction.

Demonstrating the local concern for the quality of life of its neighbors, the care center was built entirely with contributions from the New Canaan community. The care center is among an elite, nationwide group of

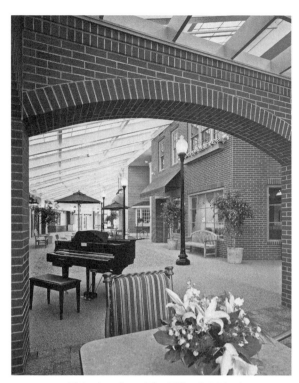

FIG. 15-3   This view down The Village's Main Street offers visual variety   *Courtesy RLPS Architects/Larry Lefever Photography*

long-term care facilities that have earned prestigious accreditation from the Joint Commission on Accreditation of Healthcare Organizations, whose standards exceed federal and state requirements. Annual expenditures are approximately $10 million and the organization's total assets exceed $10 million.

The Village shows its innovation and creativity immediately upon entry into the building. The adult day care and administrative support functions are located on the entry side of the addition, with a "Main Street" separating the two-story assisted living households from the adult day care. Visitor access to the households is controlled by this initial entry sequence and the fact that one must cross Main Street to get to the "front doors" of the households. Main Street becomes a destination in the same sense as its New Canaan downtown inspiration. When one is fully immersed in the environment of the Village, the design is as natural and as comfortable as fleece-lined gloves against a New England winter wind.

However brief a time that residents live at the Village, or however infrequent the visits of the adult day care clients, the built environment works to ease the disorientation and agitation of dementia. The environment

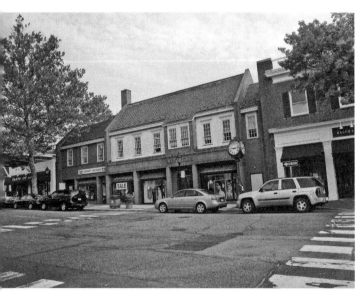

FIG. 15-2   This downtown New Canaan streetscape provided inspiration for the design of The Village   *Photograph by Jeffrey Anderzhon*

also indicates the quality of design necessary to diminish the anxiety of family members. When contrasted with other environments offering similar care, the Village provides a measuring stick against which to gauge creation of community.

Designers' and Operators' Stated Objectives and Responses

OBJECTIVE: Create a vibrant, active, and charming "downtown" or Main Street to promote a sense of freedom, wandering, and socializing.

DESIGN INTENT: Main Street, the heart of the project, recaptures many of the wonderful elements and qualities of the local town of New Canaan. (See Figure 14 in the color insert.) Many of Waveny's dementia residents still have fond, distant memories of the downtown area and growing up there, even though their short-term mem-

ory has diminished. A 28-foot-wide by 150-foot-long "street" is defined by opposing one- and two-story building façades. Each façade is a collection of smaller building fronts clad in brick or clapboard siding of varying colors. Storefront windows, flower boxes, awnings, and even a clock tower lend authenticity to the streetscape. Program spaces such as beauty/barber shop, ice cream parlor, bakery, general store, and dining piazza are placed among the façades, and many other programmed large-group activities take place on the street itself.

The floor is patterned carpet resembling cobblestone with gray-carpeted "sidewalks" along each façade. Cast street lights, potted trees, and street benches add finishing touches to the Main Street setting. To make a main street effective, it must be properly lit. Translucent skylight panels float above the street, providing soft filtered sunlight to illuminate the entire area and diminish glare.

OBJECTIVE: Create an environment that clearly defines active versus passive and public versus private settings.

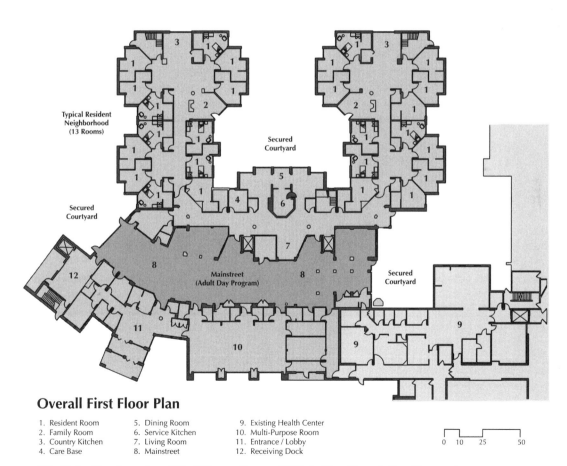

Overall First Floor Plan

1. Resident Room
2. Family Room
3. Country Kitchen
4. Care Base
5. Dining Room
6. Service Kitchen
7. Living Room
8. Mainstreet
9. Existing Health Center
10. Multi-Purpose Room
11. Entrance / Lobby
12. Receiving Dock

0 10 25 50

FIG. 15-4 First-floor plan of The Village   *Courtesy RLPS Architects/Larry Lefever Photograph*

DESIGN INTENT: A two-part design solution addresses this objective. Small, private households of 13 rooms each, with residential appointments and spaces such as open kitchens and small dining and family rooms, provide the passive or private settings. Resident rooms are all private and each is equipped with its own bath and shower to provide a more dignified bathing experience.

The second part of the solution, Main Street, captures much of the local charm of downtown New Canaan. Main Street becomes the active or public setting designed to stimulate the senses and provide "social electricity" for residents, while triggering distant memories of their younger years spent in New Canaan.

OBJECTIVE: Create a home-like environment in the residential wings.

DESIGN INTENT: The four 13-room households are organized to avoid any corridors. When moving through the facility, there is the sense of passing through furnished rooms similar to a home rather than traveling down an endless institutional corridor. Indirect lighting diffusing through ceiling coves creates a warm and inviting ambience throughout the building. An open country kitchen that doubles as a staff desk, along with a dining room setting and an adjacent family room with fireplace, further define "home." All rooms are private, but a large, built-in dresser and wardrobe cabinet that faces the corridor allows the residents' personalization of the area to be part of the overall experience when moving through a household.

OBJECTIVE: Provide an environment with seamless connections to the outdoors.

DESIGN INTENT: Strong connections to nature and the outdoors are essential to a successful program and residents' overall well-being. Each end of Main Street is a full glass wall with private, secured gardens beyond. Many of the interior street patterns, lights, and accessories carry through to the outside as if the street continued. Residents are free to wander into the gardens and explore independently. Exterior materials such as brick were also brought into the building to further emphasize the seamless inside/outside relationship.

OBJECTIVE: Provide a relaxed, comfortable, and familiar adult day care setting for local residents with memory loss.

DESIGN INTENT: Adult day care participants are dropped off, oriented, and prepared for the day's activities in a large, subdivided, multifunctional room or "home base" adjacent to the main lobby. Each of the subdivided areas

has a distinctly detailed entrance to Main Street, where the day care clients commingle and participate in the same daily activities and programs as the residents living at the facility. Adult day care residents can always return to their "home base" rooms for downtime. Main Street is designed to be large enough for the 52 on-site residents along with 40 adult day care clients.

Field Observations: Meeting the Objectives

OBJECTIVE: Create a vibrant, active, and charming "downtown" or Main Street to promote a sense of freedom, wandering, and socializing.

FIELD OBSERVATIONS: The design inspiration for Main Street is taken directly from Main Street in downtown New Canaan. The target market for the facility is residents from the immediate geographic area, particularly for the adult day care program. In this regard, Main Street's design provides a memory foundation for residents; as a secondary effect, it does the same for the staff and visiting public.

Residents and day care clients are free to roam the Main Street area during structured times. The residents can visually take in the variety of detail, peer into "shop" windows, or simply rest and absorb the activities going on around them. The attention to design detail and the execution of scale and proportion provide a new experience each time an individual enters the area. Natural but diffused light filters in through the insulated, translucent roof panels. An abundance of light-absorbing surfaces softens the area, and the mix of colors draws attention away from the faux sky.

OBJECTIVE: Create an environment that clearly defines active versus passive and public versus private settings.

FIELD OBSERVATIONS: The created environment does indeed distinguish between active and passive settings, but the line between public and private settings is somewhat less clearly defined. Main Street is the active and public area of the addition, and there is an attempt to replicate the community experience of residential space versus community space. The defined community space takes its visual foundation from the existing village vernacular and aims to create a "memory foundation" for both permanent residents and day care clients.

The entry sequence, at least from a first-time visitor perspective, is very controlled and does not impart an immediate understanding of the separation between public and private spaces. Entrance to private spaces or awareness of the separation comes only with a complete tour of the addition or a detailed review of the floor plan. The secured reception area controls access to the adult day care multipurpose room, the administrative office suite, or the Main Street area. However, to access any of the assisted living households, one must traverse the Main Street area and select one of two secured elevators or one of two secured entry doors into the assisted living residential area. Neither of the entry points to the assisted living areas is clearly apparent as a residential entry; in fact, each is intentionally hidden and difficult to access from the Main Street area.

The four households have two entry points that open into a elongated vestibule, which leads to the household living areas and the common household dining rooms. Because of a lack of a definitive delineation between spaces, it is easy to become confused and not know which area you have entered or left until you are completely inside.

The two households on the lower level have direct access to Main Street. The two upper-level households require the use of either of the two available elevators for Main Street access. Although the two-story solution is a result of the restricted site area, entry to these households detracts from the residential or home-like aesthetic. Furthermore, it confuses the public and private by introducing a purely public, mechanical device on the private side of the building. Residents and family members are not given "monumental" or visual access to stairs, which might have reduced the intrusion of the elevators. Exit stairways are secured with alarmed doors and are located at the corner of each household opposite the entrance.

OBJECTIVE: Create a home-like environment in the residential wings.

FIELD OBSERVATIONS: Each of the four households is identical in layout and finish, with only minor variations. On each of the two floors, the households are placed in a U shape, with the resident rooms located in the legs of the U and the entry and common dining areas within the connecting leg. Each household has a living area as well as a country kitchen complete with casual dining space.

The two resident room designs, though small, allow for the placement of a resident bed and occasional chair, which work to increase the residential nature of the rooms. The bed lies along an angled wall and blocks clear visual access to the window, the exterior, and the toilet in the resident toilet room. This is an intentional design

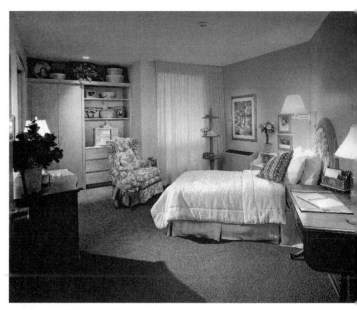

FIG. 15-5 Good visual cues to the bathroom and to the outdoors are typical for resident room design *Courtesy RLPS Architects/Larry Lefever Photography*

feature that provides visual cueing for the memory-impaired resident but restricts the furniture arrangement. The tradeoff between visual cueing and freedom for the resident to choose furniture location must be weighed on an individual basis.

Each resident room is single-occupancy with its own full bathroom, which does drive home the residential feel of the facility. However, an accordion-action door, chosen for convenience of operation and to maximize room area without interference of door swings, does not further the residential aesthetic in the resident room. Common bathing areas are not included in any of the households.

Kitchens and living rooms are classically residential; any home would be incomplete without them. The country kitchen and living and dining areas enhance the residential nature of the Village, although the appliance and cabinet finishes are contemporary and may be not be as warm as what residents are accustomed to. Nevertheless, the finishes are easy to maintain, and it is visually clear that the space is to be used as a kitchen and dining area.

The family room provides a location for the ubiquitous television and a few pieces of lounge furniture. The fireplace and a built-in wooden bench separate the circulation space from the family room, but both restrict the area for socialization and limit flexibility in furniture arrangement. This is further complicated, at least on the lower level, by an access door to the exterior courtyard, which necessitates circulation through the space to reach the door.

OBJECTIVE: Provide an environment with seamless connections to the outdoors.

FIELD OBSERVATIONS: At both the north and south ends of Main Street, the design opens to the exterior secured courtyard spaces by means of a full-height curtain wall of glass. The glass provides ready, visual access to the fenced and secured courtyards. Contemporary detailing of the walls, however, is somewhat incongruous with the established vernacular of the Main Street. In lieu of providing a seamless connection with the exterior, the incongruity actually punctuates the transition between Main Street and the exterior. This is further accentuated by the necessity of controlled access to the courtyards, for the clients' and residents' protection.

The two households on the lower level have physical connections to a secured courtyard that is well landscaped and inviting. Although it appears that residents can access the courtyard directly from the family room, the connecting doors are secured and alarmed, and do not appear readily accessible by residents without staff supervision.

Regarding the two upper-level households, convenient access to the exterior environment does not exist; access is available only via programming and staff intervention. Although relatively good visual connections to exterior spaces exist throughout the building, actual physical accessibility to the exterior spaces is not entirely seamless.

OBJECTIVE: Provide a relaxed, comfortable, and familiar adult day care setting for local residents with memory loss.

FIELD OBSERVATIONS: Clients can quickly enter the day care area through the main entry doors, allowing almost immediate engagement in activities. As the entry sequence is repeated by a client, sometimes on a daily basis, the setting becomes familiar and friendly. The space specifically designated for day care is large, with three clerestories providing excellent natural lighting. The room can be divided into three sections so that several activities can occur at once. Each section has views to the entry drive, has independent access to Main Street, and is equipped with counter space, storage, and toilets. Although the space is appropriately sized for the original intent of the program, shifting participants from Main Street to the day care space for lunch is challenging because frequent furniture rearrangements are required to do so. This daily shuffle

also tends to make the space seem more crowded than intended, according to staff.

Field Observations: Themes and Hypotheses

Creating Community

Residents and families both note that the familiarity of Main Street is a positive ingredient in the Village atmosphere and an important generator of community connection. Activities for residents within Main Street are varied and are both structured and unstructured. Spontaneity is encouraged, often manifesting itself in staff members' playing old standards on the piano while residents sing along. The country kitchens, dining rooms, and family rooms are the centers of social activity in each household, and effectively develop the sense of community within the Village.

Additionally, the emphasis on the New Canaan community aesthetic and the strong presence of New Canaan natives helps to build the community of the Village. The Village draws directly from the surrounding village—for both its building design and resident population—to strengthen the connections amongst residents and to encourage them to feel at home.

An unforeseen benefit of the Village has been the ability of up to 20 rehabilitation and skilled nursing residents to join Main Street activities. For these individuals, the Village is a definite benefit to their stay at Waveny, and their participation helps to integrate community activities for all residents at Waveny.

Making a Home

Main Street reminds residents of their past and instills the Village with a neighborhood feeling meant to make residents more at home. Residents are engaged by Main Street and are able to use the space on a scale that is neither overwhelming nor overpowering. Residential icons, including flower boxes, awnings, and divided-pane windows, make the space familiar and accessible. Residents can adapt Main Street to their own use, explore at their own pace, and enjoy the space as they see fit.

The single-occupancy rooms with private, full bathrooms do give residents their own "homes," but the setup of the rooms can make them difficult to personalize. The built-in shelving and adjacent built-in wardrobe, in combination with an angled wall and intrusive HVAC cabinet unit, provide few options for bed placement or room for the residents' own furniture.

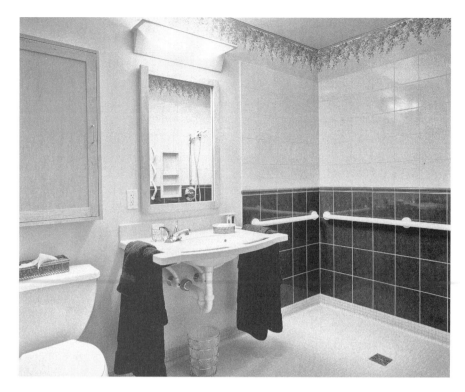

Personal choice is sacrificed to visual cueing of the bathroom and built-in structures.

The "European" showers in the bathrooms were chosen to allow full accessibility and staff assistance while maintaining a maximum amount of resident privacy. However, the European concept is certainly foreign to most individuals who are used to a single-family or even a congregate residential setting, and the unfamiliarity may dissolve feelings of being at home.

Regional/Cultural Design

The design of the Village, and Main Street in particular, is directly inspired by the surrounding community of New Canaan and is at home in its environment. No one the POE team interviewed found the environment artificial; the genuine materials and faithful detailing are clearly important to this area's clientele. Families and staff say references to local architecture make the environment much less institutional than might otherwise be the case. The Village becomes "different" from home, but "comforting" nonetheless.

Environmental Therapy

Families and staff report that resident quality of life is improved in the Village. In particular, staff have noticed a reduction in sundowning behavior because of resi-

dents' active schedule during the day. Staff and family members feel that Main Street activities engage residents more than a "house-based" environment would. Staff also note that new residents, who are often withdrawn and tentative upon move-in, become increasingly sociable as they find places and activities on Main Street with meaning to them.

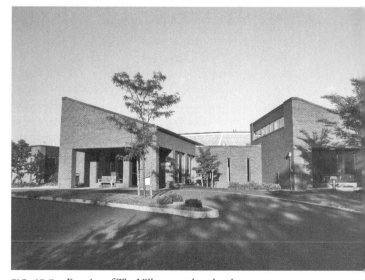

FIG. 15-7 Exterior of The Village matches the character of the existing buildings, but also imparts a dated feeling
Photograph by Jeffrey Anderzhon

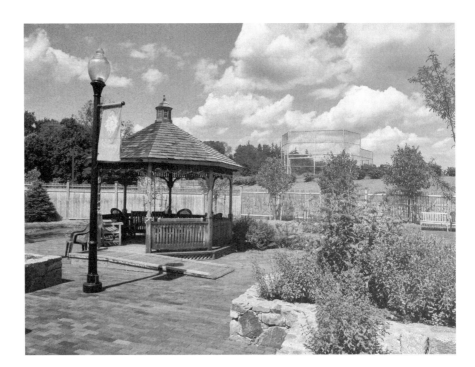

FIG. 15-8 The only shade in this secured courtyard at the end of Main Street is this gazebo, and the path to it is constructed of brick pavers, a troublesome walking surface for the elderly
Photograph by Jeffrey Anderzhon

Staff, families, and residents declare Waveny's Main Street a successful example of environmental therapy design. The lively atmosphere and accessibility of multiple activities bring residents and day participants together easily. The distinction between the semi-private resident wings and the public Main Street does not create barriers to community development.

Outdoor Environment

Several exterior spaces we intentionally created for use by residents of the Village. Two of these courtyards (the south and east) are a result of the floor-plan configuration and the addition's connection to the existing structure. They are well landscaped and visually inviting, complete with sculptures, walking paths, and seating areas. One can imagine that residents do desire to use these areas simply from having ready visual access. The courtyards are secured from elopement by attractive fencing as well as the building façades. The third courtyard (the north) is larger than the other two and is bounded by the building on the south side and security fencing on the remaining sides.

Although the evaluation team visited the site in the midst of lovely summer weather, it was somewhat disappointing to find that the courtyards seemed to be used only when other programming within the building had

become too mundane. Although this may be a result of successfully creating an intuitive interior-exterior space within Main Street, the courtyards would provide opportunities for residents to enjoy heightened sensory perceptions unobtainable on Main Street.

Within the courtyard most accessible to the north of Main Street, the selection of hard surface material (brick pavers) causes a minor inconvenience to those using walkers, as the pavers continue to settle. Additionally, there seems to be little designed opportunity for meaningful shaded areas provided by either structure or landscape material. In the end, these exterior spaces appear to be hindered by secondary design issues and, perhaps for those reasons, are only used on a secondary basis.

Quality of Workplace and the Physical Plant

Staff consider the Main Street environment to be both rewarding and challenging. Upper management notes that the multiple-venue, activity-focused daytime programming on the wide-open Main Street calls for front-line staff with outgoing personalities.

Management makes certain prospective staff watch Main Street in action and understand that Waveny gives recreational therapy equal priority to traditional caregiving. The result, according to both staff and manage-

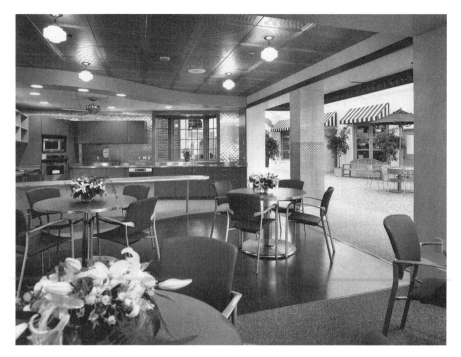

FIG. 15-9 The Main Street activity café provides a location where food-centered activities can be enjoyed by both residents and day care clients *Courtesy RLPS Architects/Larry Lefever Photography*

ment, is self-selection. Staff turnover at the Village is below regional norms and also below the turnover rate for Waveny's own rehabilitation and skilled nursing services. Frontline staff express appreciation for their work environment and seem to enjoy their daily time "on stage."

Operator Perspectives

The Waveny Care Center is extremely pleased with the Village project and shared some interesting perspectives on the first few years of operation.

Waveny feels that the Village project has been an essential part of its corporate strategy because it was the first step in broadening the scope of services offered to the community. The Village has enabled Waveny to offer assisted living, dementia care, respite stays, and day service, none of which was possible before. The success also prepared the organization for other initiatives, including the purchase of a nearby independent living community. A more complete spectrum of services gives the organization greater diversity of income and reduces the risks that fluctuations in any one market sector pose.

The Village has indeed enhanced Waveny's reputation, but licensing issues, the long-standing popularity of the nursing program, and the post-9/11

economic downturn have resulted in a different consumer profile than originally forecasted. Occupancy levels have been held down in part because Connecticut's licensing guidelines for assisted living facilities restrict how long a Village resident can remain in the assisted living environment. The high census in the nursing component, to which New Canaan residents have priority access, has discouraged some non-New Canaan consumers because Waveny cannot guarantee them a long-term care solution. The economic downturn, plus intense competition from other recently opened communities providing assisted living, have meant that residents are entering the Village frailer and with less cognitive ability than originally anticipated.

Feedback from families, residents, and staff suggest that the Village offers significant improvement in quality of life for both residents and day care participants, and Waveny's upper management strongly supports the Main Street concept. If they had the chance to do it again, Main Street would have been located with direct access to all parts of the campus, including rehabilitation and skilled nursing. Management does feel that a partial division of Main Street into smaller areas, to better control sound and other distractions, would be preferable and they intend to purchase the originally designed space dividers during the next budget cycle.

General Project Information

PROJECT ADDRESS
The Village at Waveny Care Center
3 Farm Road
New Canaan, CT 06840-6698

PROJECT DESIGN TEAM
Architect: Reese, Lower, Patrick & Scott, Ltd.
Interior Designer: Reese, Lower, Patrick & Scott, Ltd.
Landscape Architect: Stearns & Wheler, LLC
Structural Engineer: Parfitt/Ling
Mechanical Engineer: Consolidated Engineers
Electrical Engineer: Consolidated Engineers
Civil Engineer: Stearns & Wheler, LLC
Dining Consultant: Culinary Design Service, Inc.
Gerontologist: Dr. Lorraine Hiatt

Management/Development: New Life Management & Development, Inc.
Contractor: A.P. Construction Company

PROJECT STATUS
Completion date: August 2001

OCCUPANCY LEVELS
At facility opening date: 20%
At time of evaluation: 50%

RESIDENT AGE (YRS)
At facility opening: 84
At time of evaluation: 84

PROJECT AREAS

| | Included in This Project | | | | |
Project Element	Units, Beds, or Clients	New GSF	Renovated GSF	Total Gross Area	Total on Site or Served by Project
Special care for persons with dementia	52	58,500	6,130	64,630	119,130
Elder day care (clients)			Included in above		
Total net usable area (per space program):				41,109 NSF	
Overall gross/net factor (ratio of gross area/net usable area):				1.42	

DEMENTIA-SPECIFIC ASSISTED LIVING

Project Element	No. Units	Typical Size
Studio units	52	300 GSF
Total (all units)	52	300 GSF
Residents' social areas (lounges, dining, and recreation spaces):		14,010 GSF
Medical, health care, therapy, and activities spaces:		2,048 GSF
Administrative, public, and ancillary support services:		1,739 GSF
Service, maintenance, and mechanical areas:		6,754 GSF
Total gross area:		58,241 GSF

SITE AND PARKING

SITE LOCATION
Small town

SITE SIZE
Acres: 11.7
Square feet: 510,850

PARKING

| | For This Facility | | | |
Type of Parking	Residents	Staff	Visitors	Totals
Open surface lot(s)	N/A	104	23	141

CONSTRUCTION COSTS

SOURCE OF COST DATA
Final construction cost as of August 2001

SOFT COSTS
Land cost or value: Leased
All permit and other entitlement fees: $20,000
Legal and professional fees: $790,000
Appraisals: N/A
Marketing and preopening: $150,000 (first year)
Other fees: $340,000
Total soft costs: $1,300,000

BUILDING COSTS
New construction except FF&E, special finishes,
    floor and window coverings, HVAC, and
    electrical: $8,201,800
Renovations except FF&E, special finishes,
    floor and window coverings, HVAC, and
    electrical: Included in above
FF&E, and small wares, floor coverings,
    window coverings: $457,838

HVAC: $1,710,000
Electrical: $888,200
Medical equipment costs: N/A
Total building costs: $11,257,838

SITE COSTS

New on-site: $869,000
New off-site: N/A
Renovation on-site: N/A
Renovation off-site: N/A
Landscape: $100,000
Special site features or amenities: N/A
Total site costs: $969,000

TOTAL PROJECT COSTS
(include all fees and costs, except financing)
Total project costs: $12,226,838

FINANCING SOURCES
Nontaxable bonds with significant public contributions

"Old age is no place for sissies."

BETTE DAVIS, 1908–1989

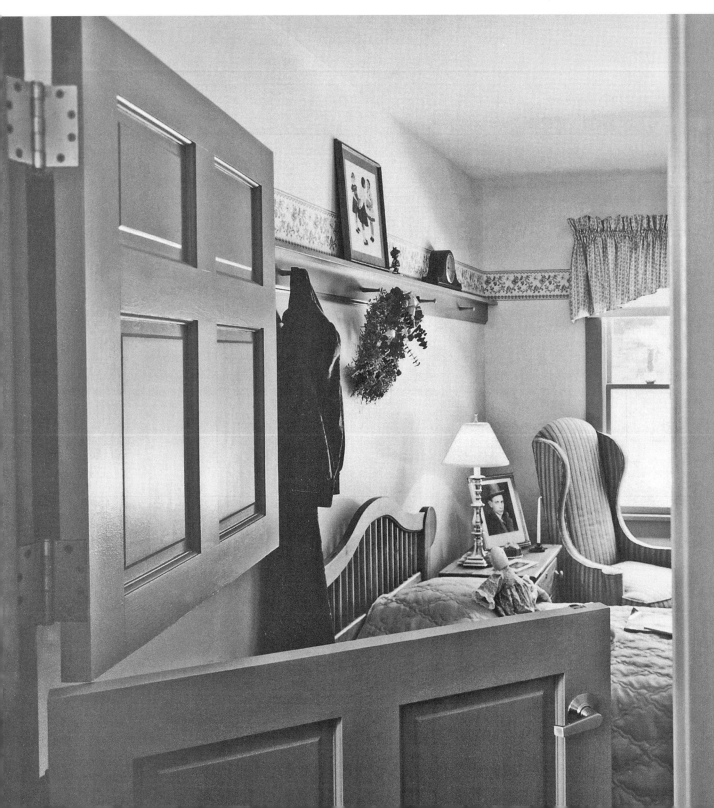

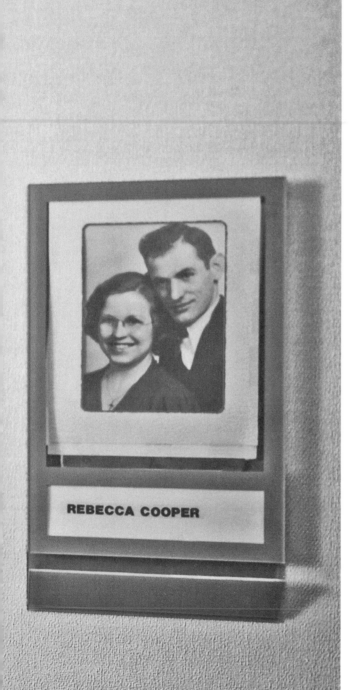

Chapter 16

Woodside Place of Oakmont

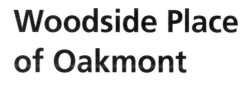

EVALUATION SITE: Woodside Place of Oakmont

COMMUNITY TYPE: Assisted Living for Dementia
* 36 assisted living residents in 30 apartments

REGION: Mid-Atlantic

ARCHITECT: Perkins Eastman Architects, P.C.

OWNER: Presbyterian SeniorCare

DATA POINTS: Resident Room: 224–440 gsf
Total Area: 649.94 gsf/resident
Total Area: 23,398 gsf
Project Cost: $106.85/gsf
Total Project Cost: $2,500,000
Investment/resident: $69,444.44
Staffing: 4.10 care hours/resident/day
Occupancy: 100% as of October 2005

FIRST OCCUPANCY: 1991

DATE OF EVALUATION: October 2005

EVALUATION TEAM: Mitch Green, AIA, Jeffrey Anderzhon, AIA; Ingrid Fraley, ASID; Leslie Moldow, AIA; Eleanor Alvarez; Thomas Hauer

FIG. 16-1 Rooms at Woodside Place are very residential in design and incorporate visual cues for residents with dementia
Photograph by Robert Ruschak

AUTHOR'S NOTE: *Environments for the aging can have a profound effect on resident family members in addition to the residents themselves. Lauren Whitehead, a teenager, intuitively knew this and eloquently expressed it during our site evaluation of Woodside Place.*

By Lauren Whitehead

One of the greatest things I think a child can experience is time with their grandparents. So many of my memories involve my grandparents; they are a major influence in my everyday life. I truly miss the time we spent together and realize the positive effect it had on me. My grandparents always wanted to spend time with my sister Michelle and me. When we were young and needed a babysitter, it meant going to Grandma's house. There was always something to do. Whether it was baking cookies or playing outside, Grandma was always playing with my sister and me. When we got older, every Saturday morning my father, sister, and I would go to Grandma and Pap's for lunch.

Just as my sister and I were getting older, so were my grandparents. The first change we noticed with age was that it was no longer safe to ride in the car if Pap was driving. His eyesight was getting worse, and his reaction time was slower. Soon our Saturday lunches were not as reliable as before. We were skeptical about the quality and freshness of their food. Then my father heard from my grandmother's beautician that she came in every other day because she could not remember her appointments and that the man who cut their grass said they would try to pay him more than once for the same job.

My Grandma had always managed the money, but that last year even simple math was troubling her. My father began to help them, but they accused him of stealing their money. We know now that paranoia is one of the symptoms of Alzheimer's disease. Another sign that a change was needed was when my Pap fell and needed 26 stitches in his head. My Grandma also fell, but it did not result in her needing medical care. Our Saturday visits became a dreaded occasion because my grandparents were no longer the same.

To relocate my grandparents from their home of over 50 years was a very hard process. After visiting other care facilities, my father decided Presbyterian Senior Care Center in Oakmont, Pennsylvania, was the right place for my grandparents. My grandparents first lived in the assisted living facility, which gave them freedom in a safe environment. They were able to walk around without obstacles like stairs. My grandparents also received better personal care, three healthy meals each day, and there were people to do the laundry and cleaning. If one of them fell, there were nurses to help them.

Because of their different levels of Alzheimer's, my grandparents were soon moved to different facilities within the Presbyterian Senior Care Center. My Grandma was moved to "The Gables" within "Westminster Place." My sister and I soon caught on as to what to say and what not to say to Grandma to not upset her because of her Alzheimer's disease. We took her for walks around the facility, and in the summertime we would go to the gazebo or courtyard. In the cold months, we went to a certain living room where my sister would play the piano and my Grandma was able to enjoy this too. We would usually visit in the morning because she was most pleasant then, but on a few of our evening trips, we found her participating in activities. On one visit, she was playing bingo, and the aides were quick to include my sister and me, which was very memorable. Sometimes we just spent time in her room because it had a home-like feel, and I think the facility worked hard to make the senior care home as home-like as possible. When we said goodbye, there was also a right and wrong way. We did it quickly and we always said we'd be back soon.

The room where my Pap stayed in Woodside Place was very accommodating and comfortable. There were activities for him to participate in, and the aides would try their best to convince him to participate. Holiday dinners were some of my favorite memories. My Grandma would be picked up, and we would all be able to be together at our own table, which was relatively secluded and made for a memorable holiday.

The social workers tried to get my grandparents to spend time together. It was arranged that they would have lunch together during the weekdays, and it worked out to be the perfect amount of time together. It was nice to know that for the period of time they got to spend with each other, it was special to them. I do not know what we could have done about my grandparents and their condition without the help of the people that work there. They were so helpful to my family throughout this big change in our life. I am so grateful that I had the opportunity to see that there is something for people who are in need of special care.

Introduction

Woodside Place of Oakmont sets the design standard for senior living environments specializing in Alzheimer's care. The designers of this remarkable facility created a paradigm of care based on a radically different philosophy: caring for dementia patients in a home-like environment will improve standards of care and overall quality of life for residents.

A diverse collective of experts, including geriatricians, nurse practitioners, researchers, architects, educators, licensing administrators, and department of aging officials, used their experience and vision to refine Woodside's philosophy and apply it to a physical layout that continues to have a positive impact on the lives of residents, their families, and caregivers.

In the late 1980s, residents with dementia were often mixed three or four to a room with the general skilled nursing population, in buildings reminiscent of hospitals rather than homes. Seeking an alternative to institutional care, in 1988 Charlie Pruitt visited a residential-based facility in Birmingham, England, called Woodside. That facility espoused home-like care of the elderly rather than an institutional layout that relied heavily on medication and physical restraints. The original Woodside's unconventional approach was not only a breath of fresh air, but also served as the impetus for Mr. Pruitt to envision a new model of care in the United States. The design of Pruitt's Woodside Place is still valid 14 years later. Numerous communities have replicated and benefited from Woodside Place's model, and new programs have expanded upon and refined its concepts.

The project is located on a campus operated by Presbyterian SeniorCare in Oakmont, a suburb of Pittsburgh, Pennsylvania. As you drive into the campus, the large, multistory 200-bed SNF and 120-bed personal care facility are the first and most prominent buildings to come into view. Woodside Place is past the parking lot and at the back of the site, in a wooded setting. The building itself is a large one-story home with a steep and significant roof. A clean white picket fence frames the front lawn, residential-style front porch, and entryway.

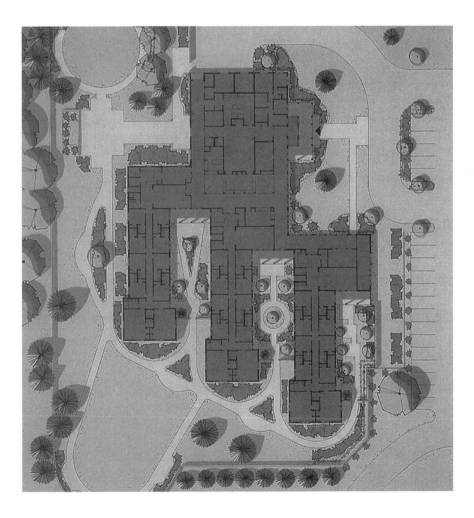

FIG. 16-2 The Woodside Place floor plan provides for three residential neighborhoods and a community gathering area that connects the neighborhoods *Courtesy of Perkins Eastman Architects, PC*

On the day of the evaluation, little pumpkins and other early autumn decorations placed around the porch enhanced the residential quality of the facility.

Woodside is described as "a non-profit, residential Alzheimer facility specially designed to provide a secure, flexible living environment for the care of 36 persons with dementia. Its purpose is to provide a quality of life which maximizes individual strengths and capabilities." The core care philosophy is tightly integrated with the environmental design. The optimum size for the facility is 36 residents, because that is the smallest number of units that can be maintained economically. It also makes sense, from a sociological perspective, to create three clusters of 12 residents to reduce the scale and further enhance the residential atmosphere. Additionally, the building runs an adult day care program for dementia-qualified attendees. The day care participants are integrated into the daily programs in the building and eat within the different homes.

As one of the first facilities to break away from the standard nursing home care model, Woodside's ground-breaking ideas, standard-bearing status, and award-winning design made it an essential part of this collection of post-occupancy evaluations.

Designers' and Operators' Stated Objectives and Responses

OBJECTIVE: Integrating the environment into the program—along with staffing, resident care, and activities—can affect residents' behavior positively by maintaining dignity and promoting self-care.

DESIGN INTENT: The design process involved an interdisciplinary approach to develop the building and program criteria. These criteria were developed from research, observation, and experience. For example, a deliberate goal is stated at the beginning of the design planning, such as "a discrete staff entrance limits resident agitation at shift changes." The implementation of the goal is reviewed after the fact to determine validity.

OBJECTIVE: There should be a common area that ties the three homes together and provides a place for activities attended by the entire group. These spaces should be designed in a manner that is both physically and programmatically flexible.

DESIGN INTENT: The common area includes a country kitchen, a great room where all residents can gather, a craft room, a sitting area, a library with fireplace, a TV room, and a music room. The rooms were designed in a

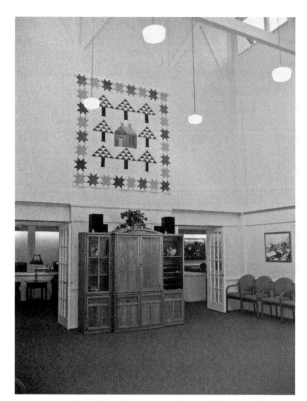

FIG. 16-3 The Great Room provides a well-lit space for large gatherings, but is acoustically challenged with its high ceilings   *Photograph by Jeffrey Anderzhon*

range of sizes to allow staff to alter group sizes to minimize agitation and unwanted stimulation. The range also permits adaptation of use over time as the need arises.

OBJECTIVE: Light and connection to the outdoors, visually and actually, are important to the well-being of residents.

DESIGN INTENT: Floor-to-ceiling windows line the interior corridors to give residents a view of the gardens and to bring in daylight. Corridors along the wandering path and doors off of each "house" provide access to secure gardens. Doors to the gardens are always unlocked, except after dark or when the temperature is below 40 degrees.

OBJECTIVE: Create opportunities for engaged wandering.

DESIGN INTENT: Threading through the major activity spaces in the common area is a wandering loop that residents frequently use. Along the course of their walk, the residents interact with staff and other residents involved in different activities. The path connects to the garden, then to wandering paths that lead into secure house courtyards and back into the building. (See Figure 15 in

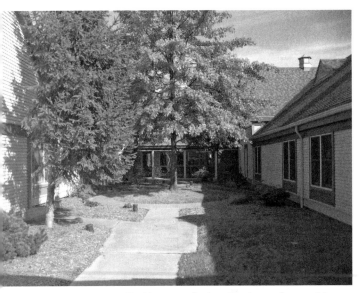

FIG. 16-4 Residents can freely enjoy the outdoors, with easy access to these secured areas from the neighborhoods and community spaces *Photograph by Jeffrey Anderzhon*

the color insert.) Baskets and shelves along the route provide various rummaging opportunities.

OBJECTIVE: Residents living in groups of 12 or less who develop familial relationships with their caregivers and fellow residents, who dine together, and who share an identifiable home will adapt well to their new environment.

DESIGN INTENT: The building is designed as three houses with 12 residents each. The homes are comprised of eight private rooms and two double bedrooms, each room with its own sink and toilet. Just as in any house, there is a residential-style kitchen and a living/dining area, in this case overlooking a gated courtyard. There is also a shared shower room and small laundry. The residential focus on care allows residents to identify with staff on a more individual basis and permits staff to monitor residents while interacting in normal daily activities.

OBJECTIVE: The homes should be laid out in the typical residential fashion, from the most public, to semi-public, to the most private spaces.

DESIGN INTENT: After passing through the entry of the home from the common area, each home's shared activity spaces are clustered together. On the other side of the kitchen/dining area, there is a corridor leading to the 10 resident rooms. The layout is meant to draw the rooms together around common spaces, as in a typical home.

OBJECTIVE: Cueing on a variety of levels helps residents orient themselves to their environment.

DESIGN INTENT: Black-and-white photographs of old Pittsburgh hang in the common area as a memory touchstone. Each home carries a distinct symbol or theme (e.g., trees, houses, stars) and has an associated color to assist wayfinding. These themes appear in the artwork, quilts, décor, and even the color of the staff's clothing. Along the resident corridors, photograph boards at unit entries display pictures with a unique meaning to residents, helping each resident to identify his or her own room. Each room has a Dutch door that allows the top half to open independently of the bottom. The resident rooms have unique décor and a high shelf for personalization that hangs in a visible, cueing position.

OBJECTIVE: Create an environment that honors staff and encourages retention.

DESIGN INTENT: The staff members have a personal stake in making residents' lives more meaningful. Each staff member is given three weeks of intensive training on working with people affected by dementia. The staff is

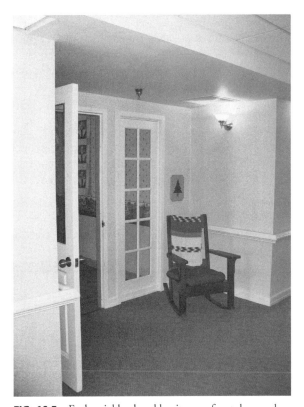

FIG. 16-5 Each neighborhood has its own front door and identification enhanced by graphics and furniture styles *Photograph by Jeffrey Anderzhon*

cross-trained to provide care, serve meals, and engage in activities, many spontaneously generated by the residents themselves.

Field Observations: Meeting the Objectives

OBJECTIVE: Integrating the environment into the program—along with staffing, resident care, and activities—can affect residents' behavior positively by maintaining dignity and promoting self-care.

FIELD OBSERVATIONS: A three-year study performed by the University of Pittsburgh's Graduate School of Public Health and School of Medicine and Carnegie Mellon University's Department of Architecture concluded that the population at Woodside Place had a slower decline in functional capacity, for 66% of the original group, than for comparable nursing home residents with Alzheimer's disease. Also, in their activities of daily living (ADLs), the Woodside residents are able to be more independent.

Some of these results likely come from the smaller scale of the facility and the home model of caregiving. The attention paid to detail in the design deserves credit as well for enhancing the well-being of residents. For example, within the resident room closets there is open basket shelving so residents can see their clothes and, with some help, dress themselves; additionally, the residential kitchens allow residents to assist with serving their own meals.

OBJECTIVE: There should be a common area that ties the three homes together and provides a place for activities attended by the entire group. These spaces should be designed in a manner that is both physically and programmatically flexible.

FIELD OBSERVATIONS: The common areas are generally well used. However, we did find that many of the spaces are not necessarily utilized in the way the initial design intended. For example, the great room, originally used for dining, has been adapted to a new use because of the poor acoustics of the high ceilings and lack of direct views to the exterior. It now serves as a multipurpose room for social events.

Additionally, the commercial kitchen is not used, because it is less expensive to produce meals in the main campus kitchen and drive the prepared food to the building. The food is transferred into steam carts, rolled into the houses, and plated home-style. The commercial kitchen was initially installed in an attempt to prove that

a stand-alone care facility for 36 could be economically viable. This proved to be the case upon opening, but the administration subsequently determined that the monetary savings in dietary care would be better allocated to other resident-care initiatives.

The range in room size allows some flexibility in redesigning spaces and adapting rooms for new uses; for example, the conference room is now used for exercise and music activities. However, the radiant flooring in portions of the building will make some renovation more difficult.

OBJECTIVE: Light and connection to the outdoors, visually and actually, are important to the well-being of residents.

FIELD OBSERVATIONS: At the time of design, there was a common conception that windows were bad for residents with Alzheimer's, because in the evening the sight of their own reflections makes them nervous. The previous paradigm also held that a view of the outside increased residents' agitation, because they cannot go out. Woodside Place's design partly debunks these notions. Walls of windows let in light and connect residents with the outside. The staff pull the window shades in the evenings and Woodside residents can generally go into the garden whenever they want, thus preventing this sort of agitation.

The greater lesson learned from the execution of this objective is the garden's ability to generate a sense of calm and purposeful activities for residents. Even in less-than-ideal weather, the outdoor garden sees plenty of use and improves residents' behavior. The staff and families report that the risks the residents face when venturing independently into the garden are worth the positive experience that the sunshine and exercise provide. The garden is a lovely space for families to visit and for residents to interact with children who visit from a local day care facility.

OBJECTIVE: Create opportunities for engaged wandering.

FIELD OBSERVATIONS: Rummaging boxes, Velcro-covered wall quilts, and a full circuit of wandering paths with open activity spaces along the way effectively engage residents. Doors were removed from the cabinets in the common spaces to reveal the contents of the shelves and allow increased rummaging. Adding a handrail on at least one side of the major walking path would assist residents.

OBJECTIVE: Residents living in groups of 12 or less who develop familial relationships with their care-

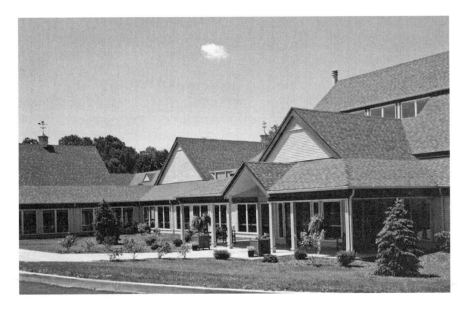

FIG. 16-6 The main entry is on a residential scale and belies the building's size with a welcoming porch
Photograph by Robert Ruschak

givers and fellow residents, who dine together, and who share an identifiable home will adapt well to their new environment.

FIELD OBSERVATIONS: The scale of the space has a definite residential quality and allows for a meaningful exchange among residents and staff. The heart of the house is the kitchen, which includes a sink, refrigerator, high-temperature dishwasher, range, and coffee pots. The space is open to residents at any time to serve themselves snacks when they are hungry. They have not had a problem with residents hurting themselves.

Just as in any home, dishes are stored in each house, washed there, and returned to the cabinets. The food arrives in a steam cart and is plated by staff and occasionally by residents who also help to serve the plates in the dining room at mealtime.

Care stations are also built into the kitchen area. While we were there, residents were assisting staff to fold towels at the care station, and later helped to serve dessert. In the low counter/desk, there is a separate drawer for files that can be locked for charting. This area maintains a residential feeling while meeting the needs of both staff and residents. The dining room has space for each resident, some adult day care participants, and family members. It is used as an additional activity space.

OBJECTIVE: The homes should be laid out in the typical residential fashion, from the most public, to semi-public, to the most private spaces.

FIELD OBSERVATIONS: Although it makes sense to place the shared areas near the entry to the common areas, the long corridor of resident rooms that results makes it more difficult for the staff to casually view residents outside of the shared areas. In future designs, shorter hallways and more centrally located shared spaces might be beneficial.

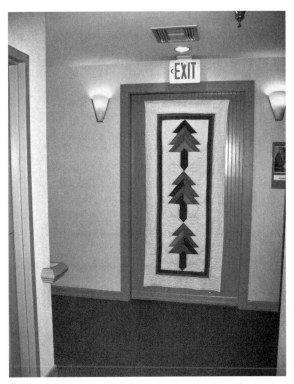

FIG. 16-7 A unique artistic quilt is hung at the end of each neighborhood corridor to help identify an individual's home
Photograph by Jeffrey Anderzhon

OBJECTIVE: Cueing on a variety of levels helps residents orient themselves to their environment.

FIELD OBSERVATIONS: Generally it is better to have people, rather than the physical environment, provide orienting clues but if one does rely on environmental clues, personalized items such as photos are more likely to be recognized than colors or other abstract symbols. Staff wished the colors of the homes were more distinctive because the blue and green have caused confusion.

Dutch doors allow residents to preview a resident room before entering to determine if it belongs to them. Closing the bottom half of the doors discourages residents from rummaging through rooms and possessions that do not belong to them. Unfortunately, staff and residents use this feature inconsistently. There are pictures by each door that serve to remind residents of their rooms; these were a precursor to memory boxes, now a very popular and common feature in many dementia-care facilities.

OBJECTIVE: Create an environment that honors staff and encourages retention.

FIELD OBSERVATIONS: There is reportedly a higher level of staff satisfaction in this facility than within a conventional nursing facility, which is most likely due to the ability of resident-oriented care to encourage personal relationships between residents and staff. The turnover rate is 8%, which is dramatically lower than the national average and lower than the rest of the campus.

Field Observations: Themes and Hypotheses

Creating Community

The country kitchen, great room where all residents can gather, the craft room, sitting area, library with fireplace, TV room, and music room are all wonderful group areas within the central common area. There is no separate living-room space in the households, although a couch has been included in each dining room, and some staff mentioned that a TV area in each house would be nice to have so the residents could enjoy it together. Currently, some residents watch TV in their rooms or in the TV room off the common area between the three houses.

Shared outdoor spaces for walking, gardening, and group activities draw residents into the gardens to interact with one another. The wandering path allows residents to interact with staff and other residents who are involved in different activities. The staff report that the outdoor spaces are not only popular, but have had a positive impact on resident well-being. Increasing well-

FIG. 16-8 Residents can bring furniture and memorabilia to their rooms to make the rooms their homes
Photograph by Robert Ruschak

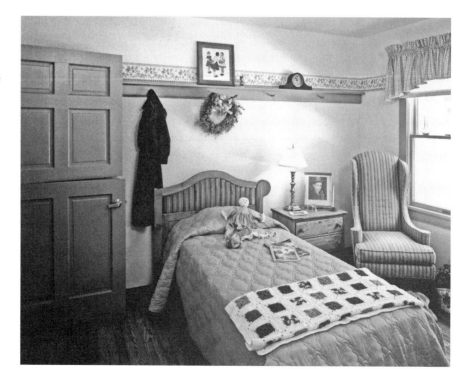

being and social interaction should help to further enhance the community spirit of Woodside.

Making a Home

Ideally, a facility comprised entirely of private resident rooms would overcome the difficulties of managing shared rooms among strangers and would create a more home-like experience for the residents of Woodside. Despite this obstacle, there are some very home-like and comforting features at Woodside. Residents can generally use the outdoor spaces as they please, and are able to participate in activities in the common kitchen area, such as folding napkins, preparing snacks, and helping staff with everyday tasks. Staying active and involved in this way will help to normalize the experience and to make living at Woodside more like being at home.

The photo boards along the corridors at each unit help to signify that resident's room as his or her own. Features such as photo boards or memory boxes are wonderful for personalizing the space and letting residents exert some control over their surroundings. Hanging pictures as in one's home will, it is hoped, make residents feel more comfortable.

Although toileting and bathroom design may not win architectural awards, proper design of toileting and bathing spaces has a huge impact on the dignity of residents' lives and the ease of care for the staff. More than 60 to 70% of the residents are incontinent, but the staff are able to manage them to the point of continence, a strategy that is greatly supported by the availability of 40 toilets. Despite the number of toilets for residents, initially there was not a designated visitor toilet. Woodside has since dedicated one of the resident common toilets for visitors.

Staff was very articulate about their desires for improvements in future toilet room designs. For example, the staff wish that showers had been included in resident bathrooms. They were not originally installed because there was concern that residents would clog the drains, create a mess, and possibly hurt themselves. However, it would be less frightening for residents to take a shower if they could do it in their rooms rather than down the hall. It would also give residents who have soiled themselves more dignity to wash in the privacy of their rooms.

As mentioned before, there is no TV room for residents to enjoy together within each home. A central living room might help residents feel more at home. Always watching TV in their rooms must be a little confining at times—not to mention that sharing a room with another resident would require them to compromise—and surely

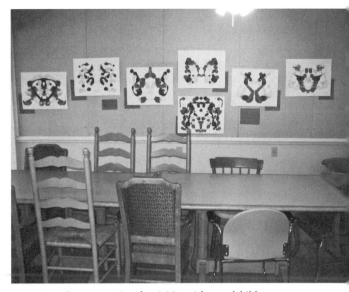

FIG. 16-9 Intergenerational activities with grandchildren and great-grandchildren abound in the community center
Photograph by Jeffrey Anderzhon

there are times when residents do not want to walk out to the shared living room.

Environmental Therapy

The program integrates the concept of flexibility and adaptability both with residents on a moment-by-moment basis and with the environment, which has been modified a few times since the facility opened. The space has proven to be adaptable to the evolving programming. For example, the original music room was too small for the popularity of the program, so it is now dedicated to the adult day care program and is sometimes used as a conference room. Exposing contents of the shelves, rummaging stations, and Velcro wall quilts are all strategic elements of the environmental therapy and work successfully to satisfy increased rummaging.

Several renovations have taken place in an open meeting room with a large table. Currently there are no walls, and residents are confused about how to enter the room. Walls are being added so that families will have privacy and a place to meet outside of the residents' rooms. The door to the beauty shop was originally located around the corner from the main circulation path, but was moved to be more visible and easier to find from the path, thus reducing resident anxiety.

The prominent main entry, which is typically a positive feature in most buildings, causes a number of difficulties for a resident population with dementia. Family members report difficulty leaving the facility because the residents can watch them walk out the door but cannot accompany them. Residents see the exit and often follow people undetected. Views of the adjacent parking lot also agitate residents, because they cannot leave. In hindsight, it might have been better to design a more indirect entryway without any views to the parking lot.

Outdoor Space

On all accounts, the most significant space for resident well-being has been the outdoor space used for walking, gardening, and group activities. Each house has its own garden directly accessible from the home's dining room. Walkways made up of different shapes and patterns, as well as varied plantings, were initially used to aid cueing and distinguish the character of each garden.

The staff report that residents do not identify the geometry of the walkways. Initially, each home had its own gate and fence, but the gates were removed to allow residents to walk throughout the entire complex freely. Although the idea of the identifiable house gardens did not pan out, the overall space is used throughout the year.

The planting was initially more complex and extensive, but over time portions were removed to create a lawn or were replaced with lower-maintenance plants. Costs for maintenance were cut in half, allowing more money to go to the care of residents. There is a raised planter box, which is frequently used by residents, and an awning over the gathering area protects the residents from the intensity of the sun.

Some wish-list items for Woodside Place include security cameras, the addition of which would allow residents to be outside on their own longer. Currently, the staff check residents about every 45 minutes. They also expressed a desire for a putting green or other activity for the men. There was a car for washing and waxing, but it proved not to be of interest to the residents and so was removed.

Quality of Workplace and the Physical Plant

There is limited staff space. A staff bathroom was added and is helpful, but it is far from the main work areas and inconvenient to reach. A staff toilet within each house would be ideal, and the staff would also appreciate a break room and their own outdoor space in locations that prevent residents' physical or visual access. The job is a stressful one and sometimes staff members "need a place to scream." Staff facilities such as the laundry areas and soiled and clean utility spaces are inadequate. There is no medication room allocated to each home.

Staffing levels appear to be generous for the population served, with direct-care daytime staffing ratios of one to five from 9:00 a.m. to 6:00 p.m., and one to nine in the evenings. The unit has one nurse per shift. The dementia unit shares several administrative staff members with the rest of the main campus, including the administrator, social worker, art therapist, and two half-time activity directors.

The building was designed with wood siding rather than a more permanent material such as brick. Although this may have been a conscious choice to highlight the residential quality of the building, in contrast to the larger brick SNF on campus, the care needed to maintain the wood siding is excessive. Light levels were initially low, which agitated residents who had a hard time seeing and were afraid of falling. Although fixtures and more efficient, better-quality bulbs have been added since the opening, some areas still lack sufficient lighting. Also, stops have been added to the windows because residents were climbing out into the garden at night.

The building has a radiant-slab heating system that was installed to allow residents to walk comfortably without their shoes on and to improve stability. Although generally comfortable, the system was not zoned, so the level of available heat is inconsistent throughout the building. Residents tend to walk around in shoes.

The staff also wish that private showers had been included in the building design. Perhaps this design would not have made their jobs easier, but it would improve the bathing experience for residents. Since opening, a high shelf has been added over the toilet for shampoos and liquids that are not good for residents to handle. A cabinet integrated into the design would have been a better choice.

Operator Perspectives

Money for the project was raised primarily through donations. The foundation community was very excited about the project, and when it came to setting a budget, they told the development advisory committee to "do the right thing" and not cut corners. As noted, maintenance and staff have suggested a few building construction improvements in retrospect.

The facility originally had a housekeeper, a dietician, a cook, and a maintenance staff dedicated to its needs alone, but now shares their services under the umbrella of the campus system. Dedicating a staff to the houses was initially done to test the model as a standalone facility so that, if successful, it could be modeled by others. This is no longer necessary, and the consolidation saves resources and money for the campus.

Psychotropic medications exclusive of depressants are used minimally to control behavior. The program and the environment play a large part in minimizing the use of medication, and the physicians support the philosophy of Woodside Place and appreciate the change in their patients.

The philosophy seems to incorporate the idea that the activities are resident focused and generated. If residents want to go outside, they can and they do. Family members are educated to understand the risks and benefits of such a policy across a wide spectrum of activities. The resident's behavior improves, but the risk of personal injury increases. Weighing of risks and benefits is a sensitive issue that tends to come down on the side of resident choice at Woodside.

Although most facilities of the 21st century strive to embrace culture change, Woodside Place has implemented this philosophy of care for the past 20 years. The small scale of the home, and the dedication of staff to each house has had a significantly positive impact on residents' lives. The success and reputation of Woodside relies on tight integration of the philosophical program, operations, and the environment. Woodside Place has earned its standing as the original role model for individualized and personalized dementia care. Many new programs have emerged that have expanded and refined the concepts that were launched here.

General Project Information

PROJECT ADDRESS
Woodside Place
1215 Hulton Road
Oakmont, PA 15139

PROJECT STATUS
Completion date: July 1991

OCCUPANCY LEVELS
At facility opening: 100%
At time of evaluation: 100%

RESIDENT AGE (YRS)
At facility opening: 83
At time of evaluation: 85

PROJECT DESIGN TEAM
Architect: Perkins Eastman Architects, P.C.
Interior Designer: Perkins Eastman Architects, P.C.
Landscape Architect: N/A
Structural Engineer: Astorino
Mechanical Engineer: Astorino
Electrical Engineer: Astorino
Civil Engineer: Gateway Engineers, Inc.
Dining Consultant: N/A
Gerontologist: N/A
Management/Development:
Contractor: Mistick Construction

PROJECT AREAS

DEMENTIA-SPECIFIC ASSISTED LIVING

Project Element	New Construction	
	No. Units	Typical Size
Private apartments	24	224 GSF
Shared-occupancy apartments	6	440 GSF
Total (all units)	30	9,466 GSF
Residents' social areas (lounges, dining, and recreation spaces):		2,262 GSF
Medical, health care, therapy, and activities spaces:		2,218 GSF
Administrative, public, and ancillary support services:		6,940 GSF
Service, maintenance, and mechanical areas:		2,512 GSF
Total gross area:		23,398 GSF
Total net usable area (per space program):		20,886 NSF
Overall gross/net factor (ratio of gross area/net usable area):		1.12

SITE AND PARKING

SITE LOCATION
Suburban

SITE SIZE
Acres: 3
Square feet: 130,680

PARKING

Type of Parking	For This Facility			
	Residents	Staff	Visitors	Totals
Open surface lot(s)	N/A	9	19	28

CONSTRUCTION COSTS

SOURCE OF COST DATA
Final construction cost as of July 1, 1991

SOFT COSTS
Land cost or value:	N/A
All permit and other entitlement fees:	N/A
Legal and professional fees:	N/A
Appraisals:	N/A
Marketing and preopening:	N/A
Other fees:	N/A
Total soft costs:	N/A

BUILDING COSTS
New construction except FF&E, special finishes,
   floor and window coverings, HVAC,
   and electrical: $2,500,000
Renovations except FF&E, special finishes,
   floor and window coverings, HVAC,
   and electrical: N/A

FF&E and small wares:	Included in above
Floor coverings:	Included in above
Window coverings:	Included in above
HVAC:	Included in above
Electrical:	Included in above
Medical equipment costs:	Included in above
Total building costs:	$2,500,000

SITE COSTS
Site costs are included in building costs

TOTAL PROJECT COSTS
Total project costs: $2,500,000

FINANCING SOURCES
$2 million funded with grants from 20 local and national
   foundations; remainder financed through Pennsylvania
   Finance Agency

Part V

Nursing Care

"If the rich could hire people to die for them, the poor could make a wonderful living."

JEWISH PROVERB

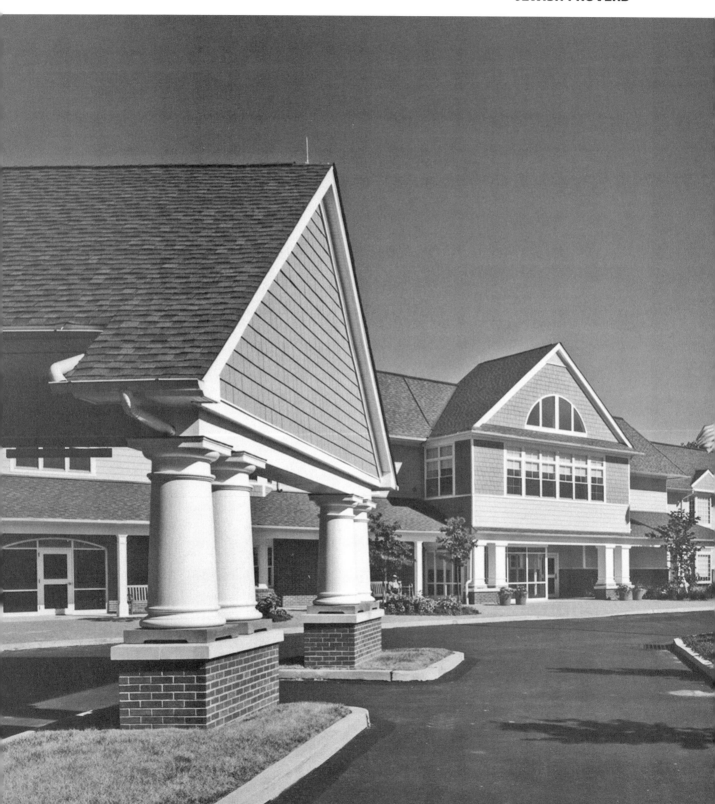

Chapter 17

Abramson Center for Jewish Life

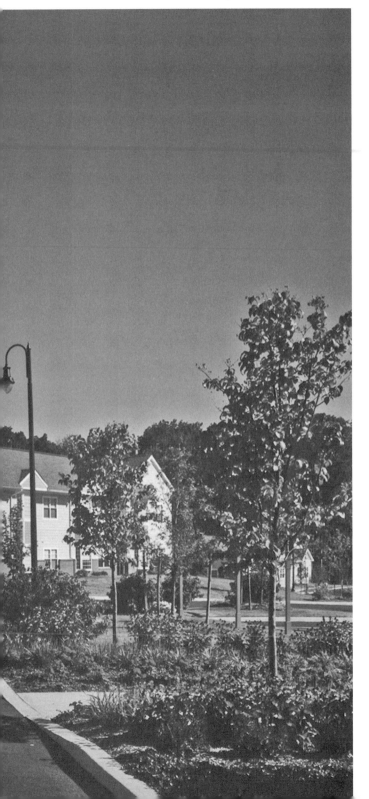

EVALUATION SITE: Abramson Center for Jewish Life

COMMUNITY TYPE: Skilled Nursing and Assisted Living Facility
- 48 assisted living apartments
- 324 nursing care beds
- Adult day care for 20 clients
- Child day care for 60 clients

REGION: Mid-Atlantic

ARCHITECT: EwingCole

OWNER: Abramson Center for Jewish Life

DATA POINTS:

Resident Room:	338–518 gsf (assisted living)
	325 gsf (nursing care)
Total Area:	989 gsf/assisted living apartment
Total Area:	47,488 gsf (assisted living)
Total Area:	1,057 gsf/nursing resident
Area:	342,362 gsf (nursing care)
Overall Total Area:	396,850 gsf
Project Cost:	$178.26/gsf
Total Project Cost:	$70,743,000
Investment/resident:	$190,169
Staffing:	3.67 care hours/resident/day
Occupancy:	99% as of June 2005

FIRST OCCUPANCY: March 2002

DATE OF EVALUATION: June 2005

EVALUATION TEAM: David Slack; Dana Barton; Melissa Strunk; Ingrid Fraley, ASID; Mitch Green, AIA; Jeffrey Anderzhon, AIA

FIG. 17-1 Although this is a very large building, the residential attributes work to reduce the scale *Photograph by Jeffrey Totaro*

Introduction

For nearly 140 years, the Abramson Center for Jewish Life and its predecessor agencies have supported the most vulnerable citizens in Greater Philadelphia with unique living environments, enlightened care, and companionship. As a private, nonprofit, Jewish-sponsored organization, their mission has remained constant: to enhance the quality of life for seniors through the highest quality of care, education, and research.

Formerly known as the Philadelphia Geriatric Center (PGC), the Abramson Center for Jewish Life has a long history of care for older adults. The center is the progeny of two 19th-century homes that provided the basic necessities of life for elderly Jewish immigrants from Eastern and Central Europe. As the facility grew and developed over the years, the need for additional services for the aged

became apparent. Seniors and their families benefit from the Center's commitment to research, as well as programs in health, rehabilitative, psychological, social, spiritual, and educational services. In fact, the Center's renowned Polisher Research Institute, founded in 1959, was the first research center in the United States sponsored by a geriatric facility, and is recognized for its research on the psychological, social, and medical aspects of aging.

Since 1997, the Polisher Research Institute has presented an annual award to honor the contributions from applied research that have benefited older people and their care. In 2002, the award was renamed in memory of the late Dr. Powell Lawton, director emeritus of the Institute. Under Dr. Lawton's guidance, the change from Philadelphia Geriatric Center to the Abramson Center for Jewish Life incorporated more than just a name change. The five-year process of moving began when it became clear that

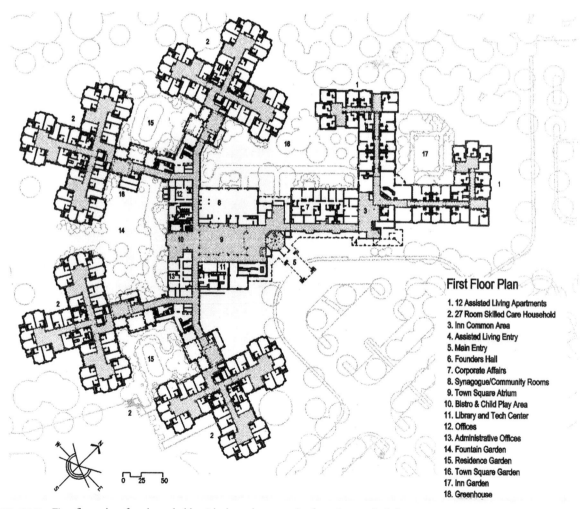

First Floor Plan

1. 12 Assisted Living Apartments
2. 27 Room Skilled Care Household
3. Inn Common Area
4. Assisted Living Entry
5. Main Entry
6. Founders Hall
7. Corporate Affairs
8. Synagogue/Community Rooms
9. Town Square Atrium
10. Bistro & Child Play Area
11. Library and Tech Center
12. Offices
13. Administrative Offices
14. Fountain Garden
15. Residence Garden
16. Town Square Garden
17. Inn Garden
18. Greenhouse

FIG. 17-2 First-floor plan: four households with three clusters each of nursing on the left, assisted living on the right, and the Town Square centered *Courtesy of EwingCole*

the Logan campus, which was in a transitional, urban neighborhood of Philadelphia, would not fulfill the future needs and goals of PGC. With tireless dedication, the CEO took on the "unthinkable" task of selling Philadelphia Geriatric Center to Temple University.

PGC's history of research and progressive care set the stage for the design of the new Abramson campus to embrace a more residential model of care. The center committed itself to encouraging staff and residents to be empowered to direct their own care program, and renewed its emphasis on privacy and dignity. The new mantra for the center became "whatever you did in your own home, you can do at Abramson."

Real estate options for new construction within the Philadelphia city limits were few and far between, because of zoning restrictions. After much searching, the facility decided on an abandoned airport in the nearby suburbs. It took two days to purchase the land and 11 months to obtain appropriate zoning. After another two years of planning and design, the beautiful 72-acre campus in suburban Philadelphia opened in October 2001; it now includes the Abramson Residence (skilled nursing), the Inn (assisted living), the Polisher Research Institute, the Weiss Senior Day Program, and Counseling for Caregivers.

The Abramson Residence's 300,000-square-foot, three-story, steel-and-concrete building includes a substantial underground complex of service corridors, elevators, and chutes that provide invisible and seamless back-of-the-house operations. All service items, food, and supplies come to the households via these passageways.

The 324 beds are divided into clusters. Nine single-occupancy bedrooms, mirroring a family home, are grouped around a sitting area and den, forming a "cluster." Three clusters form a "household," where the 27 residents enjoy a well-appointed living room, activity kitchen, dining room, and four-season porch. Two households form a 54-resident "villa." There are six villas in the Abramson Residence.

The Inn is a 60,000-square-foot, two-story, stick-built construction featuring clusters of 12 assisted living apartments that share a den and garden lounge. Two clusters form a household that shares a dining room, living room, and laundry. Residents of the Inn have access to staff physicians and medical specialists located on the Abramson Center's campus.

Town Square is the hub of social life. This two-story atrium with skylight links the Inn and the Abramson Residence to one another and houses a gift shop, kosher bistro, technology center for Internet access, library, synagogue, community room, children's play alcove, and relaxed seating for visitors, family, and residents.

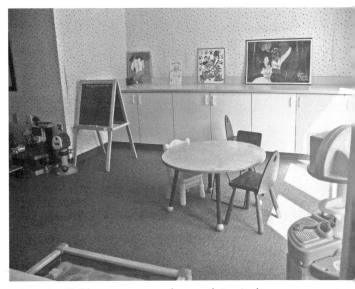

FIG. 17-3   Children are encouraged to spend time in the Town Square with appropriate activities and their own play room   *Photograph by Jeffrey Anderzhon*

The inspiring synagogue is the site of religious services, holiday services, and Jewish festivals. These events are celebrated with traditional food and programs to connect residents to their community and heritage. Two rabbis are on staff to support the religious activities and to preside over weddings and funerals. Children from the Greater Philadelphia synagogues and day schools join

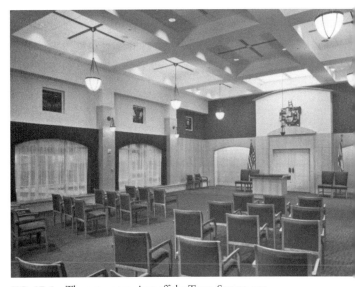

FIG. 17-4   The synagogue, just off the Town Square, provides a meditation place for residents, but can be enlarged to accommodate meetings and group functions   *Photography by Jeffrey Totaro*

residents for fun and educational programs to promote intergenerational sharing of Jewish values and customs.

Architect's Statement

The family home is the inspiration for the architecture and organization of the community. Each area of the facility—the Residence, the Inn, and Town Square—is designed to create spaces unique to its occupants while generating an overall sense of community.

The Residence design is based on a household module of 27 residents grouped in three clusters that foster privacy and independence while enabling residents to enjoy common areas. Two households form a villa of 54 residents, villas share common areas that incorporate displays of Jewish art and space for socializing. The Inn houses older adults who require assistance with the demands of daily life. It includes private studios, one-bedroom suites, access to comprehensive geriatric care, and specially designed living and dining areas.

Designers' and Operators' Stated Objectives and Responses

OBJECTIVE: Create a positive social life and milieu.

DESIGN INTENT: The Residence and the Inn offer a variety of social and gathering spaces, including dining and larger living rooms serving 24 to 29 residents, as well as home-scaled, more private dens for groups of nine to 12 residents. A clubroom, private dining spaces, and the lobby provide additional social space in the more public, main entry areas.

The atmosphere of the Town Square atrium is energized by the gift shop, tech center, art gallery, therapy areas, outpatient doctor's office, community meeting rooms, and the synagogue. The variety of spaces gives residents access to a diverse choice of social activities, as well as practical amenities such as the doctor's office.

OBJECTIVE: Blend nature and the outdoors into everyday living.

DESIGN INTENT: All circulation in the Residence and the Inn leads to destination spaces with natural light, which helps to bring the outdoors inside to residents. The building plans and massing form four garden courtyards, each with a distinct design, and the skylight atrium of Town Square provides an all-season, outdoor-scaled space easily accessible to residents and families.

OBJECTIVE: Adapt to changing needs.

DESIGN INTENT: Flexibility in floor plans allows the rooms to grow and change with the needs of residents. Adjacent resident rooms in the nursing home will have provisions for adding an interconnecting door for couples' suites, and one-bedroom assisted living apartments can easily convert to two-bedroom suites with kitchenettes and shared bathrooms.

The Residence and the Inn are anticipating aging in place that will result in a high percentage of physically frail residents with some form of dementia. The dens in each of the household clusters lend themselves to dining on a small scale, which will help the staff to better meet residents' needs as the aging-in-place model progresses. Additionally, 31 acres of the site are preserved for future development, which could be used to build a new facility for the growing dementia-care population.

OBJECTIVE: Promote health and well-being.

DESIGN INTENT: Features such as bathrooms specifically designed for elderly use, with varying levels of staff assistance and fold-down bars, help to tailor the space to the needs of residents. Corridor handrails designed for grip-

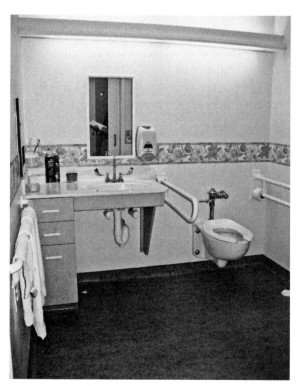

FIG. 17-5 Resident toilet rooms provide useful assistive devices and storage drawers, but residents still have to travel outside their rooms for bathing   *Photograph by Jeffrey Anderzhon*

ping and mobility as well as leaning and resting encourage ambulation. Frequently spaced furnished alcoves encourage wayfinding by providing a comfortable place for residents to rest during their walks.

Field Observations: Meeting the Objectives

OBJECTIVE: Create a positive social life and milieu.

FIELD OBSERVATIONS: Defining a household was extremely important to the design of the Abramson Residence. Initially a group of 40 residents was considered, but ultimately deemed too large. Planners decided that a smaller social scale would work better, and after much research the nine-bed cluster seemed best for the Residence. Room sizes were designed to accommodate occupancy levels in groups of nine, 27, and 54.

The initial grouping of nine neighbors provides a more comfortable and immediate "family" setting. The larger groupings of 27, especially in the household activity areas such as the dining room, promote social interaction on a larger scale and alleviate boredom.

Town Square is designed to receive residents and family members in a positive setting filled with opportunities for various activities. The bright, open space provides an uplifting experience while embracing Jewish culture. Overlooking Town Square, the second-floor balcony areas are frequently filled to capacity with residents from clusters, households, and villas gathering for concerts and special programs. It should be noted that the skylight is reportedly noisy during rainstorms and affects the acoustical quality of the Town Square, especially during scheduled events. (See Figure 16 in the color insert.)

OBJECTIVE: Blend nature and the outdoors into everyday living.

FIELD OBSERVATIONS: The flood of natural light into Town Square is dramatic and fulfilling. The connection to the immaculate courtyards is equally important, although visible only through the bistro in Town Square. The courtyards are well landscaped with seating groups aimed at promoting conversation and family visits.

Households provide consistent views to the outdoors, and the window in the cluster den is an especially commendable design concept. Some owners would see this square footage as an opportunity to add another resident room and would diminish the importance of this den with a view.

As with any multistory building, providing equal access to the outdoor environment to all residents is a challenge. It was disappointing to see that window access alone was considered adequate when one might design a small balcony or enclosed porch so residents can take in fresh air in their own households. A trip to the first floor

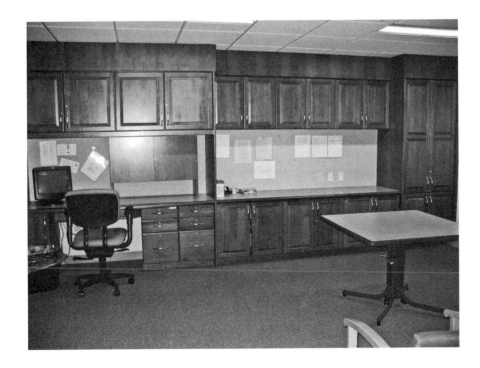

FIG. 17-6 The nurse work stations at each household are attractive but unused, as nurses prefer to congregate at a village-centered workroom *Photograph by Jeffrey Anderzhon*

has to be planned and restricts residents from spontaneous access to the outdoors.

OBJECTIVE: Adapt to changing needs.

FIELD OBSERVATIONS: The built-in flexibility of each unit design will certainly assist the Abramson Center in responding to the age-related changes of its population. Its role as a learning laboratory will also promote the addition of services in a broader context than one would normally expect.

The operators are considering expansion of the child day care center to encourage intergenerational exchange, as well as an expansion into market-rate housing for independent seniors on the additional, unused campus acreage.

OBJECTIVE: Promote health and well-being.

FIELD OBSERVATIONS: Health and well-being rely on more than just folding grab bars, correctly designed handrails, and furnished alcoves. The mission of the Abramson Center must be applauded for bringing a high level of accommodation and services to those who can least afford it. The quality of construction, the decentralization of services, and the residential scaled clusters of the Abramson Center are certainly not the norm in subsidized housing and Medicare/Medicaid health care environments.

The cluster design of nine private resident rooms seems to be a good design approach, but it is compromised by the three clusters uniting in the household living room and dining area. The dining room, with a capacity of 27 skilled nursing residents, seems institutional and as though it was designed without much thought. Additionally, there is a sight-line deficiency from the cluster of rooms to the center of activity in this larger household.

Lighting in the clusters is confusing because it consists of several different styles and types of fixtures apparently placed in random order. What appear to be wall-washers are placed at such a distance from the wall that they produce significant glare for anyone using the handrail. The number of motorized wheelchairs in use and the resulting wear on the corridor finishes was not anticipated. Additional sitting areas along the extensive corridors would be beneficial for those who are not mobile.

Vertical chutes that connect each level to the basement service level allow trash and laundry to simply drop down the chute to a holding room. Although the chute method is theoretically an interesting design, bags that are not tied securely can contaminate the chute as they fall. Decentralization of services does not eliminate the housekeeping and meds carts that crowd the corridors. Clean linen is stored in an armoire in the cluster den area and although these items are closer to the apartments, the staff still must make trips back and forth to gather or replenish linens.

Because there is no shower within the resident bathroom, bathing for all 27 residents of a household

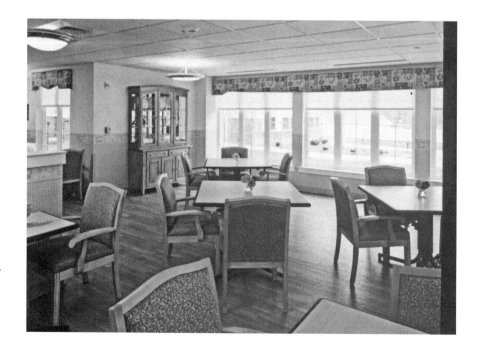

FIG. 17-7 The village dining room has wonderful natural light and durable finishes *Photography by Jeffrey Totaro*

takes place at a central bather, the logistics of which were not clear. There was no indication that any thought had been given to privacy and dignity issues of residents by incorporating individual showers in the resident bathrooms. A sliding door separates the bedroom and bathroom, offering some amount of resident privacy. Fold-down grab bars provide flexibility for staff assistance and may promote resident independence. The central bathing area is deteriorating after only a year in use. It is not at all warm and inviting, but cold and typical of central bathing rooms constructed in the 1970s. Visually obtrusive transfer chairs exacerbate the institutional décor.

All resident room entry doors feature extra-wide stiles to increase the width of the door opening. Each door is painted a neutral color, but the surrounding frame is identified by its own color. This color is then repeated on the door signage to enhance the color cueing. A nice idea; however, maintenance reported that a paint schedule with 64 different paint colors is indeed a logistical problem.

Plate rails and tack boards display a resident's personal treasures and discourage wall damage. Parallel light cornices flank the sides of the beds, providing an interesting source of nontraditional illumination. Each room features a bay window, which increases the visual spaciousness of the room and visual access to the outdoors. Cable outlets are located on both sides of the rooms for added flexibility.

Although there is a country kitchen in each household, it is generally locked and access by residents occurs only with staff supervision. It is not connected to the dining area, but has counter access through the living area. Food service to the households is via an elevator from a remote kitchen. Individual trays are currently in use; however, a plated service is under consideration pending the resolution of transportation and temperature control issues.

Field Observations: Themes and Hypotheses

Creating Community

The total environment of the Abramson Center infuses Jewish traditions and values into the daily lives of residents. Using the family home as the design inspiration, the Abramson Center for Jewish Life "draws on the cultural and religious resources of Judaism to create a strong community and to bring joy, meaning and healing to the lives of our elders." Town Square, although an attraction

to residents who are physically and mentally capable of understanding its existence, still relies on the interaction of staff and/or family members to create the community feeling and, in many cases, even to transport the resident to this area. It is neither intuitive nor generally convenient for residents.

Making a Home

Single-occupancy rooms clustered around a sitting area and den mimic a family home and invoke a residential quality, although full resident bathrooms instead of a central bather would have contributed even more to the residential quality. The three-cluster household's living room, activity kitchen, dining room, and four-season porch further enhance the feeling of a real home in the Residence, and the similar scheme of the Inn gives its residents a home of their own as well. The above-average quality of construction and the relatively successful decentralization of services at Abramson also diminish the telltale marks of an institution.

Flexibility in floor plans and the easily converted suites are also key elements of feeling at home at the Abramson Center. Couples will benefit from being able to connect two one-bedroom suites to create an apartment space that is really their own. Flexibility, the ability to personalize, and choice are critical to residents—or anyone—feeling at home in their surroundings.

Just as the suites mimic typical houses and apartments, Town Square attempts to replicate a neighborhood or community experience for residents. The well-attended events and reported popularity of the area testify to the success of Town Square. Despite the space not being entirely intuitive, as mentioned before, residents seem comfortable enough to enjoy the space and take advantage of the social opportunities it provides.

Despite the general success of the cluster design, some problems remain. The skilled nursing dining room is institutional and does not do the design justice. Smaller dining spaces, elimination of the tray service, and relatively easy access to the country kitchen would be more akin to living and dining in a residential setting. Additionally, the sight-line deficiency noted in one household creates a long, institutional corridor and is a definite deficit to the homey feel of the clusters. Poorly chosen lighting and the dismal central bathing area also hinder Abramson's attempt at creating a home.

The design alone does not create a home for residents—community and a feeling of belonging are critical to feeling comfortable in one's residence. The emphasis on Jewish values and cultural heritage unify the community at Abramson. Familiar religious iconography, a synagogue and its services, kosher meals, and a wider understanding of residents' background are invaluable comforts of home.

Regional/Cultural Design

Incorporated into the mission statement of the Abramson Center for Jewish Life is the desire and ability to welcome older adults who have no financial means and who rely on the state for medical assistance. Therefore, it would seem that this community fabric is indeed woven together with a continuous connection to Jewish heritage rather than wealth or community status. Incorporation of the kosher kitchen (the only one in the area) and the synagogue are certainly attractions for the surrounding Jewish population.

Founders Hall, with its etched glass windows and extensive display of donor plaques to honor the contributions of the Jewish community, cannot be overlooked. Artfully placed, the décor adds interest to the walls of Town Square, and the entire space becomes a testament to the commitment of the Jewish community at large for enhancing the lives of its older adults.

In examining the exterior architecture of the building, one can conclude that regional elements have been sacrificed for a more generic façade. Residential styling and scale are certainly apparent, but the overall look is one that could easily be transported to any other location without much notice.

Environmental Therapy

Layered orientation cues are central to the design, and include but are not limited to the use of furnishings, displays, colors, and patterns. Judaic artwork is strategically located to reinforce Jewish values in daily living. Perhaps the most important element of the Center is the dedication to the idea that the Abramson Residence and the Inn are "learning laboratories."

The design of all private rooms and the concept of decentralized services for a skilled nursing population are certainly commendable. Promoting a design concept that provides privacy and a residential environment throughout the entire 300,000-square-foot facility is a major accomplishment. Given these pluses, the lack of showers in resident bathrooms and the antiquated bathing facilities are all the more disappointing.

Outdoor Environment

Town Square provides an outdoor-scaled space for all-season use that is easily accessible to all mobile residents. The design of the building creates four exterior courtyards, each with a distinct character, well-appointed furnishings, and attractive landscape materials. Unfortunately, access is restricted to residents who are accompanied by staff or family members, which limits residents' ability to enjoy the outdoor spaces at will.

Because this is a multistory building, it is always a challenge to provide something aside from visual access

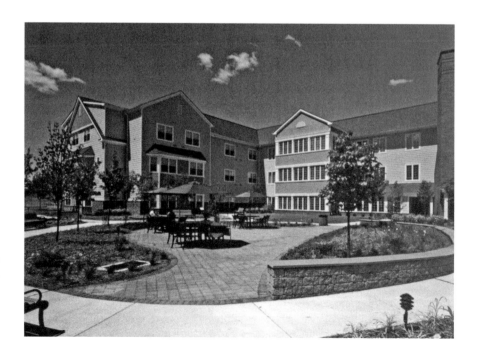

FIG. 17-8 Beautiful courtyards are easily accessed and provide special places for family and residents to gather *Photography by Jeffrey Totaro*

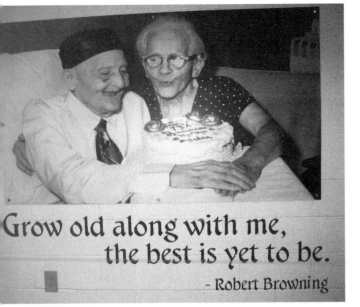

Grow old along with me,
the best is yet to be.
- Robert Browning

FIG. 17-9 The spirit of the Abramson Center is clearly defined by this poster located in the basement service corridor
Photograph by Jeffrey Anderzhon

to the community must be emphasized. There are noticeable differences in design finishes for the administrative spaces compared to those for support staff. The variable amenities and quality of workspace highlight a hierarchy among staff.

Operator Perspectives

The board, CEO, and design team were clearly faced with numerous design options and decisions that affected the outcome of the facility's design. Initially, the resident rooms were to be configured as 50 percent private and 50 percent shared-occupancy. Ultimately, they decided to move forward with all private rooms and now are certain that this was "absolutely the right decision."

Other "right decisions" for this facility include:

- No steps anywhere on the campus, with the exception of five steps into the boiler room to increase the ceiling height for equipment clearance.
- The commitment to the design and programs of spaces and activities in Town Square.

to the exterior for residents above the first floor. Alternative concepts for balconies, screened porches, or true sunrooms would have been a great addition to the design of the households.

Quality of Workplace and the Physical Plant

The home-like and small scale of the Abramson Residence and the Inn attract and help retain staff, as these elements foster positive staff and resident relationships. However, it should be noted that the extensive below-grade "mall" that houses all support spaces, and decentralizes housekeeping and food service activities, also creates a physical separation in staff functions. The above-ground staff is not necessarily connected to below-ground staff, because integration of these job functions is almost physically impossible. Maintenance has not necessarily bonded with the needs of the caregivers. Additionally, the dietary department has not necessarily picked up on residents' peculiarities and preferences.

Completely separating operations from the residential space can compromise the spirit of teamwork among staff and impede the creation of meaningful relationships with residents. Staff who work in the basement are important to the successful operation of the facility (laundry, kitchen, human resources, accounting/finance, dietary, materials management, medical records, staff training, and internal communications), and their value

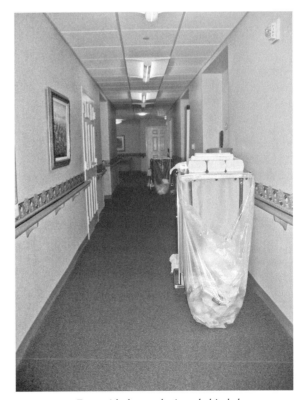

FIG. 17-10 Even with the emphasis on behind-the-scenes delivery of services, carts are evident in the corridors
Photograph by Jeffrey Anderzhon

- Occupancy sensors for up to 95 percent of the light fixtures in the facility.
- Inclusion of a children's playroom, "a brilliant idea."

Items on the center's wish list include cameras in the households (active 24/7) to show movement of residents to their families via the Internet and perhaps to be able to talk to them. Cameras could also capture information to document what operational or environmental aspects require correction as related to physical plant and operations or to further the education of legislators regarding nursing home environments.

At the time of the interview, the CEO advised that "an unfinished piece of business is the staffing program. It is now 3½ years since opening and the staff is still not solid. We turned over the Director of Nursing position three times in the first 18 months. Building the structure was easy, the program was tough."

Going back to the beginning of the facility's history will help the reader further understand these comments. Philadelphia Geriatric Center had been an established entity in Philadelphia for generations. Their programs, staffing requirements, and personnel were well estab-

lished and worked successfully with a team approach. The move had four consequences:

- The new location in suburban Philadelphia created a 20-mile commute from the Logan campus, which was nearly impossible for existing staff to undertake.
- The sale of Philadelphia Geriatric Center to Temple University included everything: furnishings, equipment, and staff.
- The 220 Logan campus residents who were transferred to the new location created an instant population; there was no opportunity to ramp up over a period of time to reach maximum occupancy or develop staff.

Because the new Abramson Center for Jewish Life opened with only a few key members from the PGC personnel, an entirely new support staff for the 324-bed skilled nursing residence and the 48 assisted living apartments had to be interviewed, trained, and exposed to the traditions of Jewish culture. Agency staffing filled many of the 400 to 500 positions available.

General Project Information

PROJECT ADDRESS
Abramson Center for Jewish Life
1425 Horsham Road
Horsham, PA 19044

PROJECT DESIGN TEAM
Architect: EwingCole
Associated Architect: Nelson-Tremain Partnership, PA
Interior Designer: Elizabeth Brawley, ASID
Landscape Architect: Carter Van Dyke Associates, Inc.
Structural Engineer: EwingCole
Mechanical Engineer: EwingCole
Electrical Engineer: EwingCole
Civil Engineer: Charles E. Shoemaker, Inc.
Dining Consultant: N/A
Gerontologist: N/A
Management/Development: N/A
Contractor: R.M. Shoemaker Company
Mosaic Artist: Jonathan Mandel

PROJECT STATUS
Completion date: March 2002

OCCUPANCY LEVELS
At facility opening date: 55%
At date of evaluation: 99%

RESIDENT AGE (YRS)
At facility opening date: 86
June 2005 average: 88

PROJECT AREAS

OVERALL PROJECT

Project Element	Units, Beds, or Clients	New GSF	Total Gross Area (GSF)	Total on Site or Served by Project
	Included in This Project			
Senior living/assisted living/personal care (units)	48	47,488	47,488	48
Skilled nursing care (beds)	324	105,300	105,300	324
Common social areas (people)	372	43,735	43,735	372
Kitchen (daily meals served)	1116	9,300	9,300	1116
Elder day care (clients)	20	3,500	3,500	20
Children's day care (clients)	60	3,500	3,500	60
Retail space (shops/restaurants, etc.)	2 spaces	2,150	2,150	2 (spaces)
Fitness/rehabilitation/wellness (daily visits)	N/A	7,180	7,180	N/A

ASSISTED LIVING

Project Element	No. Units	Typical Size
	New Construction	
Studio units	24	338 GSF
One-bedroom units	24	518 GSF
Total (all units)	48	20,544 GSF
Residents' social areas (lounges, dining, and recreation spaces):		10,520 GSF
Medical, health care, therapy, and activities spaces:		0 GSF
Administrative, public, and ancillary support services:		1,440 GSF
Service, maintenance, and mechanical areas:		3,180 GSF
Total gross area:		47,488 GSF
Total net usable area (per space program):		33,095 NSF
Overall gross/net factor (ratio of gross area/net usable area):		1.43

SKILLED NURSING

Project Element	No. Beds	Typical Room Size
	New Construction	
Residents in one-bed/single rooms	324	325 GSF
Totals	324	105,300 GSF
Social areas (lounges, dining, and recreation spaces):		43,800 GSF
Medical, health care, therapy, and activities spaces:		7,180 GSF
Administrative, public, and ancillary support services:		30,800 GSF
Service, maintenance, and mechanical areas:		28,000 GSF
Total gross area:		342,362 GSF
Total net usable area (per space program):		223,763 NSF
Overall gross/net factor (ratio of gross area/net usable area):		1.53

OTHER FACILITIES

Project Element	New Construction No. Clients	Size
Adult day care	20	3,500 GSF
Child day care	60	3,500 GSF
Total gross area:		7,000 GSF
Total net usable area (per space program):		5,185 NSF
Overall gross/net factor (ratio of gross area/net usable area):		1.35

SITE AND PARKING

SITE LOCATION
Suburban

SITE SIZE
Acres: 41
Square feet: 396,850
Area of entire campus: 73 acres

PARKING

Type of Parking	For This Facility Residents	Staff	Visitors	Totals
Open surface lot(s)	165	143	162	377
Totals	165	143	162	377

CONSTRUCTION COSTS

SOURCE OF COST DATA
Final construction cost as of June 2002

SOFT COSTS

Land cost or value:	$4,381,000
Basic architectural and engineering:	$3,405,000
Expanded architectural and engineering:	$780,000
All permit and other entitlement fees:	$1,440,000
Legal:	In fees above
Appraisals:	In fees above
Marketing and preopening:	Not available
Total soft costs:	$10,006,000

BUILDING COSTS

New construction except FF&E, special finishes, floor and window coverings, HVAC, and electrical:	$35,800,000
Renovations except FF&E, special finishes, floor and window coverings, HVAC, and electrical:	N/A
FF&E and small wares:	$3,000,000
Floor coverings:	$2,500,000
Window coverings:	$1,000,000
HVAC:	$9,000,000
Electrical:	$5,000,000
Medical equipment costs:	$5,815,000
Total building costs:	$62,115,000

SITE COSTS

New on-site:	$3,500,000
New off-site:	N/A
Renovation on-site:	N/A
Renovation off-site:	N/A
Landscape:	$500,000
Special site features or amenities:	N/A
Total site costs:	$4,000,000

TOTAL PROJECT COSTS
(include all fees and costs, except financing)
Total project costs: $70,743,000

FINANCING SOURCES
Taxable bond offering with cost of issuance: $2,193,000

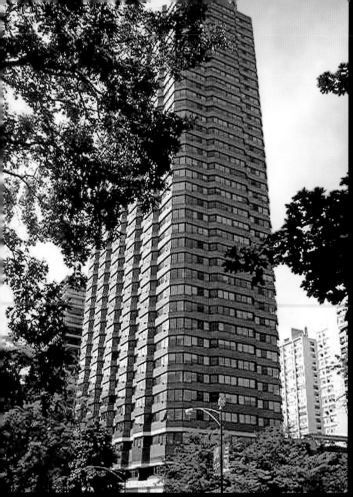

FIGURE 1 The Hallmark's independent living apartments provide spectacular views of Chicago's Lincoln Park and Lake Michigan
Courtesy of The Hallmark

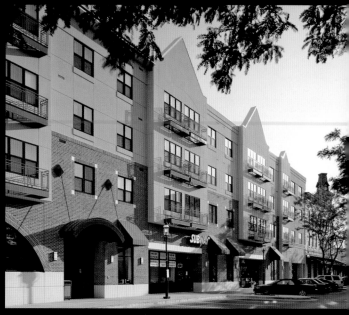

FIGURE 2 Avalon Square provides retail spaces on the first floor that offer businesses and residents an additional connection to the surrounding community
Courtesy KKE Architects, Inc.\Phillip Prowse Photography

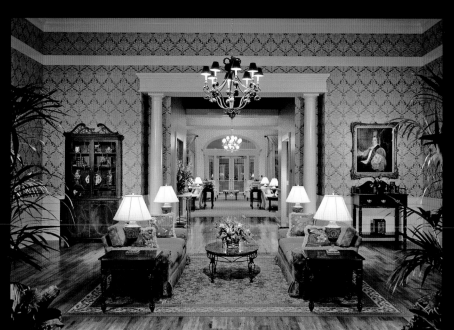

FIGURE 3 Bishop Gadsden's main entry lobby is indicative of the southern charm that is carried throughout the design of the campus
Photo by Rion Rizzo, Creative Sources Photography

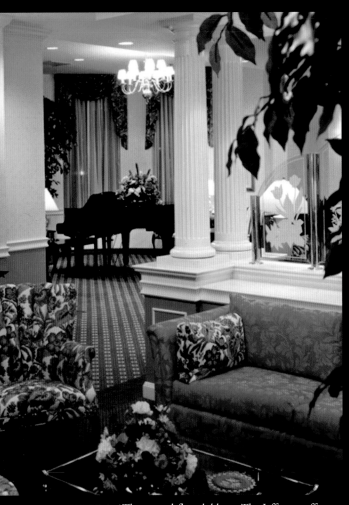

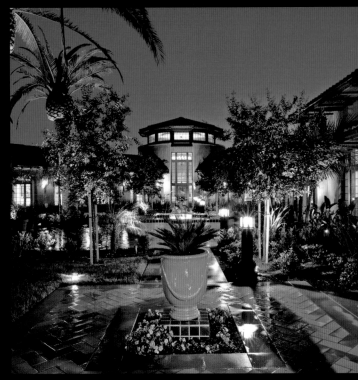

FIGURE 5   La Vida Real's entry courtyard is reminiscent of a colonial Spanish villa
www.architecturephotoinc.com

FIGURE 6   With dramatic views to the Atlantic Ocean, McKeen Towers provides an enviable setting for residents
Courtesy of O'Keefe Architects Inc.

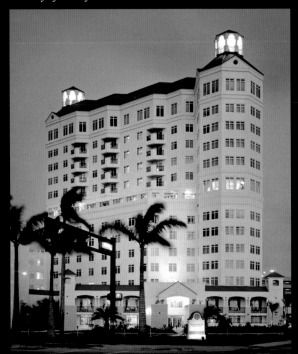

FIGURE 4   The second-floor lobby at The Jefferson offers space for residents to relax in elegance and allows them to access other community spaces
Photo by Michael Dersin Photography

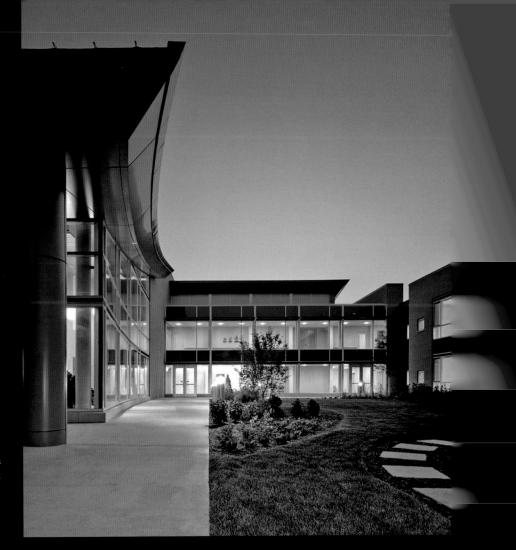

FIGURE 7 The Dominican Center at Marywood is both contemporary and inspirational
Photograph: Hedrich Blessing/Christopher Barrett

FIGURE 8 Rosewood Estate of Roseville provides a residential setting for its assisted living residents
Image courtesy of ESG Architects, Inc.

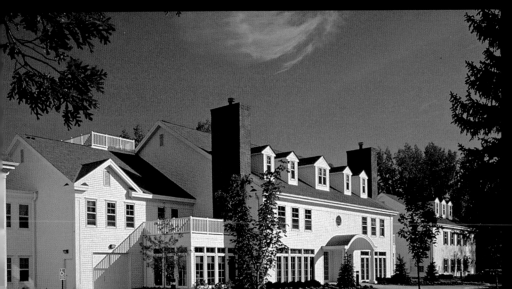

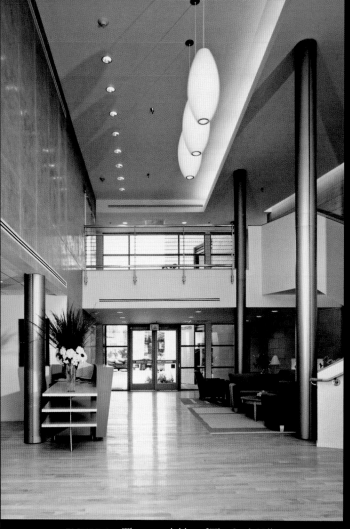

FIGURE 9 The entry lobby of The Stark Villa uses materials and design that redefine traditional assisted living architecture
Photograph by John Edward Linden

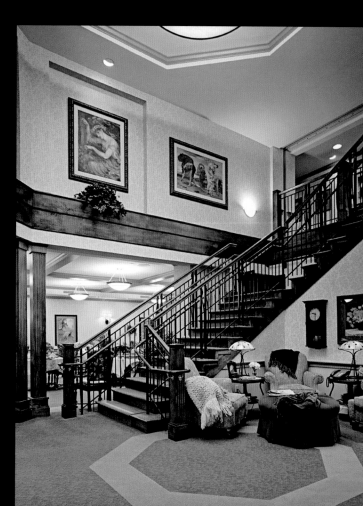

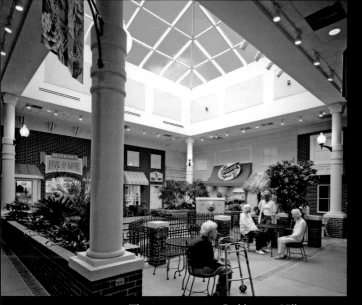

FIGURE 11 The town square at Cuthbertson Village at Aldersgate also functions as a community meeting place
Photograph by Tim Buchman

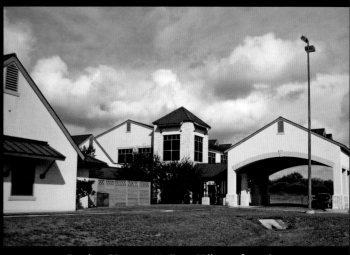

FIGURE 12 Freedom House at Air Force Village reflects the architecture of the surrounding Texas hill country
Photograph courtesy of SAGE/Society for the Advancement of Gerontological Environments

FIGURE 13 The dramatic three-story streetscape at The Forest at Duke provides visual interest in the evening light
©James West/ JWestProductions.com

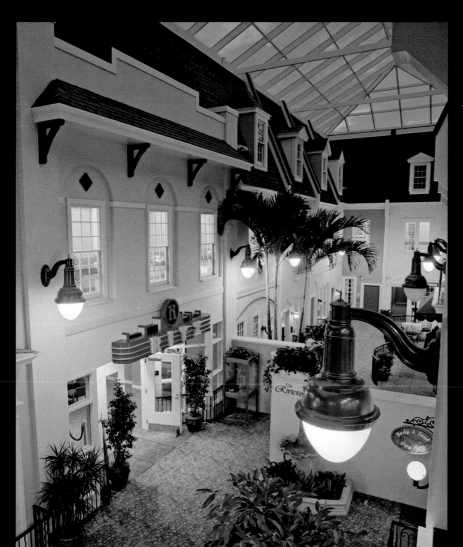

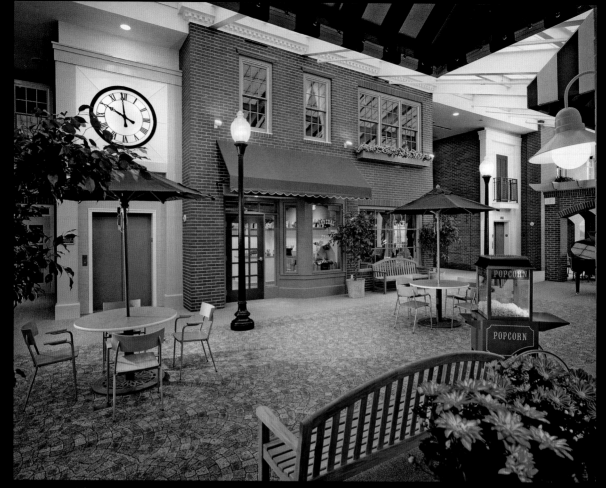

FIGURE 14 The Main Street at The Village at Waveny Care Center takes its design inspiration from the quaint New Canaan downtown streetscapes
Courtesy RLPS Architects/Larry Lefever Photography

FIGURE 15 The neighborhood configuration at Woodside Place of Oakmont includes inviting courtyards for residents
Photograph by Robert Ruschak

FIGURE 16 Town Square at Abramson Center for Jewish Life boasts a café, synagogue, computer center, and convenience store
Photography by Jeffrey Totaro

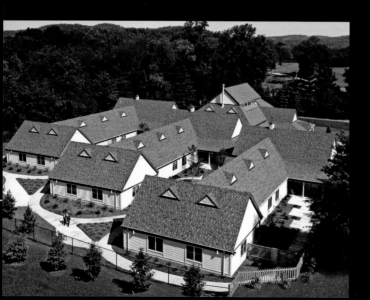

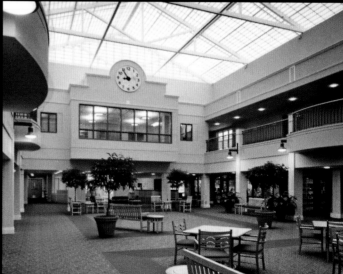

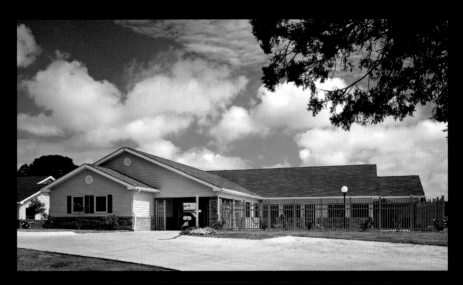

FIGURE 17 The residential design of the Green Houses™ at Traceway is reminiscent of a large, suburban ranch-style home
© 2003 Jeffrey Jacobs Photography

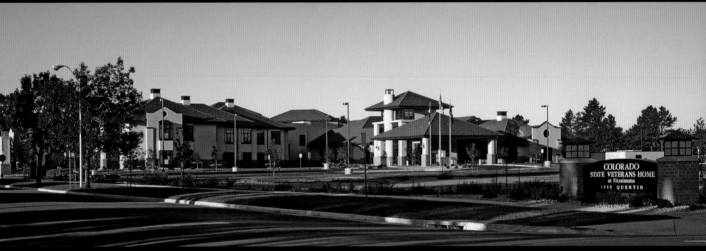

FIGURE 18 Colorado State Veterans Home at Fitzsimons takes its design inspiration from a southwestern aesthetic
©Lacasse Photography

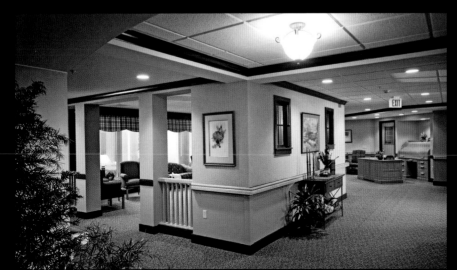

FIGURE 19 The four neighborhoods at Foulkeways at Gwynedd intersect at this well-proportioned living room
Courtesy RLPS Architects/Larry Lefever Photography

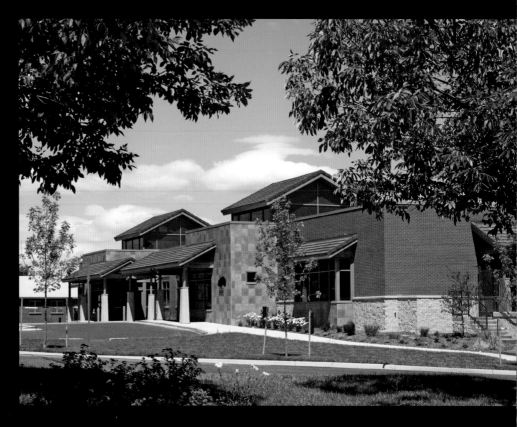

FIGURE 20 The exterior materials on Cody Day Center are grounded in earth tones commonly used in this Rocky Mountain state
©*Lacasse Photography*

FIGURE 21 The faux stream at The Tempe Health and Welfare Centre in Trondheim, Norway, creates visual interest for residents and the community
Photograph courtesy of SAGE/Society for the Advancement of Gerontological Environments

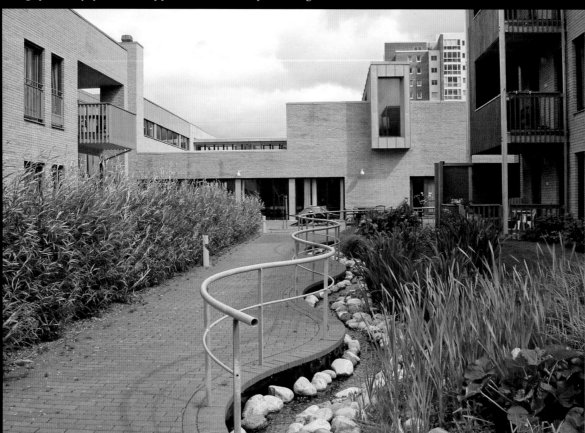

CARE COMPARISONS

Source: www.medicare.gov—July 14, 2005
SNF staffing: 3.67 care hours/resident/day
SNF occupancy: 99% (321 of 324)

Hours per Resident per Day	Abramson in PA	PA Average	National Average
Not-for-profit	Yes		
Multifacility	No		
Levels of care	Nursing		
Medicare	Yes		
Medicaid	Yes		
Licensed #	324		
# residents	321	123.5	95.3
% occ this day	99%		
RNs	0.40	0.70	0.50
LPNs	0.68	0.70	0.70
RN + LPN	1.08	1.40	1.20
CNA	2.58	2.20	2.30
RN + LPN + CNA	3.67	3.60	3.50

"Old age, believe me, is a good and pleasant thing. It is true you are gently shouldered off the stage, but then you are given such a comfortable front stall as spectator."

CONFUCIUS, 551–479 B.C.E.

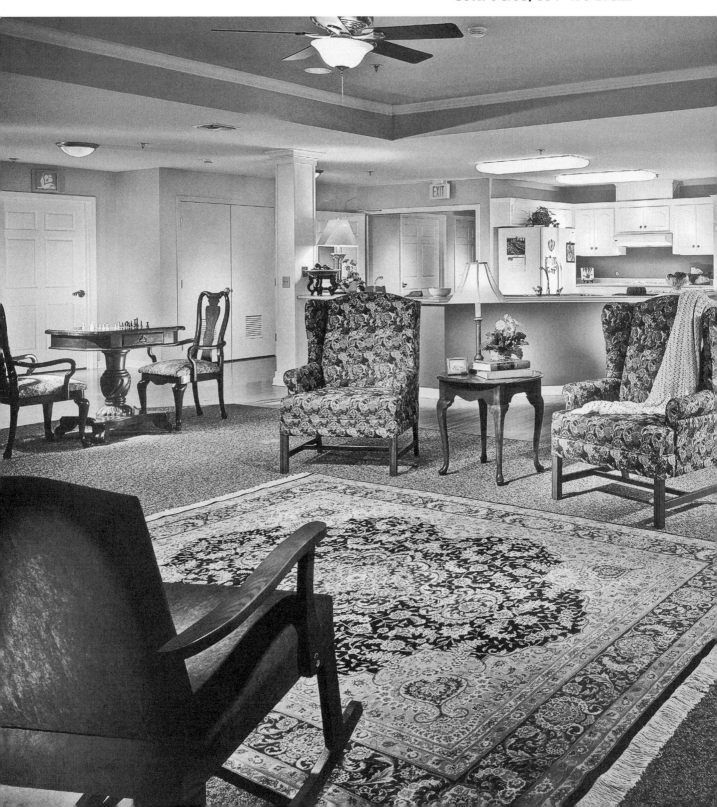

Chapter 18

The Green Houses™ at Traceway

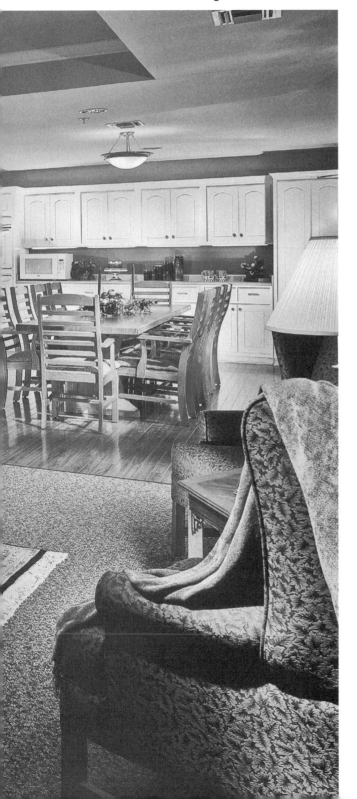

EVALUATION SITE: The Green Houses™ at Traceway

COMMUNITY TYPE: Skilled Nursing/Dementia Care
- 20 nursing care beds
- 20 nursing care beds for those with dementia

REGION: South

ARCHITECT: The McCarty Company-Design Group, P.A.

OWNER: Mississippi Methodist Senior Services, Inc.

DATA POINTS: Resident Room:	260 gsf
Total Area:	604 gsf/resident
Total Area:	24,160 gsf
Project Cost:	$131.21/gsf
Total Project Cost:	$3,170,089
Investment/resident:	$79,252.23
Staffing:	4.90 care hours/resident/day
Occupancy:	100% as of July 2004

FIRST OCCUPANCY: August 2003

DATE OF EVALUATION: July 2004

EVALUATION TEAM: Mitch Green, AIA; Jeffrey Anderzhon, AIA; James Mertz; Doug Tweddale

FIG. 18-1 The Hearth Room provides a feeling of residential warmth and visual access to the kitchen and dining room
© 2003 Jeffrey Jacobs Photography

Introduction

Tupelo, Mississippi, was the birthplace of an artist destined to change the culture of American music. Perhaps it is only fitting that the same community that brought us Elvis Presley would also be the birthplace of a progressive, challenging model of elderly nursing care built on the vernacular of the family home.

Decentralizing nursing services and grouping resident rooms in "households" have been celebrated throughout the care profession over the past few years. This culture-change approach has been embraced by care provider and designer alike, because it takes a more personal approach with individuals in need of nursing care. When successfully implemented, this approach also provides staff with more diversified tasks and, at least theoretically, promotes a higher level of interaction between staff and residents. Extended to its logical and perhaps inevitable evolution, this approach will ultimately result in stand-alone, smaller structures that are indeed structured more like large houses.

The Green Houses™ at Traceways are essentially large, single-family homes that are intended to evoke a familial aesthetic through design and a family feel through the care provision program. The facility is located on a 50-acre retirement campus that includes traditional nursing and assisted living structures, as well as aesthetically dissimilar retirement cottages. The Green Houses™ seem to be the latest "suburb" of the campus and take on the typical suburban disconnection of design to their neighboring structures.

The religiously based, not-for-profit sponsor of the Green Houses™ demonstrated no small amount of bravery in undertaking this project. Breaking new ground in skilled nursing care provision is difficult in and of itself, but doing so in a built environment and expecting regu-

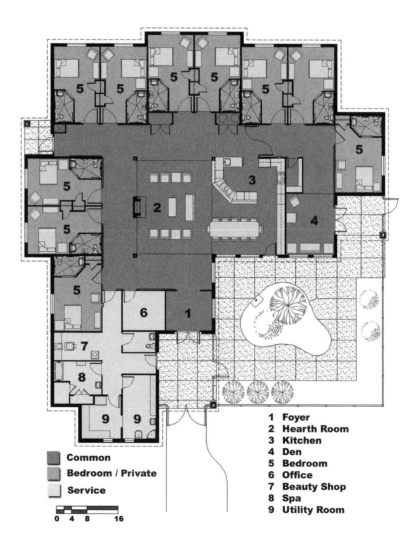

FIG. 18-2 Floor plan; resident rooms organized around the Hearth Room and kitchen *Courtesy of The McCarty Company-Design Group, PA*

Common
Bedroom / Private
Service

0 4 8   16

1 Foyer
2 Hearth Room
3 Kitchen
4 Den
5 Bedroom
6 Office
7 Beauty Shop
8 Spa
9 Utility Room

latory agencies to endorse culture change is an added challenge. The designers and administration of the Green Houses™ created a project that courageously asked regulators to expand and alter their codified views of nursing care.

Although the environment is a critical element of success, the staffing approach within that environment and the interaction between the two is equally important. To increase the chance for success, the community adopted a true universal worker concept that creates not only a small family of residents, but also a consistent "family" of staff members in each house. On this southern campus in the heart of Elvis country, the design and care provision approaches work together in a harmony that provides opportunity for both staff and residents to thrive.

Designers' and Owners' Stated Objectives and Responses

OBJECTIVE: Create a small-home environment where frail elders can live and grow while receiving skilled care.

DESIGN INTENT: At approximately 6,000 square feet, each building is a warm and friendly home with an open-plan living space called "the hearth." The home includes a fully functional kitchen and a long, family-style dining table for 12 residents. The windows provide an abundance of natural light and views of the wooded surroundings across the accessible patio/garden. Beyond the electric fireplace, wood trim, and comfortable furnishings lies the cleverly concealed

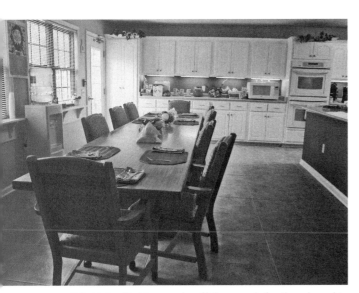

FIG. 18-3 Residents and staff share meals family style at this long dining table *Photograph by Jeffrey Anderzhon*

technical and clinical functionality of a licensed skilled nursing environment.

OBJECTIVE: Provide each elder with a private room and bath.

DESIGN INTENT: Opening directly onto the hearth are 10 private rooms with private bathrooms complete with showers. The privacy of the individual rooms gives dignity back to each elder, and an open door or short walk provide varied levels of participation in the social activities of the hearth.

OBJECTIVE: Protect the natural habitat of the site.

DESIGN INTENT: Smaller buildings and limited parking help to retain the natural feel of the wooded site. All buildings, drives, and underground utilities are strategically located to protect trees and the natural landscape.

OBJECTIVE: Develop a project that ensures financial support through current Medicaid reimbursement and encourages replication.

DESIGN INTENT: The designers met their goals of simple building systems and low costs by using residential wood-frame construction and by examining each design decision with an eye to cost. Though modest in its use of materials and architectural detailing, each home has an abundance of space and light, as well as the complete clinical functionality of a licensed skilled care environment. Enhanced communication between the design team and construction professionals was essential to the design-build project delivery and to the cost-control measures.

OBJECTIVE: Meet all state regulatory requirements.

DESIGN INTENT: With the concept being somewhat unusual by nursing home standards, strict compliance with all licensure requirements was a clear objective even in this "home" environment. The project team explored creative ways to meet the intent of each requirement and received much support and cooperation from the State Department of Licensure; no variances were requested or required.

Field Observations: Meeting the Objectives

OBJECTIVE: Create a small-home environment where frail elders can live and grow while receiving skilled care.

FIELD OBSERVATIONS: At the north edge of the continuing care retirement campus, four Green Houses™ were constructed in what can only be described as a typical suburban subdivision. The four houses are similar in

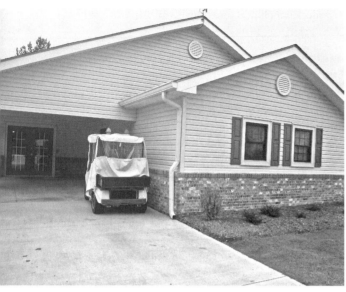

FIG. 18-4 Bulk food delivery arrives by golf cart at the front entry *Photograph by Jeffrey Anderzhon*

appearance, with modifications in exterior finishes and slight differences in appearance due to mirrored floor plans.

Each of the four houses is home to 10 residents and is designed on the model of a single-family residence, albeit somewhat larger than most suburban homes because of the somewhat larger "family." The covered entry with doorbell, the large, open-plan hearth room, and kitchen area create feelings of home.

Like so many homes, activity centers on food, its preparation, and its consumption. The kitchens of the Green Houses™ are clearly meant to be, and in fact are, a central location of both resident and staff activity within the house. Family members and other visitors share coffee and baked goods prepared by the staff in the kitchen and the adjacent dining area. Conversations and small-group socialization take place in this area as well. This space is also where the staff spend most of their time, because, as universal workers, they are responsible for all meal preparation.

Although natural light flows into the dining area through windows facing the secured courtyard, the light is fairly minimal, diffuse, and somewhat unusable within the kitchen and hearth room areas. These two spaces require artificial lighting and suffer somewhat due to the lack of visual connection to exterior spaces.

The four houses are a replacement for a more traditional skilled nursing facility on the campus, and it is fairly easy to advocate the Green Houses™ as the better environment in which to live. From observations of residents during the course of a typical day, it appears that

this small-home environment provides an improved setting for the residents and one in which their lives have at least an opportunity to improve. Growing in life, however, also means remaining connected to a community while participating in activities within that community. Although the Green Houses™ have many praiseworthy features, they fall short on connection to community.

OBJECTIVE: Provide each elder with a private room and bath.

FIELD OBSERVATIONS: The building has been specifically designed to provide each of the 10 private-occupancy resident rooms with its own full bathroom, complete with accessible shower. The location and layout of the bathroom allow the overhead lift system to transport nonambulatory residents into their bathrooms. However, this cannot be accomplished without staff assistance and the removal of a solid bathroom door. Thus, the privacy gained by providing individual bathrooms is lost once a resident reaches the point of needing transfer.

The resident rooms, each about 260 square feet, allow only a minimal amount of personal furniture in the room. Additionally, the room proportions and the location of the overhead lift system significantly restrict the placement of furniture.

OBJECTIVE: Protect the natural habitat of the site.

FIELD OBSERVATIONS: Although it appears that the natural vegetation grew unchecked around the site for the

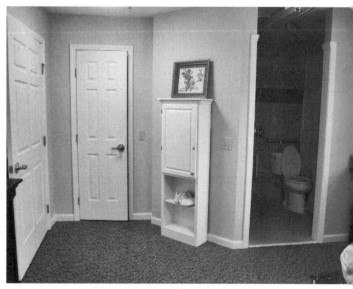

FIG. 18-5 Resident room entry, closet, and medication storage are all located in a confined space *Photograph by Jeffrey Anderzhon*

buildings, there is very little mature or specimen-quality vegetation. With few exceptions, the sites for the buildings were clear-cut without regard for existing vegetation, and were graded to the building levels required. Some larger trees were saved from what appears to have been a fairly dense young forest; however, these trees are of questionable visual value and perhaps were spared only because of their size.

The landscaping is minimal: little has been done except seeding of areas around the buildings. Within the fenced courtyard, the landscaping is still lacking and certainly would not engage any resident who might enjoy gardening.

OBJECTIVE: Develop a project that ensures financial support through current Medicaid reimbursement and encourages replication.

FIELD OBSERVATIONS: The approach of designing smaller buildings or houses certainly reduces the cost of construction by moving into the realm of residential building. (See Figure 17 in the color insert.) This type of construction can be accomplished by a wider variety of contractors and is not necessarily relegated to those who specialize in nursing home or health care construction.

Replication of this model is a goal that has been and continues to be met. Whether the popularity of the Green Houses™ concept comes from promotion by the developers or from the actual appeal of the design, it has attracted interest around the country and spawned the construction of numerous replications.

The residential methods, means of construction, and staffing approach have minimized the costs of care delivery within this model of facility, making it attractive for maximizing any reimbursements from governmental sources. It is prudent to note, however, that our discussion of minimizing the costs of care refers to providing care to the maximum number of individuals—we do not address the quality of that care in this evaluation.

OBJECTIVE: Meet all state regulatory requirements.

FIELD OBSERVATIONS: The Green Houses™ are a striking example of an unconventional nursing facility that is able to meet existing state regulations. Collaboration with state regulators was essential in this case, and this objective should serve as an example to all designers in the field. Moving the creativity of the design beyond the ordinary medical-model nursing facility, and doing so within established regulatory codes and with the cooperation of regulators are all commendable accomplishments. The results of what must have at times been a frustrating effort provide an example that is both daunting and encouraging.

Field Observations: Themes and Hypotheses

Creating Community

Within each small house there is a small community created by residents and staff. The universal-worker approach to staffing increases the amount of interaction time between staff and the residents, and the familiarity among staff and residents enhances the overall sense of community.

Community, however, goes beyond a house's four walls. The location of the Green Houses™, at the extreme end of the retirement campus, and the intervening undeveloped property create an underlying feeling of isolation not only from the larger community of Tupelo, but also from the rest of the retirement campus. All resident participation in campus activities outside of the houses begins with a bus or van ride to the location of the activity. The distance is too great for resident ambulation even if sidewalks had been provided for residents' use. Likewise, all goods are brought to the house on carts from the main campus central delivery.

One of the stated goals of the Green Houses™ concept is for the small nursing homes to be easily integrated into any community fabric. Perhaps the isolation of the homes upon the larger campus is an indication that, from a community standpoint, the homes can operate independently. In fact, if these homes were across the city, their connection to the larger campus would change very little. However, to provide the services necessary for a skilled nursing facility, they must rely on support staff and services provided in another location.

Interactions between the adjacent homes have created a sense of community amongst the residents and staff of the four Green Houses™. The interactions take place in a structured setting and generally revolve around holidays or special events. Usually one house hosts a party in its secured courtyard and invites all the other households to the event.

Making a Home

The Green Houses™ at Traceways are essentially large homes that build a family environment through the design of the building and goals of the care plan. The small group of 10 residents makes it easier for residents to feel like part of a family and to accept the facility as their new home. The kitchen, family-style dining table, and the hearth all try to give residents the amenities of any suburban home and encourage social interactions. Despite the few drawbacks in design, private rooms and

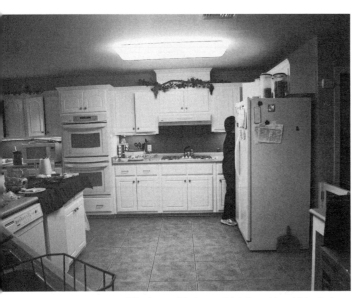

FIG. 18-6 The house kitchen, which is residential in design, is also the hub of resident and staff activity   *Photograph by Jeffrey Anderzhon*

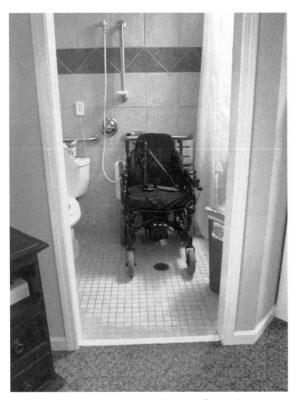

FIG. 18-7 Open showers provide privacy for residents, although this design with the shower in the center of the room is inconvenient to use   *Photograph by Jeffrey Anderzhon*

bathrooms further replicate a single-family home experience, while preserving resident dignity and privacy.

The universal-worker approach inherently encourages more lengthy interaction between residents and staff and within a wider variety of care-provision contexts. Because each house has only 10 residents, it is easy for them to connect with one another and the staff and to consider themselves family members.

More flexibility in the arrangement of furniture would allow residents to feel even more at home in their surroundings: personalization and control of the environment are a key part of making a house a home. One other drawback to the community is the disconnect from the larger community. Perhaps residents would benefit from more involved interaction with residents from other parts of the campus.

Regional/Cultural Design

The houses would fit into many middle-class suburban neighborhoods without revealing that they contain a licensed nursing facility. There is, frankly, nothing outstanding about the architectural aesthetic that serves the purpose of the selected design approach: to blend into a common residential vernacular. Even the interiors take their inspiration from middle-class family rooms, complete with fireplaces, overstuffed recliners, neutral finishes, and high-end kitchen appliances. Every element of the design allows it to fade into and become a part of the landscape of 21st-century suburban America.

Environmental Therapy

There is little doubt that the environment has positively contributed to the residents' quality of life. The improvement was particularly evident as the initial residents of the houses transferred from the more traditional and very institutional nursing facility to their new surroundings.

Residents clearly attested to the benefits of their new environment, often using the word "home" during our interviews. Residents and staff shared anecdotal evidence testifying to the increase in cognitive abilities for some of the residents who were moved into the houses. Of course, the improvements could indicate the benefits of the new environment or reveal the detriments of the old institutional environment.

The efficacy of purely universal workers can be problematic, particularly when the staff is responsible for meal preparation. The time available for resident interaction can be compromised by the time needed for meal preparation and other essential activities.

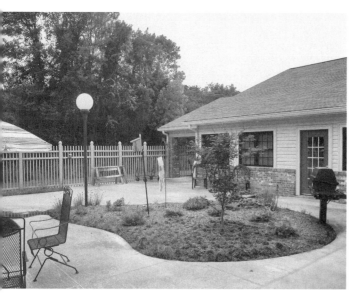

FIG. 18-8 The secured courtyard, though well used, lacks natural shading, and access to the center planting area requires wheelchairs to roll off the hard surface *Photograph by Jeffrey Anderzhon*

Outdoor Environment

The exterior spaces for residents are limited, difficult to access, and lacking in inviting amenities. Residents cannot directly access the exterior, fenced courtyard from the hearth room, but instead must take a circuitous route toward the back of the house and through the den. Residents might use the outdoor spaces more if there were readily available views and clearly accessible routes to the courtyards.

Quality of Workplace and the Physical Plant

Finding available staff for the workplace was not an issue, because of the unique staffing approach and new building. Interviews with both staff and administration indicate that when the new universal-worker approach was presented to the existing staff, there was great clamor to work in the Green Houses™. The quality of the workplace environment is demonstrably higher because of the residential nature of the environment and a kind of natural lessening of stress that accompanies a noninstitutional setting.

Some questions remain regarding the universal-worker concept and its relationship to quality of care. The staff within the households spend much of their time preparing and serving meals. Generally, residents spend a lot of time in the dining and hearth rooms and are within view of staff, but they occasionally need assis-

tance in their own rooms at a time when staff members are occupied preparing meals. Attending to those resident needs requires careful attention so as not to cross-contaminate food after providing care. The staff must also make sure that the task they left unattended does not endanger the residents in the common areas.

Operator Perspectives

There is little question that the owner is quite pleased with the Green Houses™ design and accompanying care-provision approach. The approach to care provision and the design of the Green Houses™ germinated from the care perspective and are deeply connected to one another—the program was thoroughly developed, then followed by an accommodating environmental design.

In conjunction with a national initiative, the Green Houses™ have received a large amount of attention for innovation. They have a firm foundational belief that their unique approach to care provision is more humanistic, and they are willing to share their belief with any visitor. To this extent, the construction of this facility has been highly successful in the eyes of the owner/operator.

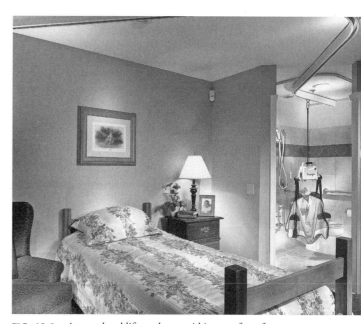

FIG. 18-9 An overhead lift track may aid in transfer safety, but adds an undesirable institutional appearance
© *2003 Jeffrey Jacobs Photography*

General Project Information

PROJECT ADDRESS
The Green Houses at Traceway Retirement Community
2800 West Main Street
Tupelo, MS 38801

PROJECT DESIGN TEAM
Architect: The McCarty Company-Design Group, P.A.
Interior Designer: The McCarty Company-Design
    Group, P.A.
Landscape Architect: Philips Garden Center
Structural Engineer: N/A
Mechanical Engineer: The McCarty Company-Design
    Group, P.A.
Electrical Engineer: The McCarty Company-Design
    Group, P.A.
Civil Engineer: Site Engineering Consultants
Dining Consultant: N/A
Gerontologist: N/A
Management/Development: N/A
Contractor: The McCarty Company-Construction
    Group, Inc.

PROJECT STATUS
Completion date: April 2003

OCCUPANCY LEVELS
At facility opening date: 100%
At date of evaluation: 100%

RESIDENT AGE (YRS)
At facility opening date: 82
At date of evaluation: 85

PROJECT AREAS

SKILLED NURSING

Project Element	New Construction	
	No. Beds	Typical Room Size
Residents in one-bed/single rooms	40	260 GSF
Total	40	10,424 GSF
Social areas (lounges, dining, and recreation space):		10,104 GSF
Medical, health care, therapy, and activities spaces:		772 GSF
Administrative, public, and ancillary support services:		2,496 GSF
Service, maintenance, and mechanical areas:		364 GSF
Total gross area:		24,160 GSF
Total net usable area (per space program):		18,872 NSF
Overall gross/net factor (ratio of gross area/net usable area):		1.28

SITE AND PARKING

SITE LOCATION
Small town

SITE SIZE
Acres: 13.9
Square feet: 608,563
Area of entire campus: 51.2 acres

PARKING

Type of Parking	For This Facility			
	Residents	Staff	Visitors	Totals
Open surface lot(s)	0	6	17	23

CONSTRUCTION COSTS

SOURCE OF COST DATA
Final construction cost as of August 15, 2003

SOFT COSTS

Land cost or value:	$48,000
Basic architectural and engineering:	$174,715
Expanded architectural and engineering:	$23,883
All permit and other entitlement fees:	$4,964
Legal:	$1,373
Appraisals:	$3,500
Marketing and preopening:	N/A
Total soft costs:	$256,435

BUILDING COSTS

New construction except FF&E, special finishes, floor and window coverings, HVAC, and electrical and medical equipment:	$1,162,573
Renovations except FF&E, special finishes, floor and window coverings, HVAC, and electrical:	N/A
FF&E and small wares:	$47,655
Floor coverings:	$130,216
Window coverings:	$1,050
HVAC, plumbing, fire protection:	$547,781
Electrical:	$351,483
Medical equipment costs:	$114,555
Total building costs:	$2,355,313

SITE COSTS

New on-site:	$454,672
New off-site:	$99,739
Renovation on-site:	N/A
Renovation off-site:	N/A
Landscape:	$3,930
Special site features or amenities:	N/A
Total site costs:	$558,341

TOTAL PROJECT COSTS
(include all fees and costs, except financing)
Total project costs: $3,170,089

FINANCING SOURCES
$2.8 million was raised from the local community; interim bank loan for 18 months to be converted to permanent financing using tax-exempt revenue bonds

CARE COMPARISONS

Source: www.medicare.gov—July 15, 2005
SNF staffing: 4.90 care hours/resident/day
SNF occupancy: 140 of 140 = 100% (total for entire campus)

Hours per Resident per Day	Traceway in MS (Cedars Health Center)	MS Average	National Average
Not-for-profit	Yes		
Multifacility	Yes		
Levels of care	CCRC		
Medicare	Yes		
Medicaid	Yes		
Licensed #	140		
# residents	140	85.7	95.3
% occ this day	100%		
RNs	0.42	0.40	0.50
LPNs	0.88	0.90	0.70
RN + LPN	1.32	1.30	1.20
CNA	3.58	2.40	2.30
RN + LPN + CNA	4.90	3.70	3.50

"The hardest years in life are those between ten and seventy."

HELEN HAYES (AT AGE 83), 1900–1993

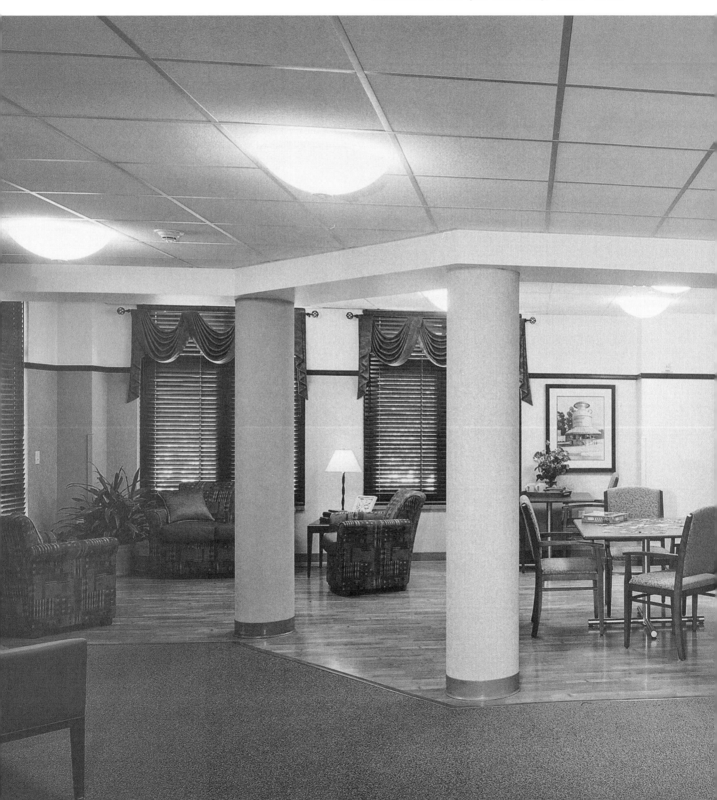

Chapter 19

The Colorado State Veterans Home at Fitzsimons

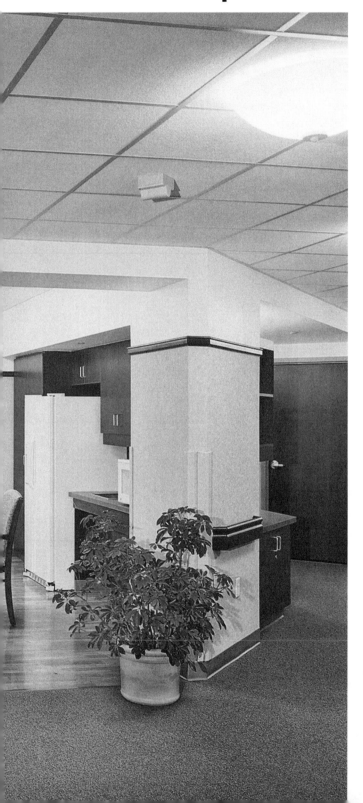

EVALUATION SITE: The Colorado State Veterans Home at Fitzsimons

COMMUNITY TYPE: Skilled Nursing
- 180 nursing care residents

REGION: Rocky Mountain Front Range

ARCHITECT: Boulder Associates

OWNER: State of Colorado, Department of Human Services

DATA POINTS:

Nursing Private Resident Room:	265 gsf
Nursing Shared-Occupancy Resident Room:	425 gsf
Total Area:	125,000 gsf
Nursing Total Area:	694 gsf/resident
Total Project Cost:	$24,835,740
Project Cost:	$198.69/gsf
Investment/resident:	$137,976.33
Staffing:	3.9 care hours/resident/day
Occupancy:	92% as of January 2006

FIRST OCCUPANCY: July 2002

DATE OF EVALUATION: January 2006

EVALUATION TEAM: Jeremy Vickers; David Slack; Jeffrey Anderzhon, AIA; Jane Rohde, AIA, FIIDA; John Shoesmith, AIA

FIG. 19-1 Each family room serves as a nourishment center and has access to the outdoors ©*Lacasse Photography*

Introduction

At the base of the Rocky Mountains, Denver is the gateway to the new West and the end of the journey across the Great Plains. It is fitting that the State Veterans Home at Fitzsimons, in suburban Denver, could be either the model for future, large veterans nursing facilities or the ultimate conclusion to the modified medical model of facilities.

The 180-resident facility is dissected into eight units—divided evenly between two floors—of either 42 or 48 residents. The facility is too small to call itself a traditional or medical-model nursing facility, but is too large to undertake a household approach to nursing care. Falling somewhere in the middle, the facility does break down the more familiar approaches of veterans nursing facilities, but does not completely adopt the philosophy of culture change through a more resident-oriented environmental design.

This nursing facility lies on a level grade in front of the mountains in Aurora, Colorado, on a medical campus that evolved from a military fort. (See Figure 18 in the color insert.) The imposing structure of the facility embraces the fort or campus by an angled bedroom wing toward the east, and turns its back on the security fence separating the campus from the surrounding one-story residential neighborhood. The two-story, stuccoed structure contradicts the notion that land is an abundant commodity west of the Mississippi River and adds an inner-facility, vertical connectivity component.

Arriving at the facility by vehicle is somewhat confusing, as one must enter the campus fully, traverse around the building, and backtrack to the main building entry. Adult day care was originally included in the building program, and its separate entry (along with employee entry and vendor deliveries) is on the back side of the building. The entries are somewhat difficult for first-time visitors to discover and can be disorienting. There is an underlying feeling as you enter that you are

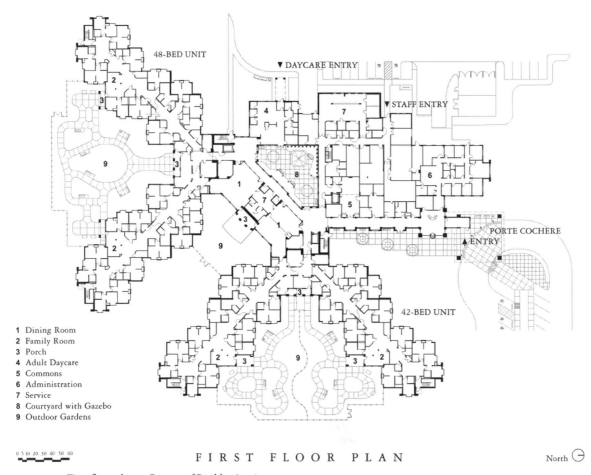

1 Dining Room
2 Family Room
3 Porch
4 Adult Daycare
5 Commons
6 Administration
7 Service
8 Courtyard with Gazebo
9 Outdoor Gardens

0 5 10 20 30 40 50 60

FIRST FLOOR PLAN

North

FIG. 19-2 First-floor plan   *Courtesy of Boulder Associates*

straying into unwelcome territory and trespassing on guarded territory.

Architect's Statement

The program called for a state-of-the-art, 180-bed, skilled nursing facility that would provide maximum independence for the veterans while optimizing staffing and other operational aspects to minimize expenses. Two 42-bed and two 48-bed nursing units were developed in a crenellated cluster design that features decentralized alcoves for nurse aides. Using a flexible, pager-enabled call system, cluster sizes are adjusted to fit staffing needs at each shift. Only 20 of 180 beds are private, so biaxial and L-shaped double rooms with dividing walls were developed. Each resident has equal access to the corridor, to the toilet room, and to the windows. Bay windows with window seats increase usable space without exceeding maximum allowable room sizes. Resident toilet rooms feature oversized accordion doors, extra maneuvering space, and folding grab bars flanking the water closet for functional accessibility exceeding ADA requirements.

Designers' and Owners' Stated Objectives and Responses

OBJECTIVE: Create a design that maximizes staffing efficiency and recognizes that 80% of life-cycle operating costs for a facility are staff-related.

DESIGN INTENT: The facility's 180 beds are divided into two 42-bed units and two 48-bed units. Each unit is further divided into six equal clusters, each with a CNA work area to allow one CNA per seven or eight residents during the day. The units reconfigure into four clusters in the evening (1:10/11/12) and again into three clusters at night (1:14/16). Sizing the units this way ensures that there are no unnecessary full-time employees on any shift. Support and social areas are decentralized on the units to reduce travel and transportation time. Dining rooms are also decentralized, one per unit, to reduce travel distances and are paired so that a single serving pantry supplies food to two dining rooms.

OBJECTIVE: Empower and enable residents to be as independent as possible.

DESIGN INTENT: Because the cluster design and decentralized family and dining rooms reduce travel distances, it is easier for residents to travel freely throughout the build-

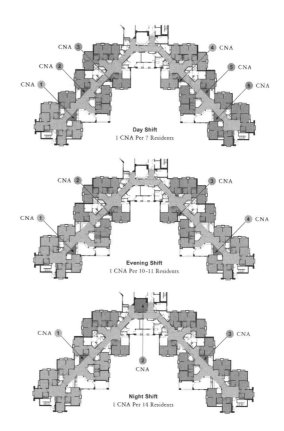

STAFFING | 42-BED SKILLED NURSING UNIT

FIG. 19-3 The staffing plan that efficiently locates staff on different shifts *Courtesy of Boulder Associates*

ing. Resident rooms are designed for flexibility in bed and furniture placement and allow residents to customize their rooms. The customization is not only beneficial in terms of resident choice and independence, but it is especially helpful for residents who may be weaker on one side due to stroke or other injury. The toilet rooms, with grab bars, plenty of space for maneuvering, and wide doorways, also enable independence for residents.

OBJECTIVE: Maximize privacy for residents.

DESIGN INTENT: Despite the double-occupancy rooms, all resident rooms were designed to give each resident his or her own space. Neither resident passes through the other's personal space to reach the vestibule, corridor, or toilet room. The individual bay windows and thermostats further eliminate the need for residents to intrude into their roommate's space. Toilet-room doors within the resident rooms are oversized accordion doors, made easier to operate for privacy by adding two extra accordion panels so that the door need not be pulled taut.

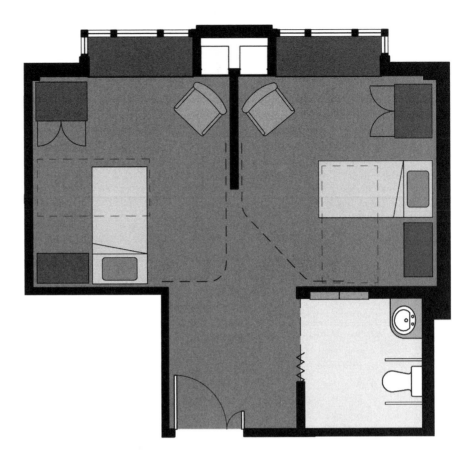

FIG. 19-4 Shared-occupancy resident room plan *Courtesy of Boulder Associates*

Bathing suites are located near the midpoint of each leg of a unit, minimizing travel distances and avoiding the need for residents to pass major public areas such as dining or activity rooms to reach the suites. Although it was hoped that only one resident at a time would use the bathing suite, each area (grooming, toilet, shower, and tub) is separated from the others by full-height privacy curtains or accordion doors. The shower area has a separate drying area.

OBJECTIVE: Provide functional accessibility that exceeds the Americans with Disabilities Act (ADA) and the Uniform Federal Accessibility Standards (UFAS) requirements.

DESIGN INTENT: We believe that ANSI A117.1 establishes minimum accessibility standards that work well in many situations. However, when designing for seniors, some areas require larger clearances and alternative designs to enable residents to remain as independent as possible. Federal ADA and UFAS regulations reference ANSI A117.1, which mandates an 18-inch dimension from the centerline of a water closet to the sidewall and horizontal, wall-mounted grab bars. Although this design provides good accessibility for a younger wheelchair user

with good upper body strength, it does not work as well for an older person, and it does not allow space for aides to assist with transfers. The federal Veterans Administration (VA) recognizes this and has changed its standards for VA nursing homes but not for state veterans homes.

The Paralyzed Veterans of America helped to advocate for the water closets to be moved away from the sidewall and to include flanking fold-down grab bars in all resident toilet rooms. This provides better accessibility and flexibility to move the bars out of the way for staff-assisted transfers.

Vertically split room doors give residents a normal-size, lighter entrance door with easy maneuvering on the pull side and a wider path when the other leaf is held open by a hold-open closer. Bedrooms are sized to allow adequate clearances for wheelchairs and walkers around the beds. The available combinations of furniture configurations allow rooms to be configured for optimal accessibility for each resident.

OBJECTIVE: Design universal resident units to allow for future flexibility.

DESIGN INTENT: The four nursing units are universally designed to allow special populations, such as short-term rehabilitation or dementia-care clients, to be housed together if desired. Because many residents suffer from some level of dementia, all resident wings are designed to avoid overstimulation yet feel comfortable to family, staff, and residents alike. Each unit can be divided into as many as four sections, using smoke-barrier and area-separation doors to create subunits as small as 10 or 11 beds. The pager-enabled call system allows customization in keeping with varying unit sizes and types. As the resident population changes, and as new therapies for dementia care become available, the building design will support the inevitable changes needed in unit sizes and types.

Field Observations: Meeting the Objectives

OBJECTIVE: Create a design that maximizes staffing efficiency and recognizes that 80% of life-cycle operating costs for a facility are staff-related.

FIELD OBSERVATIONS: It is commendable that concerns related to staffing are given status equal to other, more traditional design decisions. Perhaps the design team's decision to approach the new facility with staffing squarely in mind signals a shift in the issues that will be critical to designers of the future. A design approach that places staff use and patterns paramount to other decisions certainly makes sense given the significant portion of operating resources devoted to employees. This design layout pays particular attention to the location of staffing within the parameters of particular shifts, and makes sense, at least on paper.

Success on paper does not always hold water in reality. Unfortunately, this is the case at Fitzsimons, but not out of neglect for the design. The amount of time spent on the environmental design was wasted because the management and the staff who use the building on a daily basis do not use it as planned and have allowed their care provision to evolve in a natural fashion that ignores the design. This is in no small part due to significant turnover in upper-level management following the opening of the facility.

The frontline caregivers have been given neither training nor an explanation of the intended use of the environment. Although training would have helped at first, it is possible that, despite consistent reinforcement about the environment and its intended use, the staff still would have adopted the current model. They have overridden the intentions of the designers and work in a manner most convenient to them personally. Generally, staff work at a location where the resident charts are filed, where fellow staff members seem to congregate,

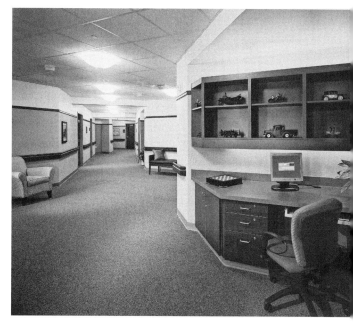

FIG. 19-5 The view along a household corridor with nursing desk   ©*Lacasse Photography*

and where the communication technology is located, as opposed to the alcoves provided in certain staffing areas.

OBJECTIVE: Empower and enable residents to be as independent as possible.

FIELD OBSERVATIONS: The design of the resident clusters, with individual kitchen and activity areas, was a good beginning to the decentralization of services and a step in the right direction for the creation of a more cohesive and identifiable household. Each of these neighborhoods contains either 21 or 24 residents situated along a diagonal circulation spine terminating at the centrally located dining, activity, social, and main circulation portions of the building. Two diagonal households create a nicely sized, fenced courtyard.

The inclusion of 21 residents within this arrangement creates a fairly lengthy distance from the furthest resident room to the central portion of the building. Although the design—which includes niches for staff desks and widened areas for resident room entries—diminishes the visual length of this corridor, it does remain a fairly long corridor bereft of natural light or visual connection to the exterior. The considerable traffic to and from the central dining and activity areas simply exacerbates the unmistakably institutional feel of the corridor.

The family rooms located near the center of the households each include a limited kitchen with a refrigerator. The location of these rooms seems to be somewhat arbitrary and does not provide either a visual or physical destination. The areas appear to be underutilized by residents and do not appear to be used at all for meal service or other significant activities. The centrally located dining rooms provide all regularly scheduled meals but incorporating flexible mealtimes would empower residents to eat when it is convenient and desirable for them, not staff. The kitchenette in the family room would provide that flexibility, but the design is not used as intended and fails to aid in empowering residents' meal choices.

Although the central dining room relies on scheduled meals, space originally allotted for an adult day care program has been taken over by a creative dietary staff as a dining space that provides a limited menu and short-order dining for residents and staff. The popularity of the program and the resulting interactions between staff and residents prove the success of this amenity and show that it deserved to be a part of the original design.

OBJECTIVE: Maximize privacy for residents.

FIELD OBSERVATIONS: Design parameters allowed a maximum of 20 private resident rooms, and as a result maximizing resident privacy became more difficult and more important. The privacy issue is addressed in the design by incorporating "toe-to-toe" bed arrangements divided by a solid wall. The bed arrangement, along with bay windows for each resident, does enhance privacy and personal space, especially compared to a more traditional, medical-model resident room design; although the rooms are a step up from the shared rooms

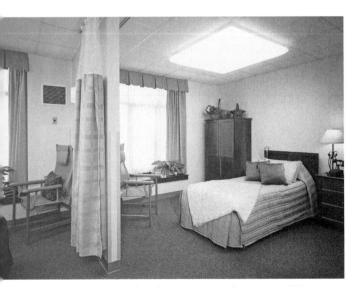

FIG. 19-6   A shared-occupancy resident room   ©*Lacasse Photography*

in many nursing facilities, this compromise still falls short of fully private rooms, particularly because the resident toilet rooms are shared by two individuals who may or may not be compatible. The design does provide definable individual space and individually identifiable visual access to the exterior in a way that visually enlarges the resident room area. It is also commendable that the resident room design includes individually controlled mechanical units so that each resident can maintain personal air comfort levels.

OBJECTIVE: Provide functional accessibility that exceeds ADA and UFAS requirements.

FIELD OBSERVATIONS: The standards set forth in the ADA and the UFAS were derived for a "stereotypical" individual who needs assistive devices for the activities of daily living. Unfortunately, individuals who require such devices cannot be stereotyped. It is commendable that this design considers the population living within the environment rather than blindly prescribing to the existing standards, thereby relieving staff and residents of the inconvenience of heavy, institutional resident room doors and grab-bar locations that hinder more than they help.

Although the design most likely does not exceed ADA and UFAs requirements, it does provide functional accessibility for an elderly population and for staffing assistance. As with the consideration of staff interaction with the environment, the design explores alternatives and details that allow residents more independence even when they require physical assistance.

OBJECTIVE: Design universal resident units to allow for future flexibility.

FIELD OBSERVATIONS: A truly universal design would allow a resident to age in place and remain within the environment with little or no modification even as the resident's needs change. The resident rooms were designed for some, though not much, versatility. However, the introduction of a large bay window in each resident space and the minimal length of the wall dividing shared rooms limit furniture arrangements for full access by both resident and staff. There is very little space for socializing or visiting with guests, and there are institutional hospital privacy curtains around the bed. The curtains do block visual access but do nothing to minimize sound transmission.

When imagining the possibilities for future adaptations and modifications of elderly congregate living communities, often the focus is upon the shift from nursing to assisted living or the adoption of an environment designed specifically for dementia-care residents. The size of the resident rooms and the double-loaded corridor configuration do not lend themselves to flexibility or adaptability. The corridor design also limits the size or subdivision of the units into different households, as one would need to pass through one household to access another. Additionally, a subdivision like this would further break down the community and isolate at least half of the subunits.

Field Observations: Themes and Hypotheses

Creating Community

A community is born when a resident population with similar interests, backgrounds, or beliefs develops a foundation for social interaction. Many elderly campuses, particularly those operated by not-for-profits, focus on a commonality of religion or other affinity group, such as military veterans. There are some complicating factors when developing a community of veterans. Although the facilities primarily serve veterans, nonveteran residents live there as well. Also, even veterans have lived lives outside of their years of service and have developed other interests and hobbies.

Creation of a community must go beyond strategically placed military memorabilia. A community requires social interaction with others within that community, shared common activities, and the ability to maintain a connection to the larger community surrounding the campus. It is the responsibility of the environmental design to meet all these requirements by providing both the space and the ambience to do so.

Over the years, the converted military base that the aging veterans call home has evolved into a combination government and health care campus, but it has retained its inwardly focused, fortress-like feeling. The Veterans Home reinforces this feeling by orienting the main entry inward toward the base and placing the delivery and back-of-house functions toward the main street to the west of the building. The architectural statement is that the facility is turning its back on the community and turning in on the base. The Home is at once isolating itself from the surrounding community and stating that it is reserved for a particular clientele—which is not entirely negative, as the community is designed with veterans in mind. However, even the military clientele lived and worked beyond the base fences and may want to preserve their connections to the broader community.

Within the building itself, there is a layering of community. Households are paired and intersect at com-

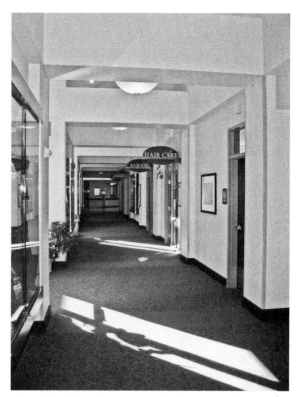

FIG. 19-7   The main entry corridor "main street" with natural light, display cases, and shops   *Photograph by Jeffrey Anderzhon*

mon dining and activity areas, so it seems natural for each of the pairs to intersect with the adjoining pair of households on the same floor. Unfortunately, this does not occur, and is in fact discouraged by the design of the building.

Within the administrative and support portion of the building, a sort of "main street" has been included that houses a library, barber\beauty shop, and ice cream parlor. The corridor from the main entry leads to this social area, with "stores" on one side and ample glass with appealing visual access to the exterior on the other. This is a pleasing area that is underplayed in design, does not fully take advantage of the exterior space, and has undersized spaces for main-street activities.

Although not a part of the building program or planning, the space originally dedicated to the discontinued adult day care program was successfully converted to community use. The room is fairly easy for the residents to access and is big enough for large gatherings without being cavernous. The dietary staff's successful implementation of a dining option in this space allows residents to order breakfast and lunch from a limited menu. The space has access to the central courtyard for barbecues in good weather or for refreshment and gatherings after the band concerts that occasionally take place in the courtyard. The uses for the space will undoubtedly expand as the imaginations of staff and residents explore further options. It is fortunate that the space is now available, especially given that the original design and building program did not include a multipurpose space that could accommodate a fairly large number of residents for community gatherings.

Making a Home

Individual thermostats, bay windows, and wardrobes are commendable attempts to give residents their own space, even in shared rooms. However, by necessity the design forces residents to share a portion of the room and the toilet room, which certainly diminishes the aspect of individual ownership and correspondingly diminishes any feelings of home. Accordion doors in the toilet rooms, no matter how they have been modified for ease of use, create an institutional aesthetic and further exacerbate the diminished feeling of home.

The size and proportion of the resident's private area and the use of wardrobes rather than distinctive closet areas for clothing restrict furniture arrangements to only two realistic configurations, and further limit resident choice in this regard. The selection of a large and visually overpowering overhead lighting fixture provides lighting levels appropriate for elderly eyes, but does so in a manner that is almost completely overwhelming to the individual entering the room. Because the fixture is the only light in the room, and because the level of light cannot be faded or dimmed, care after dark rudely awakens both residents.

Regional/Cultural Design

The design of the Colorado State Veterans Home arguably takes its inspiration from a southwestern aesthetic. Faux stucco and faux accent clay barrel-tile roofs recall a southwestern architectural feel rendered in contemporary materials. Beyond the use of exterior materials, however, the design and the interior of the building pay little homage to the building location, geographically or culturally. Inside the building, visitors quickly realize that they are in a nursing facility that could be anywhere in the country—which is disappointing given that the entire resident population hails from Colorado.

The homogeneous space and apparent assumption—conscious or unconscious—that all veterans share similar health needs not only demean the space but also underestimate the staff and residents living and working

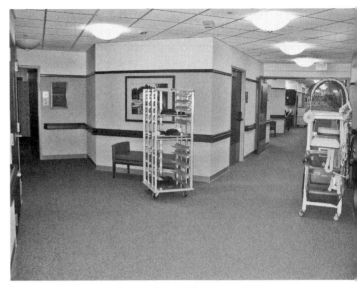

FIG. 19-8   The offset design of the resident room entry provides a place for carts, but does not eliminate them from the corridors   *Photograph by Jeffrey Anderzhon*

within the building. The design inadvertently drives the care program and the environment toward institutionalization and neglects a regional design vernacular that the occupants are most likely accustomed to. The exterior design of the building comes closer to achieving that success than does the interior. This is not to say that the interior is not pleasing or well done; it just fails to trumpet its geographic location and culture of the residents.

Despite shortcomings in regional design, the interior spaces are accommodating, warm, and charming. The pleasing environment surely lowers the anxiety levels naturally experienced by residents moving into a congregate living facility. With the glaring exception of the dining areas, acoustics are well controlled and provide a sort of contemplative feeling throughout the facilities.

Environmental Therapy

A great deal of attention was paid to the environment's ability to assist staff in everyday care provision and ensure that a heightened, more personal level of care is provided to residents. This approach was not fully implemented and the environment falls short of fully realizing its potential regarding resident therapy. Although disappointing, the failure is not on the part of the architects or the constructed environment, but is a result of the unfortunate disconnection between the design and the way the staff was trained—or more appropriately, not trained—to use the space.

This facility is clearly a preliminary step in a long journey of environmental change for a bureaucratically bound client. The design cracked the door to a less institutional approach to long-term care for a very institutionally inclined client. It attempts, through design, to create an environment that encourages independence for residents and efficiency for staff. When compared to older veterans homes, Fitzsimons succeeds, but it falls a bit short when compared to contemporary standards in long-term care. The disparity is not because the designers did not attempt to push the envelope, but because the client pushed only as far as its comfort level would allow.

In the end, an environment that provides a comparatively more meaningful and therapeutic atmosphere for residents was achieved. Choices, though limited, are provided to both resident and staff to enhance care provision and provide a less institutional environment that has yet to achieve its full potential.

Outdoor Environment

Well-defined and accessible exterior areas between the resident households naturally expand in width as the resident wings extend outward and away from each other. The areas are visually accessible from each of the resident rooms along the courtyard, but are physically accessible from the family rooms through two covered porches, one off of the family room and one adjacent to the activity room. Unfortunately, neither of the access points is readily visible by either staff or residents unless they are fully

within the family or activity rooms. As a result, the space is underused, and staff are less likely to allow residents full access to the space because they are not able to watch the residents without being in the courtyard or adjacent rooms. Additionally, reaching the activity rooms and navigating through the furniture and tight spaces can be difficult for residents, particularly those using ambulation assistance devices.

The courtyards have concrete walkways and decorative fencing to deter resident elopement. Park-bench seating staggered along the walkways provides rest areas along the way for residents exercising or walking in the area. However, there is only very sparse landscaping, no shade, and the only obvious activity is walking. There are no resident-accessible planting beds, structured shading devices, or devices for resident-directed, passive activities. The courtyards are visually attractive, with an expanse of green that seems to grow and widen when viewed from the building. Unfortunately, the spaces are difficult to reach and can be somewhat boring.

Opposite the central dining areas and across a corridor, there is a courtyard fully surrounded by the structure of the building. This small area is mostly surfaced with concrete, but has landscaped areas and shade trees. A nicely detailed and scaled gazebo is also located in this courtyard, along with several tables and movable chairs. The courtyard is easy to see from the adjacent corridor through which all visitors and staff must traverse to access the resident areas.

The inner courtyard is shaded by the surrounding building and gazebo structure and is attractive, inviting,

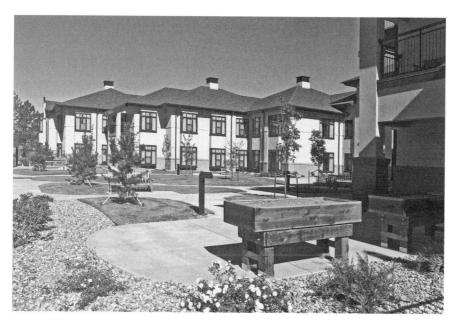

FIG. 19-9 Secured courtyards are large and without intimacy, and thus limit resident social activity
©*Lacasse Photography*

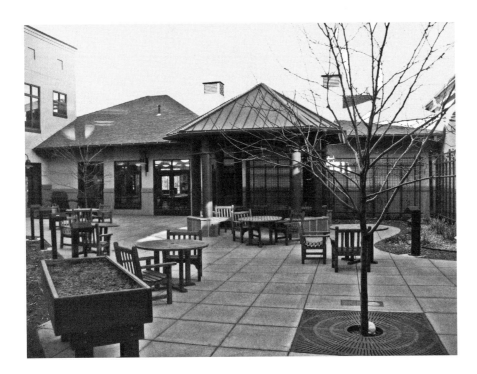

FIG. 19-10 The central courtyard hosts military band concerts, barbecues, and other outdoor activities for the entire facility *Photograph by Jeffrey Anderzhon*

and secure from resident elopement without overt staff supervision. It is somewhat confining, but this in fact adds an element of vibrancy and activity that draws residents to the space. It appears that residents prefer to spend their time outdoors in this courtyard and that it serves to promote community social interaction. Compared to the other available exterior spaces, it is little wonder that this courtyard is in constant demand.

Quality of Workplace and the Physical Plant

The failure of the attempts to tailor the design to the needs of staff has in actuality complicated the delivery of care. Discussions with frontline staff and department heads revealed consistent surprise that the shape of the corridors and the inclusion of niche desks for staff were intended to encourage staff efficiency. The building is certainly not used as intended by the design efforts. The staff and administration indicate that the inset resident room doors and desk niches in the corridors actually increase staffing needs because there is less direct physical communication to the rooms.

Operator Perspectives

Although significant design resources were devoted to coordinating the environment and work locations for the staff, in the end the purpose of those spaces was not communicated to staff or to the current administration. The centralized dining and activity rooms have challenged operations. The administration would prefer to move closer to a true household concept, but this would require decentralized dining and would render the larger dining room and supporting commercial pantries unnecessary. Furthermore, in the case of decentralized dining, the location of the commercial kitchen would become even more remote and would further increase staff inefficiency.

The administration is also convinced that the environmental design, particularly the location of spaces and the niches in the corridors, contributes to a diminished level of activity by residents. They tend to stay in their rooms, either fearful of the lengthy walk to an activity space or disoriented by the numerous angles and niches along the corridor.

General Project Information

PROJECT ADDRESS

The Colorado State Veterans Home at Fitzsimons
1919 Quentin Street
Aurora, Colorado 80010

PROJECT DESIGN TEAM

Architect: Boulder Associates, Inc.
Associate Architect: Luis O. Acosta Architects, PC
Interior Designer: Boulder Associates, Inc. with SOdesign
Landscape Architect: Valerian, LLC
Structural Engineer: J.C. Baur & Associates
Mechanical Engineer: McGrath, Inc.
Electrical Engineer: BCER Engineering, Inc.
Civil Engineer: Rocky Mountain Consultants, Inc.
Gerontologist: Lorraine G. Hiatt, Ph.D.
Dietary Consultant: Systems Design International, Inc.
Cost Consultant: Hanscomb, Inc.
Contractor: Roche Constructors, Inc.

OCCUPANCY LEVELS

At facility opening date: 6%
At time of evaluation: 75%

RESIDENT AGE (YRS)

Upon initial opening: 76
At time of evaluation: 71
(Note: Approximately 70% of residents were male at time of evaluation)

PROJECT STATUS

Completion date: July 2002

PROJECT AREAS

PROJECT AREAS

Project Element	Included in This Project			Total On-site or Served by Project
	Units, Beds, or Clients	New GSF	Total Gross Area	
Skilled nursing care (beds)	180	101,550	101,550	180
Common social areas (people)	180	14,350	14,350	180
Kitchen (daily meals served)	660	3,850	3,850	660
Elder day care (clients)	24	2,150	2,150	24
Fitness/rehabilitation/wellness (daily visits)	40	3,100	3,100	40

SKILLED NURSING

Project Element	New Construction	
	No. Beds	Typical Room Size
Residents in one-bed/single rooms	20	265 GSF
Residents in two-bed/double rooms	160	425 GSF
Totals	180	39,300 GSF
Social areas (lounges, dining, and recreation spaces):		13,400 GSF
Medical, health care, therapy, and activities spaces:		7,200 GSF
Administrative, public, and ancillary support services:		19,500 GSF
Service, maintenance, and mechanical areas:		13,900 GSF
Total gross area:		125,000 GSF
Total net usable area (per space program):		84,470 NSF
Overall gross/net factor (ratio of gross area/net usable area):		1.48

SITE AND PARKING

SITE LOCATION
Urban

SITE SIZE
Acres: 15.0
Square feet: 653,400

PARKING

Type of Parking	For This Facility Residents	Staff	Visitors	Totals
Open surface lot(s)	0	98	22	120

CONSTRUCTION COSTS

SOURCE OF COST DATA
Final construction cost as of July 2002

SOFT COSTS

Land cost or value (land conveyed to state by federal government, no appraisal available):	$0
Basic architectural and engineering:	$1,528,993
Expanded architectural and engineering:	$666,707
All permit and other entitlement fees:	$307,993
Legal:	$0
Appraisals:	$0
Marketing and preopening:	$33,872
Total soft costs:	$2,537,565

BUILDING COSTS

New construction except FF&E, special finishes, floor and window coverings, HVAC, and electrical:	$13,646,199
Renovations except FF&E, special finishes, floor and window coverings, HVAC, and electrical:	$23,451
FF&E and small wares:	$1,402,227
Floor coverings:	$547,814
Window coverings:	$134,500
HVAC:	$2,444,470
Electrical:	$1,727,098
Medical equipment costs:	$533,327
Total building costs:	$20,459,086

SITE COSTS

New on-site:	$1,648,413
New off-site:	$0
Renovation on-site:	$0
Renovation off-site:	$0
Landscape:	$190,676
Special site features or amenities:	$0
Total site costs:	$1,839,089

TOTAL PROJECT COSTS
Total project costs: $24,835,740

FINANCING SOURCES
The Federal Veterans Administration provided 65% of construction costs, FF&E, and some soft costs. The state funded the remaining 35% plus all other costs not funded by the VA.

CARE COMPARISON

Source: www.medicare.gov—January 30, 2006
SNF staffing: 4.80 care hours/resident/day
SNF occupancy: 152 of 180 = 84.4%

Hours per Resident per Day	Colorado Veterans Home	CO Average	National Average
Not-for-profit	Yes		
Multifacility	No		
Levels of care	SNF		
Medicare	Yes		
Medicaid	Yes		
Licensed #	180		
# residents	152	82.8	95.3
% occ this day	84.4%		
RNs	0.98	0.70	0.50
LPNs	0.98	0.70	0.70
RN + LPN	1.98	1.40	1.20
CNA	2.80	2.20	2.30
RN + LPN + CNA	4.78	3.60	3.50

"Age is an issue of mind over matter. If you don't mind, it doesn't matter."

MARK TWAIN, 1835–1910

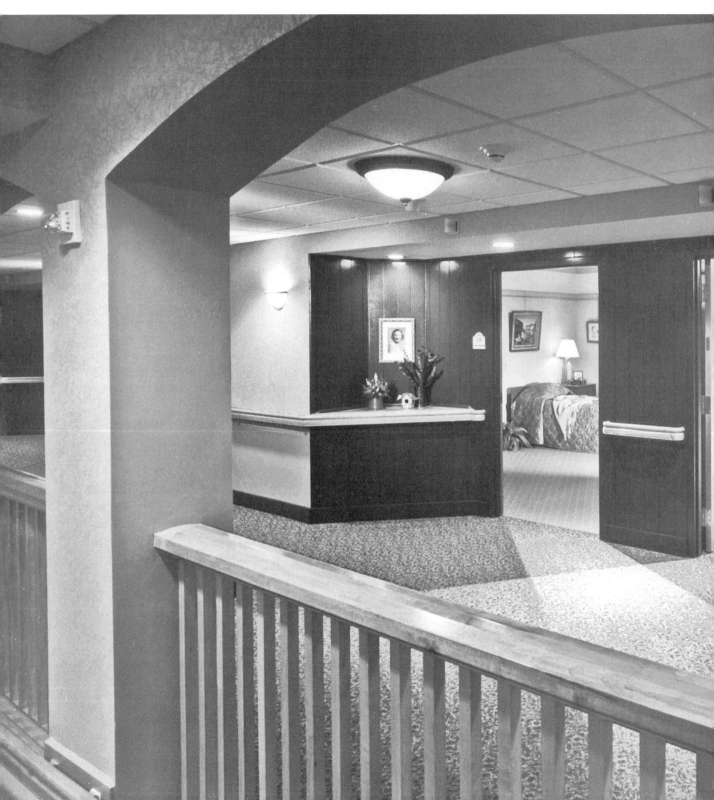

Chapter 20

Foulkeways at Gwynedd

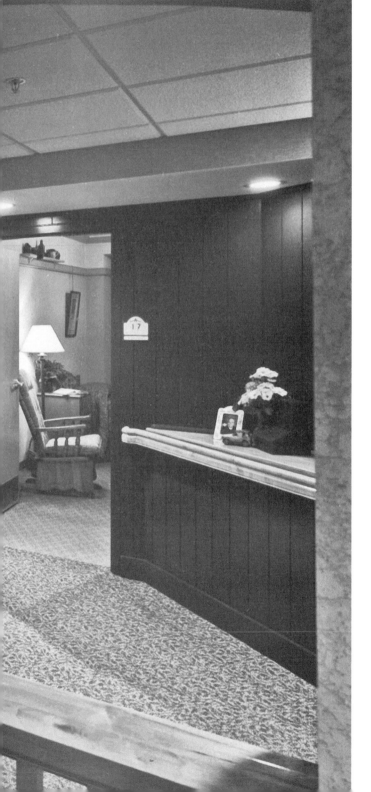

EVALUATION SITE: Foulkeways at Gwynedd

COMMUNITY TYPE: Skilled Nursing Component of CCRC
• 40 nursing care beds

REGION: Mid-Atlantic

ARCHITECT: Reese, Lower, Patrick & Scott, Ltd.

OWNER: Foulkeways at Gwynedd, Inc.

DATA POINTS: Resident Room: 350 gsf
Total Area: 1,306 gsf/resident
Total Area: 52,223 gsf
Project Cost: $205.47/gsf
Total Project Cost: $10,730,072
Investment/resident: $268,251.80
Staffing: 5.20 care hours/resident/day
Occupancy: 95% as of June 2005

FIRST OCCUPANCY: August 2001

DATE OF EVALUATION: June 2005

EVALUATION TEAM: David Slack; Dana Barton; Melissa Strunk; Ingrid Fraley, ASID; Mitch Green, AIA; Jeffrey Anderzhon, AIA

FIG. 20-1 Simple contrasts highlight resident room entries from the single-loaded corridor *Courtesy RLPS Architects/Larry Lefever Photography*

Introduction

Setting excellent standards since 1967, the Foulkeways at Gwynedd retirement community honors the Quaker values of respecting the equality and dignity of each individual. Notably, the facility was the first continuing care retirement community established in Pennsylvania and the first in the nation affiliated with the Religious Society of Friends (Quakers). The community came to fruition through the dedicated efforts of the Gwynedd Meeting of the Quakers, and provides its residents with a "community of life for older persons who want to maintain or improve their quality of life and security under a framework of mutual caring."

Located in a wooded, suburban setting of 106 acres just 20 miles from Center City, Philadelphia, Foulkeways offers cottages and apartments for independent living. It has a proactive focus on the maintenance of good health and mobility through good nutrition, exercise, and—above all—an enjoyable community life.

To accommodate an illness or the normal changes that come with age, a continuum of care, including residential health care, assisted living, and skilled nursing, is available to all residents. In the late 1990s, Foulkeways restructured its existing levels of care and with new construction in mind created a "future care committee" comprised of two board members, five staff members, and 13 residents who worked together to establish the "ideal" environment. With more than five years devoted to the research, planning, and execution of this premise, Foulkeways was able to restructure its existing levels of care by phasing out old nursing and assisted living beds into new accommodations. In August 2001, Gwynedd House opened to provide care for those individuals requiring skilled nursing; in July 2003, Abington House was added to the continuum to provide assisted living. Both buildings incorporate distinct, state-of-the-art designs and health care concepts which, in partnership with the dedicated staff, provide a range of health care services to residents in need of additional support.

This engaging lifestyle, filled with warmth and friendliness, is easy to slip into. Although mission statements and a philosophy of care can be easily expressed in words, the creation of this vibrant community was not

FIG. 20-2 Overall floor plan: The four households, containing 10 residents each, come together at the shared living and dining rooms *Courtesy RLPS Architects*

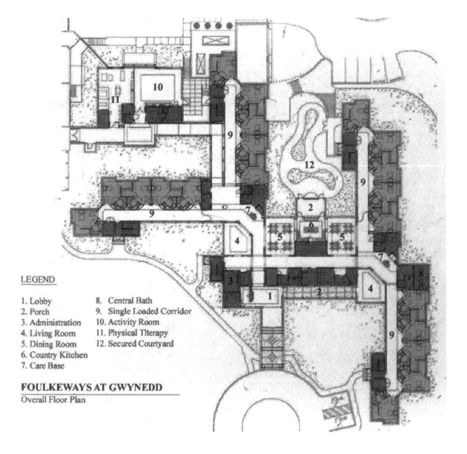

LEGEND

1. Lobby
2. Porch
3. Administration
4. Living Room
5. Dining Room
6. Country Kitchen
7. Care Base
8. Central Bath
9. Single Loaded Corridor
10. Activity Room
11. Physical Therapy
12. Secured Courtyard

FOULKEWAYS AT GWYNEDD
Overall Floor Plan

an accident. The planners set their own standards of quality and, with strong community involvement and extensive research, Foulkeways initiated its own model of care based upon the following goals:

- Integration of the community population by avoiding perceptions of "us and them."
- Blurring the distinctions in the built environment between independent living and higher levels of care.
- Decentralization of all services.
- Incorporation of the universal-worker concept.
- Development of a health care-lifestyle strategy.

Although the list is certainly commendable, it pales in comparison to Foulkeways' commitment to force a change in culture and behavior and to understand that the built environment does foster a way of life. To that extent, barriers of resistance had to be eliminated. *Visiting* the health center was not acceptable; instead, *being* in the health center had to be routine and a normal way of life. In short, the design sought to create an environment that enhanced resident participation by focusing campus activity within the health center. A successful health center would be unavoidable by residents—they would be compelled to participate out of a desire to join in on the action.

Thus, the "community of life" was established and housed within a new community center. Located in the middle of the campus, this dynamic building has it all: mail center, casual or elegant dining, activity-driven classrooms, extensive library, pharmacy, swimming pool, greenhouse, beauty salon, wellness center, and ample public space for the Lobby Art Show, which features diverse artists each month.

The community center is the place where all residents meet for information, intellectual stimulation, and social recreation. Because it is also the entrance to Abington House (assisted living) and Gwynedd House (skilled nursing), residents from all levels of care enjoy the center together and experience the full sense of community in all its vibrancy.

Architect's Statement

Foulkeways, which was the first Quaker community and the first campus-style care facility in Pennsylvania, approached its new skilled care facility with three objectives:

- Use simple forms and materials
- Create a home-like setting
- Build a strong connection to the outdoors

These directives inspired a design that uses single-loaded corridors throughout, resulting in "transparent" corridor walls that connect one to nature in a bright and uplifting interior. Corridors are further animated with illuminated display niches at each resident room entry. All 40 private rooms include tiled European-style showers, as well as a large walk-in closet used by residents and staff for personalized resident supplies. All social and dining spaces are central to the open plan for staff efficiency and are monitored through four care stations consisting of a simple wood desk and rear roll-top desk where the computer is housed. An open country kitchen serves two flanking dining rooms. The stucco exterior is reminiscent of an old Quaker meeting house, utilizing strong chimney forms, lower scaled room elements, simple brackets, and stone veneer at the "front porch." The single-loaded corridors translate into an exterior that is neither institutional nor repetitious and provides a transparent view into the building in the evening.

Designers' and Operators' Stated Objectives and Responses

OBJECTIVE: Create a noninstitutional aesthetic consistent with the Quaker philosophy of simplicity.

DESIGN INTENT: Simple materials of stucco and stone, varying roof heights, porches, and distinctive chimney elements, along with overhangs and wood brackets, all translate into a simple but beautiful style reminiscent of a Quaker meeting house. The single-loaded corridors translate well to the exterior, creating a nonrepetitious and varied elevation not typically associated with skilled care facilities.

OBJECTIVE: Diminish the traditional, dark, and institutional double-loaded corridors in resident wings.

DESIGN INTENT: Each resident corridor was designed to be single-loaded, with only five rooms per wing. The explosion of natural light and connection to the outdoors immediately breaks down the institutional medical-model stigma. The outdoors becomes part of the interior décor. Pocketed resident room doors, along with illuminated display niches, further animate each corridor.

OBJECTIVE: Decentralize the plan from a nursing care standpoint to diminish the institutional overtones associated with skilled care facilities.

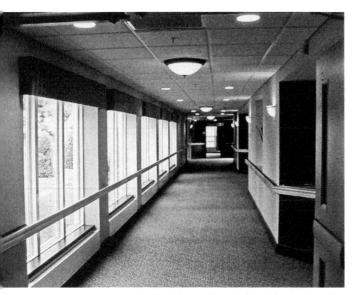

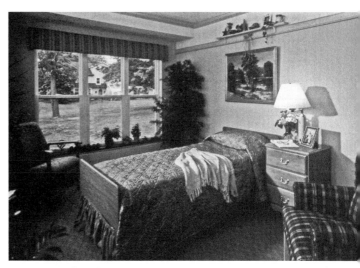

FIG. 20-3 Single-loaded corridors are flooded with natural light and offer outstanding seasonal views to the garden areas
Courtesy RLPS Architects/Larry Lefever Photography

FIG. 20-4 All resident rooms are private and provide ample space for personalized furniture arrangements
Courtesy RLPS Architects/Larry Lefever Photography

DESIGN INTENT: Two wings of five rooms radiate from a simple wooden staff desk that also directly views the living and dining rooms. Charting and other medically related functions occur in an adjacent back room, out of sight. The decentralization and residential detailing create a quieter, home-like setting.

OBJECTIVE: Design a facility that makes resident dignity and privacy paramount to the success of the project.

DESIGN INTENT: In the new skilled care facility, all 40 resident rooms are private. Each room is spacious and includes enough floor area for additional pieces of furniture belonging to residents. Each room also includes a large walk-in closet rather than the standard 2′ × 3′ wall closet, which allows residents to store more of their belongings nearby, and functions as an area for staff to stock supplies needed by that individual resident. Medications are also stored in a double-locked drawer within each closet. A tiled, European-style corner shower is provided within each private bathroom to allow residents the dignity and comfort of bathing in their own rooms.

OBJECTIVE: Create a facility that is flexible enough to address any changes in the marketplace or industry.

DESIGN INTENT: The design of the paired resident rooms allows a simple conversion from two skilled care rooms to a large, one-bedroom, assisted living apartment. The conversion includes removing one wall in a walk-in closet, creating a passageway, and renovating one private bath into an L-shaped kitchen.

Field Observations: Meeting the Objectives

OBJECTIVE: Create a noninstitutional aesthetic consistent with the Quaker philosophy of simplicity.

FIELD OBSERVATIONS: High marks must be awarded to the design team for the outstanding incorporation of native materials, predominantly stone and wood, in the simplest of forms. Simplicity here is defined by quality and the masterful use of color and texture to combine exterior and interior materials that complement each other and create a genuinely home-like atmosphere. Painted wood-paneled walls and trim, natural-finish handrails, and Shaker-style cabinetry reflect the Quaker philosophy of simplicity. A sense of comfort and calm abounds in every room.

OBJECTIVE: Diminish the traditional, dark, and institutional double-loaded corridors in resident wings.

FIELD OBSERVATIONS: With the exception of one or two small hallways, each corridor is single-loaded and faces an immaculately landscaped courtyard. The feeling of the outdoors is present throughout the building and the uplifting quality that natural light induces is evident. Staff and residents clearly benefit from the exposure to the outdoor environment: during our visit, one immobile resident enjoyed watching the birds play in the courtyard.

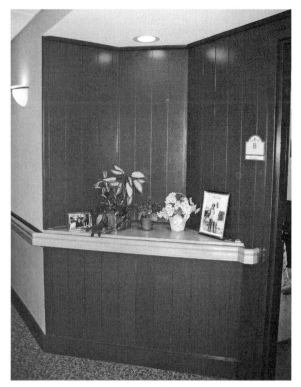

FIG. 20-5 Personalization of resident room entries takes many forms *Photograph by Jeffrey Anderzhon*

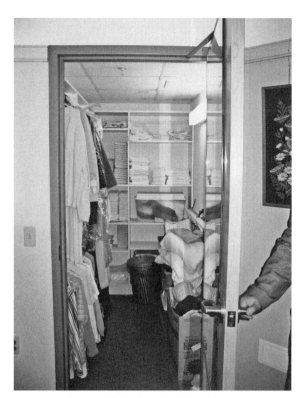

FIG. 20-6 Large, walk-in closets in the resident rooms serve a dual purpose: storing personal belongings as well as daily necessities that support a decentralized supply system *Photograph by Jeffrey Anderzhon*

OBJECTIVE: Decentralize the plan from a nursing care standpoint to diminish the institutional overtones associated with skilled care facilities.

FIELD OBSERVATIONS: The design of the building reflects and supports the resident-centered care program. No housekeeping, maintenance, or medication carts were observed. With an underground system of tunnels, residents are separated from the delivery of their services, keeping corridors and neighborhood spaces free of clutter and institutional equipment. The home-like atmosphere is provided continuously without interruption. The only exception is the delivery of meals, which are prepared in a remote kitchen and delivered to the neighborhood kitchens for service to residents.

The decentralization system is also evident in the resident rooms, where all housekeeping and personal supplies required by the resident are stored within the room. It should be noted that this system of decentralization also required additional training of staff in nonmedical alternatives in caregiving.

OBJECTIVE: Design a facility that makes resident dignity and privacy paramount to the success of the project.

FIELD OBSERVATIONS: The square footages in the resident units—areas of 350 square feet in the skilled care rooms and 480 square feet in the assisted living rooms—were chosen to remove some of the stigma of moving from one level of care to another. In fact, the assisted living apartment is just a bit smaller than the smallest independent studio apartment. The skilled nursing rooms were designed with plate rails and display shelves to accommodate resident furnishings and personalization.

OBJECTIVE: Create a facility that is flexible enough to address any changes in the marketplace or industry.

FIELD OBSERVATIONS: Foulkeways was one of the first providers to embrace the concept of achieving behavior changes through the environment and of removing barriers between levels of care. To a large extent, this effort has been successful, as residents are more willing to move from independent to assisted living, thus increasing the turnover rate in independent housing. With the added square footage in assisted living, more couples are willing to move, specifically those with one partner who is frailer than the other. As administration noted at the time of the evaluation, residents are "vot-

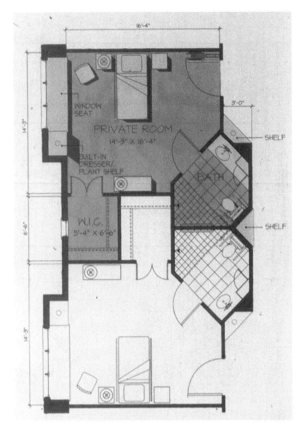
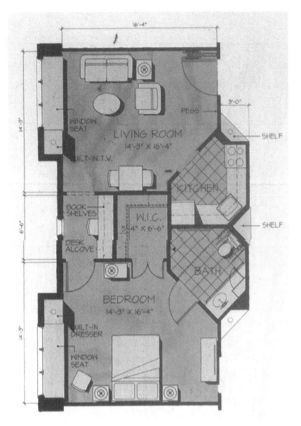

FIG. 20-7 + **FIG. 20-8**   Versatility in design allows resident rooms to be modified from private nursing care rooms to assisted living suites   *Courtesy RLPS Architects*

ing with their feet" and readily accepting the assisted living lifestyle.

Part of the early planning process included scenarios to protect Foulkeways from changes and spikes in supply and demand from their residents for appropriate levels of care. As a result, the initial design of the skilled nursing rooms included the flexibility to easily combine adjacent units and provide additional one-bedroom assisted living apartments.

Field Observations: Themes and Hypotheses

Creating Community

The dedicated board of directors, whose vision and planning are responsible for the successful integration of the new community and health center into the existing campus, have done the impossible by initiating culture change and thereby modifying resident behavior. The newly constructed community center functions as the heart of the campus. Abington and Gwynedd House

raise the bar on design and architectural criteria for supportive housing for older adults. As comfortable as home, the architecture is a reflection of the warmth and friendliness of the Foulkeways lifestyle.

Making a Home

Ease of access and human scale are hallmarks in the household design of Foulkeways. Two small wings of five apartments each shorten the distance to the core area. The single-loaded halls with opposing window walls frame the view to the immaculate gardens and are absolutely delightful—these corridors are definitely meant for strolling and create a pleasing home-like environment for residents and staff.

Living room, kitchen, and dining spaces are well appointed, and all three spaces incorporate a significant number of windows and garden views and bring nature into the building each day. (See Figure 19 in the color insert.) Screened porches maximize garden exposure, although on the day of the evaluation the adjacent electric generator happened to be running and disrupted the serenity of the garden.

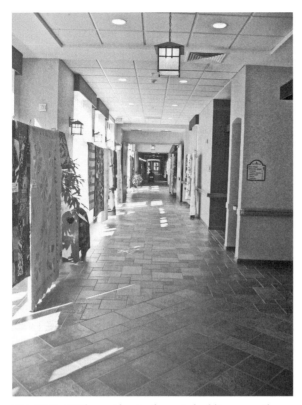

FIG. 20-9 Wide corridors in the main building are easily transformed into gallery space for quilt shows and other exhibits *Photograph by Jeffrey Anderzhon*

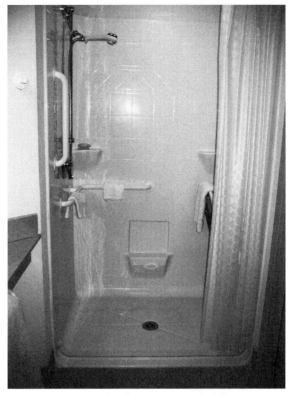

FIG. 20-10 A vertical grab bar at each ALF shower is a simple way to enhance resident safety *Photograph by Jeffrey Anderzhon*

The kitchen is well planned. The obligatory steam table is nicely enclosed by an elevated knee wall and extensive solid-surface countertops that are durable and attractive. Cabinetry is again wood, with Shaker styling, contributing to the country-kitchen atmosphere. The windows keep the kitchen light and airy.

Designed with concern for resident needs, each room features a bed wall with direct views to the bathroom and a bay window seat with generously sized windows overlooking manicured outdoor spaces. Plate rails within the resident room and package shelves just outside the resident room door encourage resident personalization.

A large, walk-in closet accommodates personal belongings, including medications, which are stored in a double-locked drawer. Decentralization means that linens and housekeeping supplies are also stored in this closet, via a well-designed shelving system that does not conflict with the resident's personal space.

Designed with a European shower concept, the bathroom spaces work very well for more independent residents as well as those who require additional assistance. Small tiles on the floor create more grout lines to

clean, but the tradeoff is additional slip resistance. Grab bars included on the front of the large vanity make for a handy addition in terms of safety as well as towel storage. Shaker-style cabinetry provides adequate space for toiletries and additional capacity for products required as a result of the decentralization of supplies.

Although residents can shower in the comfort and privacy of their own rooms, a charmingly appointed central spa is available for those residents wishing to pamper themselves in warm and comforting surroundings.

Regional/Cultural Design

The architectural styling and material composition are ideally suited for the wooded Pennsylvania location. Simplicity and quality are the hallmarks of both interior and exterior design, supported by thoughtful use of natural materials, including a wide variety of stone and wood products. Blending into the existing campus architecture, the community and health center maintain the framework of Quaker values in a traditional, yet state-of-the-art, design.

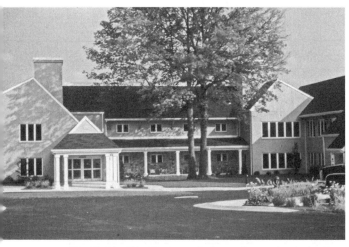

FIG. 20-11 The Quaker style that embraces simple details and finishes is evident in the exterior design   *Courtesy RLPS Architects/Larry Lefever Photography*

Environmental Therapy

Wide, naturally lit corridors with incredible views to the outdoor gardens and a genuine home-like atmosphere contribute to the emotional well-being of residents. More like a gracious boulevard than a connecting corridor, the "main street" connection to the community center amenities is *the* place where residents meet for information, intellectual stimulation, and social recreation. As one resident stated, "Life at Foulkeways provides abundant opportunities to continue to learn and grow."

Outdoor Environment

Much attention has been focused on the outstanding visual connections to the exterior environments, especially in the Abington and Gwynedd Houses; other programs also invite residents to interact with "mother nature." Greenhouse gardening and grounds beautification programs are organized by the residents' association. Woodland walking trails take advantage of the natural landscape. Fresh flowers are arranged by residents and displayed throughout the campus.

Quality of Workplace and the Physical Plant

Although the environment supports resident-centered care, the management and staff clearly contribute in large part to the success of this community. With a philosophy that promotes problem solving at all levels, each individual is committed to the mission of the organization. The caregivers have the tools and resources, as well as administrative support, to be proactive about resident care.

The Quaker influence may well have contributed to this success, but the team approach, along with personal accountability, drives the quality of care. The director of nursing commented that "the staff at Foulkeways could be transported to any other building or any other campus and continue to problem solve their way to success."

Operator Perspectives

In discussing the history of the Foulkeways campus and the direction the board took to restructure the health care component, administration was quite honest and open about the fact that in 1964, when the old health care center was built, the design clearly "missed the boat."

The original health care center was a quiet place—a place that you hoped you would not need. Based upon conventional thinking of the time, the double-loaded corridors had no natural light. The skilled nursing program included tray service to resident rooms; housekeeping, food, and med carts that cluttered the hallways; a central nurses' station; and a stainless steel bathing room purchased from a local hospital. The assisted living/dining room was tucked away in a remote corner and "had the atmosphere of a morgue."

Learning from past experiences, and combining that information with the inherent principles of Quaker tradition, Foulkeways created a "life style healthcare strategy." This was not going to be accomplished by architecture alone. The planners removed all resident resistance and in fact changed behavior and negative perceptions about higher levels of care.

Foulkeways was not afraid of tearing down architectural and cultural barriers. Four of the five original buildings were torn down to make way for the new community and health care center, and a new health care philosophy, calling for a "proactive focus on the maintenance of good health and mobility though good nutrition, exercise and enjoyable community life," was put into place. The success of the project can be read in the smiling faces of residents, staff, and family members.

General Project Information

PROJECT ADDRESS
Foulkeways at Gwynedd
120 Meetinghouse Road
Gwynedd, PA 19436

PROJECT DESIGN TEAM
Architect: Reese, Lower, Patrick & Scott, Ltd.
Owner's Architectural Consultant: Lynn Taylor Associates
Interior Designer: Reese, Lower, Patrick & Scott, Ltd.
Landscape Architect: Reese, Lower, Patrick & Scott, Ltd.
Structural Engineer: Zug & Associates, Ltd.
Mechanical Engineer: Consolidated Engineers
Electrical Engineer: Reese Engineering, Inc.
Civil Engineer: Burisch Associates
Dining Consultant: Culinary Design Service

Gerontologist: N/A
Management/Development: N/A
Contractor: C. Raymond Davis & Sons, Inc.

PROJECT STATUS
Completion date: August 2001

OCCUPANCY LEVELS
At facility opening date: 100%
At date of evaluation: 95%

RESIDENT AGE (YRS)
At facility opening date average: 83.4
June 2005 average: 88

PROJECT AREAS

SKILLED NURSING

| | New Construction | |
Project Element	No. Beds	Typical Room Size
Residents in one-bed/single rooms	40	350 GSF
Total no. of rooms/residents	40	14,000 GSF
Social area (lounges, dining, and recreation spaces):		4,900 GSF
Medical, health care, therapy, and activities spaces:		4,000 GSF
Administrative, public, and ancillary support services:		3,200 GSF
Service, maintenance, and mechanical areas:		7,040 GSF
Total gross area:		52,223 GSF
Total net usable area (per space program):		33,121 NSF
Overall gross/net factor (ratio of gross area/net usable area):		1.57

SITE AND PARKING

SITE LOCATION
Suburban

SITE SIZE
Acres: 3
Square feet: 130,680
Area of entire campus: 105 acres

PARKING

| | For This Facility | | | |
Type of Parking	Residents	Staff	Visitors	Totals
Open surface lot(s):	0	38	24	62

CONSTRUCTION COSTS

AUTHOR'S NOTE: *The following information is based on actual costs (completed).*

SOURCE OF COST DATA
Final construction cost as of August 2001

SOFT COSTS
Land cost or value:	N/A
All permit and other entitlement fees:	N/A
Legal and professional fees:	N/A
Appraisals:	N/A
Marketing and preopening:	N/A
Total soft costs:	$1,010,764

BUILDING COSTS
New construction except FF&E, special finishes, floor and window coverings, HVAC, and electrical:	$6,006,429
Renovations except FF&E, special finishes, floor and window coverings, HVAC, and electrical:	N/A
FF&E and small wares:	$100,000
Floor coverings:	$158,000
Window coverings:	$40,000
HVAC:	$1,264,000
Electrical:	$1,017,000
Medical equipment costs:	N/A
Total building costs:	$8,585,429

SITE COSTS
New:	$792,000
Renovation:	$342,000
	(electrical substation relocation)
Total site costs:	$1,133,879

TOTAL PROJECT COSTS
(include all fees and costs, except financing)
Total project costs: $10,730,072

FINANCING SOURCES
Nontaxable bond offering through Montgomery County Higher Education Authority

CARE COMPARISON

Source: www.medicare.gov—July 14, 2005
SNF staffing: 5.20 care hours/resident/day
SNF occupancy: 38 of 40 = 95%

Hours per Resident per Day	Foulkeways in PA	PA Average	National Average
Not-for-profit	Yes		
Multifacility	No		
Levels of care	CCRC		
Medicare	Yes		
Medicaid	No		
Licensed #	50		
# residents	38	123.5	95.3
% occ this day	95%		
RNs	1.88	0.70	0.50
LPNs	0.28	0.70	0.70
RN + LPN	2.17	1.40	1.20
CNA	3.03	2.20	2.30
RN + LPN + CNA	5.20	3.60	3.50

Part VI

Community-Based Services

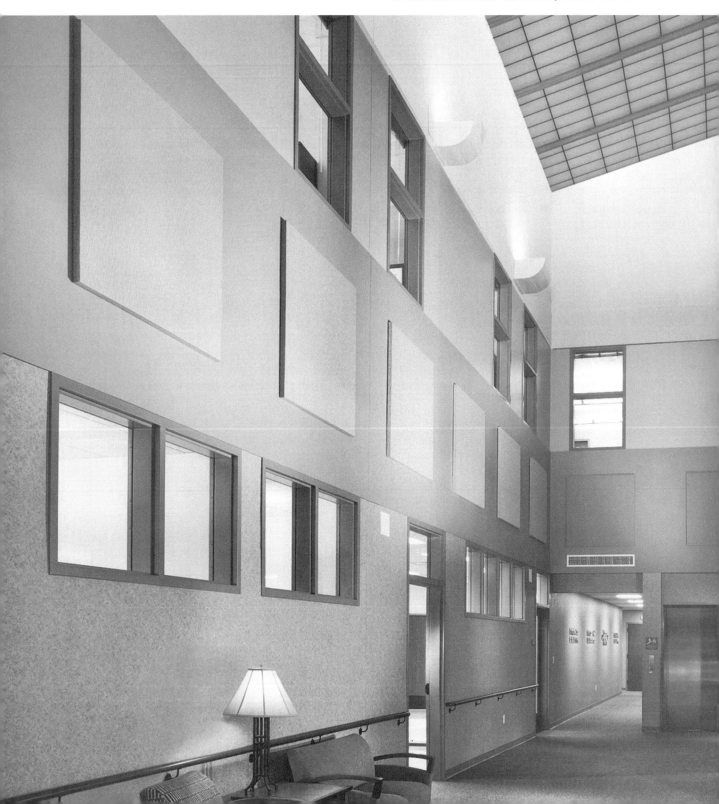

"Age considers; youth ventures."

RABINDRANATH TAGORE, 1861–1941

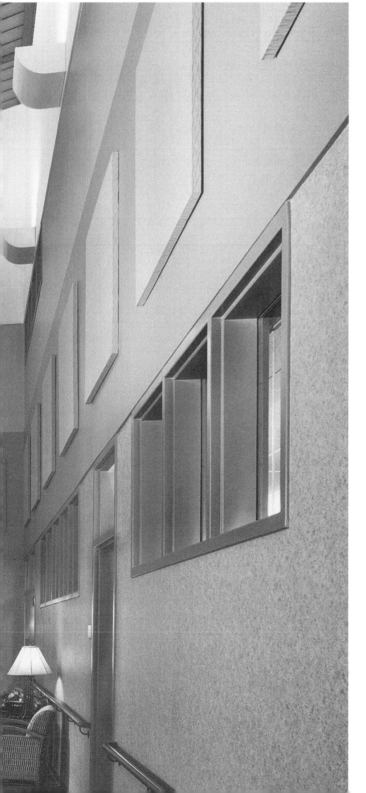

Chapter 21   Cody Day Center

EVALUATION SITE: Cody Day Center

COMMUNITY TYPE: Adult Day Care
- Adult day care (PACE program) for 404 clients
- Child day care for 25 clients

REGION: Rocky Mountain Front Range

ARCHITECT: Boulder Associates

OWNER: Total Longterm Care, Inc.

DATA POINTS:

Total Participants:	404 registered clients
Average Daily Participants:	330 registered clients
Total Area:	149 gsf/participant
Total Project Area:	49,200 gsf
Project Cost:	$8,074,000
Investment/total adult registered participant:	$19,985.15/registrant

FIRST OCCUPANCY: January 2004

DATE OF EVALUATION: January 2006

EVALUATION TEAM: John Shoesmith, AIA; Jane Rohde, AIA, FIIDA; Jeffrey Anderzhon, AIA; Jeremy Vickers; David Slack

FIG. 21-1 The two-story atrium allows natural light to flow into the lower level, which is below grade
©Lacasse Photography

Introduction

The Cody Day Center amazingly accommodates 160 to 170 PACE participants per center every day in one warm and welcoming environment. The owners, Total Longterm Care, set out to design a building plan that would conveniently allow two separate centers to share a common space and functions. The design response to the complex, dual program translated into a building that, for the most part, functions very well and is seen as a success by Total Longterm Care and the review team.

The center has two teams of staff to care for the large number of daily participants between the two centers, and a unique physical plant that is largely successful, despite a few drawbacks. The pride that management, staff, and participants of the Cody Center take in their building, and the image that it displays to the community, were readily evident to the review team.

Despite the overwhelming approval of the program and building, the owners cite three main issues with the building: inadequate office space, limited clinic space,

and parking and van circulation issues. They believe these problems arise from the fact that they underestimated the size of the building required to serve up to 500 participants.

Architect's Statement

The program called for twin senior day centers housed in a single structure in a redeveloping area of an older suburb. Capitalizing on a sloping site, the architects developed a two-story solution that provides at-grade entries for participants at the upper level and at-grade entries for staff at the lower level. The plan allows both centers to operate independently while sharing clinical, administrative, therapeutic, personal care, and service functions. Consideration of staff needs revealed the necessity of combinable conference spaces, a lounge, shower/locker rooms, a fitness facility, and a child day care center. Dayrooms share generous patio areas along the east and west faces of the building, where carefully arranged walls

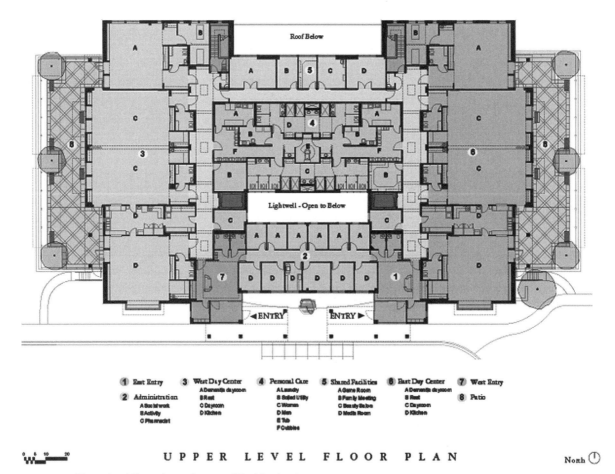

FIG. 21-2 Upper-level floor plan *Courtesy of Boulder Associates*

and curved trellises control low-angle sun. Custom-fabricated steel fencing will support climbing vines as the landscaping matures. A central atrium anchors the building, orienting staff and participants while bringing natural daylight into both levels of the building.

Designers' and Owners' Stated Objectives and Responses

OBJECTIVE: Provide functional accessibility that exceeds ADA and IBC requirements.

DESIGN INTENT: ANSI A117.1 establishes minimum accessibility standards that work well in many situations. However, in designs for seniors, some areas require larger clearances and alternative designs to enable participants to remain as independent as possible. Doors and adjacent clearances at Cody exceed code minimums and power operators are provided at all building entrances. Shower and bathing areas also exceed minimum standards, to provide improved accessibility and ample space for staff to assist participants.

OBJECTIVE: Provide a comfortable, warm, and inviting environment.

DESIGN INTENT: Colorful exterior materials that include local stone, brick, block, and tile set the tone for the interior palette. Participants, families, and staff all respond to the welcoming ambience created by the combination of warm colors, comfortable furniture, indirect lighting, and Western-themed artwork.

OBJECTIVE: Design features to attract and retain staff.

DESIGN INTENT: Careful attention was paid to creating supportive work environments for all staff members. Improved ergonomics at workstations, large exam rooms with beds rather than exam tables, and extra space for assisting participants with toileting and bathing bring greater workplace safety to employees. Indoor and outdoor break areas, generous shower/locker rooms, and a fully equipped fitness facility are provided for employees. A child care center allows staff members' children to be cared for on-site and to participate in intergenerational activities with Cody Center clients.

OBJECTIVE: Resolve the site boundary dispute with the city.

DESIGN INTENT: Because of inaccurate records and land title, the city contested the ownership of a key 50-foot-wide strip of land along the main frontage. Lengthy negotiations with the city resulted in the client retaining use of 20 feet of the land, and an administrative variance in response to restrictive parking regulations allowed the program for the facility and needed parking to fit within the confines of the site.

OBJECTIVE: Address drainage issues.

DESIGN INTENT: Because of a lack of storm sewers in the vicinity, the sloping site, and requirements for stormwater detention and water-quality treatment basins, the site appeared at first to be significantly undersized for the program. The design team found a solution for draining the upper parking lot by funneling runoff through a water-quality basin into underground stormwater detention tanks. Roof drainage joins the runoff and then is metered out to the street at historic flow rates. The lower parking lot is graded to provide detention within the lot before stormwater reaches the water-quality basin, which in turn releases stormwater to a second street at historic flow rates.

OBJECTIVE: Receive city planning and zoning approval.

DESIGN INTENT: The city's initial review of the project design identified a number of issues that demanded negotiations and compromise on behalf of both the city and Cody Day Center. Although the city planning guidelines recommended placing the building close to the street, the slope of the site from south to north would have resulted in entrances only at the lower level on the north side, where van loading and unloading would have been mixed with employee parking. Participants assisted by transportation staff would have had to use elevators to reach the dayrooms. Persistence was required to eventually convince city planning staff that the building needed adequate space for van loading at the south side on the upper level.

OBJECTIVE: Create connections to the outdoors that allow abundant daylight to enter the center.

DESIGN INTENT: Site constraints and programmatic requirements shaped the building into a deep rectangle with windowless basement walls on three sides, which made it difficult for daylight to reach much of the building. Knowing that ample light would increase staff effectiveness and participant attitudes, the architects proposed a central, skylit atrium that would bring light to the lower level and to interior offices on the upper level. Medical clinic and therapy areas are clustered around the atrium at the lower level and elevators open onto the atrium, clearly orienting staff and participants. Smaller translucent skylights are also employed in the dayroom corridors on the upper level, adding to the bright and airy atmosphere of the center.

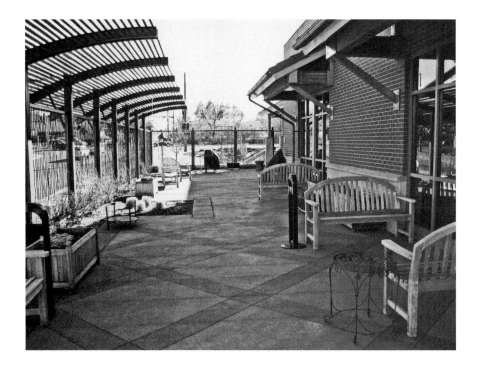

FIG. 21-3 Patios just off the dayrooms provide clients with a secure and shaded place to enjoy the outdoors *Photograph by Jeffrey Anderzhon*

OBJECTIVE: Develop a two-story solution to a traditionally single-story program.

DESIGN INTENT: Total Longterm Care's previous facilities were designed on a single level, to avoid having to move participants between levels. The need for two day centers on a relatively compact site led to the two-story solution. The dayrooms, serving kitchens, administrative areas, personal care areas, and other functions needed on a daily basis by all participants are located on the upper level where participants enter and exit the facility. Functions not utilized daily by participants, and staff-only areas, are located on the lower level where staff enter and exit the building. Hospital-size elevators are located within each day center and connect to the atrium at the lower level where the clinic and therapeutic suite are located.

OBJECTIVE: Share as many functional spaces as possible between the two day centers.

DESIGN INTENT: Departmental programming meetings revealed which functions and facilities could share space and which could not. Collectively, the client and design team determined that administrative and therapeutic areas could be shared and that staff support areas could be shared as well if sized properly. Even though there would be only one bathing tub to support both centers, each needed a separate personal care area to control the flow of personal clothing and laundry. In response, the separate personal care areas were located back to back and share access to the tub room. The medical clinics also required separate spaces, but could share the specialists' offices and medical records room. The clinics were arranged to share a few common areas and now find that the arrangement is beneficial because it allows staff members to cover for each other when it is busy.

OBJECTIVE: Although sharing space works well for some functions, others require independence.

DESIGN INTENT: The separate day centers are located on opposite sides of the building, each with its own entrance, dayrooms, outdoor patio, and elevator for quick access to therapeutic and clinic areas on the lower level. Each lobby has its own artwork to help differentiate the spaces, and each of the center's dayrooms has its own serving kitchen. Staff work areas and offices are provided in each center so that staff are close to the participants.

OBJECTIVE: The child day care facility, a late addition to the program, must meet state and county health department regulations.

DESIGN INTENT: The child day care center has its own discrete entrance from the employee parking lot. The doors are secured until released by staff using a video intercom system. Outdoor play areas with shade structures were designed for use by the three different age groups. Each indoor space is tailored to the needs of the three age groups and a serving kitchen is provided.

OBJECTIVE: Create readily available outdoor access for participants and staff.

DESIGN INTENT: In previous centers designed for Total Longterm Care, site constraints and tenant space limitations prevented meaningful outdoor spaces from being developed. Despite the relatively tight site, the designers were able to organize the two centers' dayrooms to open onto patio areas that feature stained concrete paving, landscaping, covered porches, shade-providing trellises, and custom fencing that will allow vines to enclose the area. Planters for participants to garden in and gas grilles for special lunches add to the usefulness of these patios. Staff also have their own trellis-covered outdoor patio.

OBJECTIVE: Bring confidence to the organization and express commitment and passion for the work involved.

DESIGN INTENT: The design, the quality of construction, the attention given to design of workspaces, and the flow of people through the building all work together to create an environment that truly meets this goal. Recruitment and retention of employees is easier at this center than at the earliest centers. The census has increased beyond established goals due to the response of family members and participants when visiting the facility. The interior design and themes convey the quality of care that is provided here.

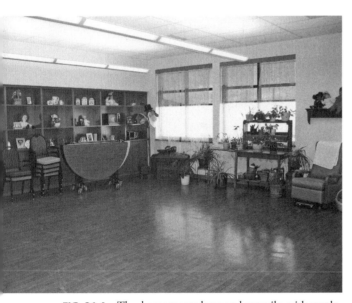

FIG. 21-4 The dayrooms are large and versatile, with ample storage and support spaces for clients and staff *Photograph by Jeffrey Anderzhon*

Field Observations: Meeting the Objectives

OBJECTIVE: Provide functional accessibility that exceeds ADA and IBC requirements.

FIELD OBSERVATIONS: Generally, accessibility issues within toilet rooms and showers were thoughtfully considered. The only exception is that the linen wardrobe is located behind the hand sink. The wardrobe extends into the floor space in some instances and this makes it hard for participants in wheelchairs to access the sink properly. Putting the cabinet elsewhere, or providing a small amount of additional space between the sink and the cabinet, would be an improvement.

The main issue for staff and participants to overcome is related less to the layout inside the toilet or shower room than to the distance required to access those rooms. Each dayroom has a single-stall toilet room within it that is constantly busy. Participants often have to use the restrooms that are centrally located by the showers. These toilet rooms provide an ample number of toilets to meet demand, but the distance to this space is too difficult for some residents to manage on their own. If the toilet/shower rooms were even more centrally located to the dayrooms, or if there were more than one toilet in the dayrooms, participants would have the needed access.

OBJECTIVE: Provide a comfortable, warm, and inviting environment.

FIELD OBSERVATIONS: The local stone, brick, block, and tile used on the Cody Center set the building apart from its neighbors in a subtle and sophisticated way. (See Figure 20 in the color insert.) The interior color palette is warm and inviting and draws inspiration from the character of the exterior material choices. Indirect lighting strategies and finish selections appear to be sound, although maintenance has reported difficulty in keeping the flooring clean. The struggle to keep the floors in good shape was evident in the worn appearance of the carpet in the staff entry corridor on the lower level, and was also reported for the VCT surface on the main floor of the building outside the dayrooms.

OBJECTIVE: Design features to attract and retain staff.

FIELD OBSERVATIONS: In general, staff appreciated the thought that went into providing adequate space to assist with showering and toileting, exam room size, and workstation ergonomics. The staff break room is more than adequately sized, nicely lit, and well outfitted. Because of this, the staff use it frequently throughout the day.

The exercise room is less spacious but very well equipped. It was reported that the exercise room is not used by many employees, but is used very often by those who do. Staff parking is generally inadequate; staff have had to resort to parking on the streets adjacent to the building. Forty percent of the children in the day care program are children of employees. Parents of children in the day care are very involved and visit during the day.

The director of the Cody Center stated that, generally, staff retention is difficult; finding an exceptional RN to staff and run the PACE clinic is the biggest challenge. Clinics create quite a bit of stress for employees—the job is definitely difficult. The director mentioned that the Cody Center building does help to attract staff, but that the crowding in the clinic and office spaces due to the large demand for services is a detriment to recruitment. The clinic overcrowding led to the relocation of a few of the larger clinics, such as podiatry, to other locations in the building, which in turn has caused inefficiency in operations.

OBJECTIVE: Resolve the site boundary dispute with the city.

FIELD OBSERVATIONS: Although this is a technical issue that had to be resolved prior to receipt of approval to construct the building, it is commendable that the dedication of the design team was at a high enough level to undertake a responsibility that is normally part of the legal process for land purchase. This objective, however, does not necessarily have either a positive or negative impact on the clients of the day care center.

OBJECTIVE: Address drainage issues.

FIELD OBSERVATIONS: Drainage is important to the success of a developed property, so that the operators can be good neighbors by keeping water runoff from damaging adjacent real estate. Appropriate drainage is critical to the operation of a building, particularly where freezing may occur, so that there is no ponding that may freeze and become a safety issue. However, this issue is resolved by appropriate engineering principles and is thus more objective than subjective. Additionally, in most communities, drainage plans require governmental approval prior to receipt of a building permit. Though this is important for a project to move forward, it has only peripheral effect on the efficacy of the building for day care clients.

OBJECTIVE: Receive city planning and zoning approval.

FIELD OBSERVATION: The architect's response demonstrates that good intentions were involved in placing the van loading area on the south side of the upper level,

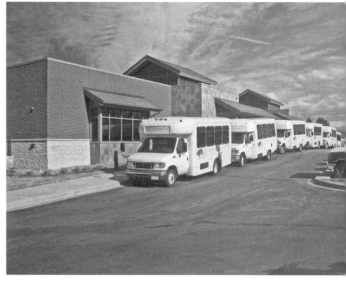

FIG. 21-5 Due to the constraints of a small site, client pickup and drop-off become a significant traffic issue
Photograph by Jeffrey Anderzhon

away from the general parking provided to the north. The southern, upper-level entrance makes sense not only in terms of separating traffic, but also for participant access to primary-use spaces inside the building. That said, the access to and layout of the van loading on the south side of the building as designed is not adequate.

For vans to access the loading area, they must circulate through a small parking area. The transportation director called the circulation into and back out of the parking area a "nightmare." It would be more efficient if vans had their own dedicated loop through the parking lot. As it is, vans must often back up to park along the building. When dispatched to the facility, emergency vehicles block all access to the building for vans and bring the transportation program to a standstill.

During the programming stage, the quantity of parking spaces was reduced. This, combined with the van circulation on the site, is the biggest challenge for the building. The Cody Center is currently negotiating with a church on an adjacent property for additional parking.

OBJECTIVE: Create connections to the outdoors that allow abundant daylight to enter the center.

FIELD OBSERVATIONS: The central atrium brings a pleasant sense of the outdoors inside and supplies ample light to the lower level of the building. Staff commented that having the light coming in through the interior windows to the atrium made the space seem much bigger, lighter, and a better environment in which to work. The physical therapy staff commented that they enjoy the atrium as an extension of the therapy gym. Handrails allow standing group exercise to take place in this space as well.

OBJECTIVE: Develop a two-story solution to a traditionally single-story program.

FIELD OBSERVATIONS: Cody is designed with a clinic on the lower level and the main entrance for clients on the upper level, where the center's buses transport elderly clients from their homes to the day care center. The travel between floors is difficult. The owners said they will never design a center on two floors again, because of the staffing and transport issues that have resulted. They feel that the two-story solution is more staff-intensive than a one-story solution when participant escort time is accounted for. The room planned as a media room on the upper level has turned into a triage room because no participants enter the building on the lower level.

OBJECTIVE: Share as many functional spaces as possible between the two day centers.

FIELD OBSERVATIONS: The building design provides an organization that allows efficient sharing of services. The centralized spaces between the day care assembly rooms contain both support for the day care programming and office spaces for staff who serve both sides of the center. The separation of the day care assembly areas was a part of the building program for a variety of noncare program reasons, but experiencing the functionality of this layout, one might wonder, had these building programmatic issues not been in place, whether this would still not have been the most effective organizational solution. The building works well and efficiently within this design.

OBJECTIVE: Although sharing space works well for some functions, others require independence.

FIELD OBSERVATIONS: The residents are divided by zip code and the only overlap between participants from the east and west occurs in the clinic. Although the duality of the building is somewhat confusing for first-time visitors, it did not seem to be an issue for staff or participants. It is questionable whether the cost of providing two receptionists and two separate reception areas is justifiable, but staff report that because the east and west sides operate as two separate centers, the dual reception is a necessary component of the design and the program.

OBJECTIVE: The child day care facility, a late addition to the program, must meet state and county health department regulations.

FIELD OBSERVATIONS: The child day care can house 41 children, but has been serving an average of 35 per day.

Forty percent of the children enrolled in the day care are children of employees, and the program is also utilized by the adjacent Kaiser Healthcare System office. The spaces are ample and well suited for the ages served. Staff report that it would be nice to have the infant and toddler spaces adjacent to each other, and that they would reconsider using the easily cleaned VCT floor in the infant room because it feels cold to the children and is unforgiving for older infants who stumble. Outdoor spaces for the children are well designed and well utilized.

OBJECTIVE: Create readily available outdoor access for participants and staff.

FIELD OBSERVATIONS: Exterior spaces are self-accessible, but because of fire-code egress requirements, securing the gates completely is not possible. This has caused an issue with elopement, as 85% of the participants have some form of dementia.

Outdoor spaces are used often in the summer and during the warmer days of spring and fall. Horticulture classes are one of the activities offered. Caregivers report that the doorways to the courtyards are not wide enough and can make it difficult for some wheelchair-bound participants to easily go in and out on their own.

OBJECTIVE: Bring confidence to the organization and express commitment and passion for the work involved.

FIELD OBSERVATIONS: Staff are very proud of their new building and treat it with pride. This feeling transfers to their care provision and their attitudes toward the day care clients. The staff are friendly and effusive in their interactions with the numerous clients and with visitors. In discussing this issue with both staff and administration, we found that Cody Day Center has become the work location of choice, with some staff from other locations operated by the owner anxiously awaiting transfer to Cody.

Field Observations: Themes and Hypotheses

Creating Community

Because of the nature of the PACE program, which reaches directly into the community to provide all-inclusive care for the underserved elderly, this facility has a significant role in the creation of at least a small part of the larger community. Cody Day Center is, for the clients it serves, their entire community—one that revolves around the staff and programming within the Center. There is an obvious benefit to clients from par-

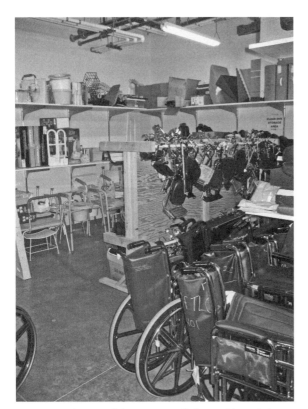

FIG. 21-6 As part of the program, Cody provides assistive devices for clients and ensures their maintenance. However, ample space to do so is an issue yet to be resolved
Photograph by Jeffrey Anderzhon

ticipation in this community, which includes cheerful, consistent, and welcoming staff, as well as a structured program that involves clients rather than simply providing the physical care they may need.

Outdoor Environment

The outdoor spaces may be physically accessible, but the risk of elopement restricts participant use. Finding a compromise between these two needs would give the residents a more readily accessible outdoor space to enjoy. Classes and structured activities, such as the horticulture classes, certainly provide opportunities to enjoy the space, but do not give clients the freedom and spontaneity to enjoy the space however they please.

Quality of Workplace and the Physical Plant

Concerted efforts to retain and attract staff, such as the child care center, exercise room, and above-average indoor and outdoor staff spaces, all contribute to a pleasant, convenient, and enjoyable work environment. However, the inefficiency of a two-level building, the separation/combination of certain functions, and the crowding in the clinics may have adverse effects on the environment.

Staff are proud of the building and take pride in taking good care of it. Because of this, they have been cleaning the floors frequently and using multiple layers of wax on the flooring. The wax layers are scratched deeply, which make the floor appear damaged when in reality only the wax is scratched. If the floor was stripped, treated with a thinner layer of wax, and received a daily cleaning instead of a large amount of wax every other day, the appearance of the VCT would improve.

Operator Perspectives

As a PACE (Program for All-inclusive Care for the Elderly) provider, we work to improve the health care of our participants by providing under one roof every type of care and support that seniors need, managed by interdisciplinary teams that meet daily to review and monitor each participant's condition. On-site physicians and geriatric nurse practitioners can intervene as soon as they detect health changes. Our program requires space to assist participants with the full range of activities of daily living.

The architects worked closely with our staff to establish a complex building program that would accommodate all of our services: home health care, personal laundry, medications, transportation, medical and dental care, physical and occupational therapy, speech therapy, meals, counseling, activities, hair care, and dementia care. Individual meetings with caregivers, therapists, drivers, home health aides, activities staff, and food service staff provided the details needed to create a building that better serves our participants, families, and staff.

General Project Information

PROJECT ADDRESS
Cody Day Center
8405 W. Alameda Ave.
Lakewood, CO 80226

PROJECT DESIGN TEAM
Architect: Boulder Associates, Inc.
Interior Designer: Boulder Associates, Inc.
Landscape Architect: Land Architects, Inc.
Structural Engineer: Structural Consultants, Inc.
Mechanical Engineer: Boulder Engineering Co.
Electrical Engineer: Boulder Engineering Co.
Civil Engineer: Sellards & Grigg

Dietary Consultant: William Caruso & Associates, Inc.
Contractor: Calcon Constructors, Inc.

PROJECT STATUS
Completed January 2004

OCCUPANCY LEVELS
At facility opening date: 321 participants
At time of evaluation: 404 participants

RESIDENT AGE (YRS)
At facility opening date (average): 80
At time of evaluation: 84

PROJECT AREAS

Project Element	Included in This Project			Total On-site or Served by Project
	Units, Beds, or Clients	New GSF	Total Gross Area	
Elder day care (clients)	400 (125 daily census)	15,600	15,600	400
Children's day care (clients)	25	2,900	2,900	25
Fitness/rehabilitation/wellness (daily visits)	75/day	2,800	2,800	
Medical clinic (daily visits)	80/day	4,800	4,800	

Project Element	New Construction, Typical Size
Adult day center	28,190 GSF
Social areas (lounges, dining, and recreation spaces)	850 GSF
Medical, health care, therapy, and activities spaces	7,600 GSF
Administrative, public, and ancillary support services	5,630 GSF
Service, maintenance, and mechanical areas	6,930 GSF
Total gross area	49,200 GSF
Total net usable area (per space program)	42,270 NSF
Overall gross/net factor (ratio of gross area/net usable area)	1.16

SITE AND PARKING

SITE LOCATION
Suburban

SITE SIZE
Acres: 2.23
Square feet: 97,200

PARKING

Type of Parking	For This Facility		
	Residents	Staff	Totals
Open surface lot(s)	86	10	96

CONSTRUCTION COSTS

AUTHOR'S NOTE: *The following information is based on actual completed costs*

SOURCE OF COST DATA
Final construction cost as of January 2004

SOFT COSTS
Land cost or value:	$450,000
All permit and other entitlement fees:	$281,000
Other:	$597,000
Total soft costs:	$1,328,000

BUILDING COSTS
New construction except FF&E, special finishes, floor and window coverings, HVAC, and electrical:	$4,358,000
Renovations except FF&E, special finishes, floor and window coverings, HVAC, and electrical:	N/A
FF&E and small wares:	$402,000
Floor coverings:	$219,000
Window coverings:	$15,000
HVAC:	$362,000
Electrical:	$461,000
Medical equipment costs:	$134,000
Total building costs:	$5,951,000

SITE COSTS
New on-site:	$557,000
New off-site:	$140,000
Renovation on-site:	N/A
Renovation off-site:	N/A
Landscape:	$98,000
Special site features or amenities:	N/A
Total site costs:	$795,000

TOTAL PROJECT COSTS
Total project costs: $8,074,000

FINANCING SOURCES
Nontaxable bonds with significant public contributions

Part VII

Scandinavian Comparisons

"To me, old age is always ten years older than I am."

JOHN BURROUGHS, 1837–1921

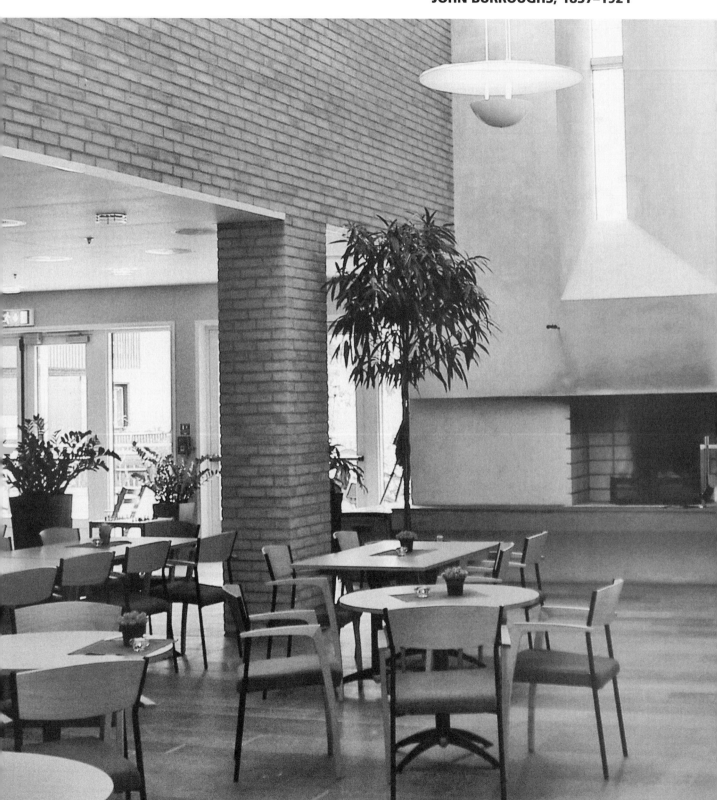

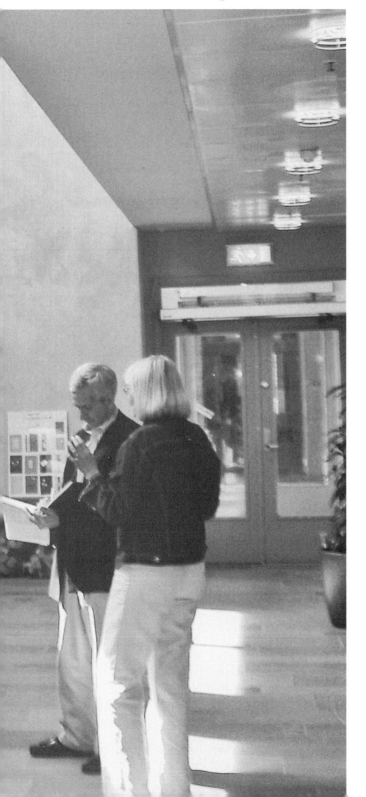

Chapter 22

Tempe Health and Welfare Centre

EVALUATION SITE: Tempe Health and Welfare Centre Trondheim Kommune

COMMUNITY TYPE: Aging-in-Place Community
- 61 sheltered housing apartments (assisted living)
- 24 assisted living apartments (nursing care)

REGION: Scandinavia

ARCHITECT: HRTB AS Arkitekter MNAL

OWNER: Trondheim Kommune, Norway

MANAGER: Trondheim Kommune, Norway

DATA POINTS:

Resident Room:	612–910 gsf (56.9—84.5 gsm) sheltered housing 306 gsf (28.4 gsm) assisted living
Total Area:	1,139 gsf (105.8 gsm)/resident
Total Project Area:	96,818 gsf (8,994.7 gsm)
Total Project Cost:	Unknown
Investment/resident:	Unknown
Staffing:	4.0 care hours/resident/day
Occupancy:	95% as of June 2005

FIRST OCCUPANCY: 2003

DATE OF EVALUATION: June 2005

EVALUATION TEAM: Knut Bergslund; David Green; Mitch Green, AIA; Robert Lagoyda; Jerry Weisman, Ph.D. (this evaluation completed in conjunction with Society for the Advancement of Gerontological Environments [SAGE])

FIG. 22-1 The community dining room is an expansive space available for use by the entire surrounding community *Photo provided by members of the SAGE POE team*

Introduction

At 58 degrees above the equator, Trondheim is one of the largest cities near the Arctic Circle. Possessed of more than 1,100 years of history and the birthplace of the legendary Norse King Olaf, Trondheim has a population of 165,000, making it Norway's third-largest city. In the gentle hills and valleys surrounding the historic town center are a variety of neighborhoods of red-painted houses with white trim, interspersed with more modern concrete structures and brick-faced institutional buildings.

Always a center of learning and a regional industrial hub, North Sea oil has invigorated Trondheim and created new opportunities. In meeting on the central government's mandate to rethink its social welfare health care system, the Trondheim Kommune took a larger view, considering what would constitute a better relationship between Kommune and citizen, and citizens and their health care system. The result is an approach that challenges traditional perceptions, especially for a metropolis that foresees a stable working population coupled to an ever-rising population of older adults.

As Dr. Tor Am, Municipal Executive for Health and Social Welfare, put it, "although the traditional health care system and private industry would look at Trondheim and see more and more dependent customers, *we* want to see more and more independent inhabitants who can cope by themselves and use our services only when necessary."

This philosophical break focuses on empowerment, health promotion, prevention, rehabilitation, and city planning with new ideas about where services are located and how they are delivered. For older adults, who constitute more than 12% of the population and consume a majority of the 35% of government and health care expenditures, the Kommune set a goal of a 50% reduction in the need for nursing homes and a 20 to 30% reduction in the need for home care.

Implementation of this policy relies on a blend of home care, outpatient health services, and facilities all organized by the concept that "the money follows the resident." Residents are classified according to 17 activities of daily living (ADL) variables, with programs designed for each resident based on functional capabilities. A single "gatekeeper" agency, staffed by doctors, nurses, therapists, social workers, and psychiatric nurses, follows the resident, adjusting the service mix as needs change.

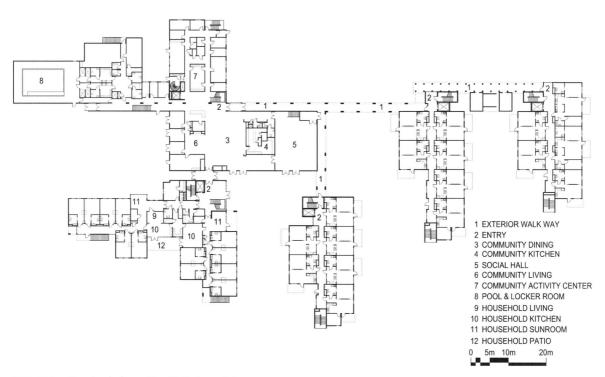

1 EXTERIOR WALK WAY
2 ENTRY
3 COMMUNITY DINING
4 COMMUNITY KITCHEN
5 SOCIAL HALL
6 COMMUNITY LIVING
7 COMMUNITY ACTIVITY CENTER
8 POOL & LOCKER ROOM
9 HOUSEHOLD LIVING
10 HOUSEHOLD KITCHEN
11 HOUSEHOLD SUNROOM
12 HOUSEHOLD PATIO

0 5m 10m   20m

FIG. 22-2   First-level plan   *Graphic by Jason Reis*

The results are impressive. Measured by acuity level, Trondheim now has more "nursing home patients" receiving care at home than in institutions. More than 50% of residents receiving three hours of care per day still live at home; even for those receiving four hours of care per day, 25% still live at home. Nursing home patients have become, increasingly, memory support residents, with an expanding network of programs designed to support both residents and their families.

But where should these narrower bands of older adults, some needing memory support and some needing ADL assistance, live when their present homes are no longer an option? The Kommune's choice is decentralization: create a new prototype of a "health and welfare center" and distribute these centers throughout the neighborhoods to keep people living where they are now. The new centers ought to have congregate housing for older adults needing ADL assistance, memory support households for frail elderly in need of 24-hour supervision, and health and welfare offices to coordinate community-based care. Recognizing that all of Trondheim's residents are their clients, the Kommune wants each project to have a community center open to all residents of the neighborhood.

This was the design brief for the Tempe Health and Welfare Centre: become the prototype for Trondheim's new concept for neighborhood-based services for older adults.

Designers' and Operators' Stated Objectives and Responses

OBJECTIVE: Decentralize housing and services for older adults in noninstitutional, home-like settings.

DESIGN INTENT: The design contains a four-part project, which includes 61 "congregate housing apartments" for older adults in need of daily living assistance but wishing to maintain an independent lifestyle, a 24-resident "memory support unit" composed of four six-resident households in a two-story building for older adults in need of 24-hour supervision at high levels of care, a health service center to coordinate daily assistance and neighborhood care programs, and a "community center" open to both on-site residents and surrounding neighbors.

OBJECTIVE: Implement a new prototype for neighborhood-based older adult service centers.

DESIGN INTENT: The four-part project is tucked into a gently sloping site between the neighborhood and the

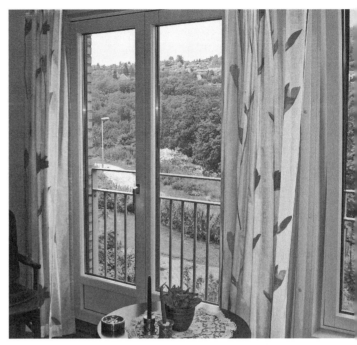

FIG. 22-3 Each apartment has large windows and a small balcony *Photo provided by members of the SAGE POE team*

river valley. The memory-care program is designed to permit area residents to stay in their neighborhood as care needs change, and the community center has a variety of spaces for older adult activities.

OBJECTIVE: Create sheltered housing apartments that can accommodate complete aging in place, including skilled and hospice care as required.

DESIGN INTENT: The 61 one-bedroom apartments are large, with full kitchens and wheelchair-accessible bathrooms. All apartments have exterior terraces or balconies and most apartments have kitchen windows overlooking the interior "street" for added community connection.

OBJECTIVE: Pioneer small-scale assisted living units based on six-person households.

DESIGN INTENT: In a two-story building adjacent to the community center, there is a memory support unit with public rooms facing south onto a private garden. Each pair of households makes up one floor, with shared offices, employee facilities, and care support areas. All resident rooms are single-occupancy with wheelchair-accessible bathrooms. Households on a floor can be separated or open to each other as required by resident needs.

OBJECTIVE: Utilize cook-chill food preparation to realize the benefits of centralized preparation with small-scale care delivery.

DESIGN INTENT: A centralized cook-chill kitchen in downtown Trondheim delivers food to all neighborhood-based care centers. Cook-chill convection ovens for each pair of households allow the households to present the food family-style to residents. Tempe meets code-mandated requirements for health, cleanliness, and food temperature through proper equipment and training.

OBJECTIVE: Integrate the new health and welfare centers into neighborhood life through location, innovative programming, and amenities open to all.

DESIGN INTENT: An open campus plan emphasizes permeability and connections across the site between the neighborhood and the river valley. The community center is located at the "100 percent corner" to maximize neighbor-resident interaction. The community center is equipped with a range of indoor and outdoor spaces

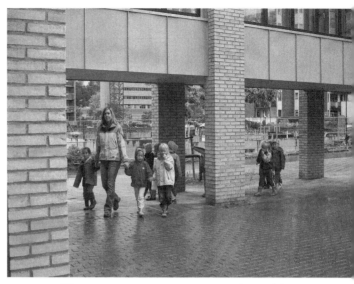

FIG. 22-5 The open campus encourages community participation and use of facilities   *Photo provided by members of the SAGE POE team*

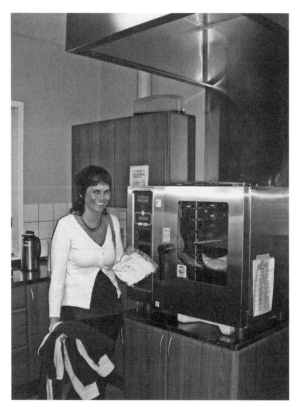

FIG. 22-4 A centralized cook-chill kitchen provides food which is then heated in a convection oven located between each pair of assisted households   *Photo provided by members of the SAGE POE team*

capable of supporting a wide range of activities. The community center has an artist-in-residence program and café that help bring people together.

Field Observations: Meeting the Objectives

OBJECTIVE: Decentralize housing and services for older adults in noninstitutional, home-like settings.

FIELD OBSERVATIONS: Tempe's site plan and scale meet the requirement for a noninstitutional design. The four components—congregate apartments, memory care, health service center and community center—each function independently while maintaining connections that do not overwhelm neighborhood accessibility. Separated into wings, the apartments minimize their own interconnection, further reducing the scale of development.

Although successful in plan, Tempe's architectural imagery is less residential than it might be. Neighborhood-facing façades tend to be brick-faced and somewhat severe, with smaller-scale windows opening on informal, garden-facing façades. The office and health service center stand between the neighborhood and the community center, restricting access and creating a more closed approach. The community center's first-floor brick wall disguises the café, atelier, and multipurpose room activities behind, and the most open passage between neighborhood and

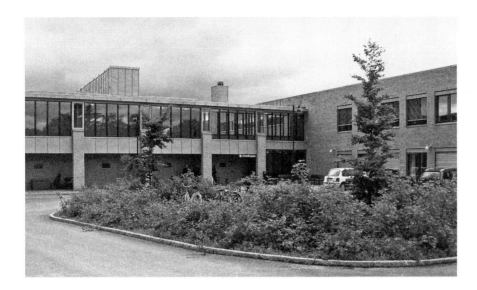

FIG. 22-6 The facility's main entry is understated and lacks residential character *Photo provided by members of the SAGE POE team*

the river bypasses the brick-paved community-center courtyard, robbing it of life.

OBJECTIVE: Implement a new prototype for neighborhood-based older adult service centers.

FIELD OBSERVATIONS: The neighborhood health service center, congregate apartments, and memory support unit implement three components of the new neighborhood-based strategy. Tempe provides the facilities; the Kommune's job is to manage marketing and occupancy to best meet individual needs while maintaining efficient operations, contributing to Kommune-wide capacity, and fulfilling the "neighborhood-based" pledge.

In this period of transition from the older centralized system to the new neighborhood-based model, it is difficult for Tempe as the prototype to meet everyone's expectations. Initial placements into the apartments and the memory support unit followed the neighborhood-basing mandate whenever possible. Outreach by the health service center to older adults in the surrounding area has been more difficult, as it has taken some time for residents to get accustomed to having this resource nearby.

OBJECTIVE: Create sheltered housing apartments that can accommodate complete aging in place, including skilled and hospice care as required.

FIELD OBSERVATIONS: The 61 one-bedroom apartments are organized in three-story blocks that run in parallel from the neighborhood toward the river valley. Second-floor enclosed corridors connect the community center to the first and second blocks. Thereafter, the connection runs on grade between block two and block three. Within each block, primarily one-bedroom apartments are organized facing east or west along double-loaded corridors. With no more than six apartments per floor, a portion of each corridor is single-loaded to allow daylight to enter the space.

OBJECTIVE: Pioneer small-scale assisted living units based on six-person households.

FIELD OBSERVATIONS: Each six-person household was designed with single-occupancy rooms, a living room/lounge, a dining room with a single-family-style table, and a country kitchen shared between two houses. Common to two houses are utility rooms, a serving pantry with the cook-chill convection oven, a laundry room, a storage room, and a staff office/lounge area. The intent was to run each house as a separate unit but with staff backup available next door.

Within a year of opening, staff and family members agreed that the six-person household was too socially confining, so operations were switched to 12-person households instead. Reasons cited focused on creating a more positive social milieu that would be less prone to disturbances from personality conflicts. As a result, one of the two dining rooms is now used as an activity lounge, while the other has several tables to seat all 12 residents. Residents cross through the country kitchen/serving pantry to pass from one side to the other, but this does not seem to create either inconvenience or a safety problem.

Resident rooms are 30 square meters each, including a large bathroom with European shower. Room

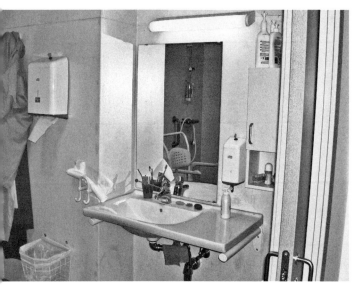

FIG. 22-7 Storage space for personal toiletries in the bathroom is very limited, and lighting levels are not bright enough for elderly eyes   *Photo provided by members of the SAGE POE team*

entries have a double-leaf door that meets local codes for bed movement, but the corridor side provides no front-door personalization for memory cueing. Tempe provides an electric bed, night table (which converts to a writing desk), and guest chair; residents are encouraged to add their own favorite furnishings. A patient

lift is located in every room, but, because it does not connect to the bathroom, it has limited utility. Each room has two windows, one a "French balcony" with in-swinging doors and a railing immediately beyond. In both the resident room and throughout the rest of the household, floor finishes are sheet vinyl, producing a high-glare environment that fails to cushion resident falls.

Resident bathrooms do not match the design standard evident elsewhere. Fixtures are isolated; counter and medicine-cabinet space for residents are minimal. The toilet does not have assistive devices nearby, and, more critically for a memory support unit, cannot be seen from the bedroom. Grab bars in the shower are minimal and the lighting produces considerable glare.

For the entire 24 residents, frontline staffing totals seven full-time employees (FTEs) on days, four FTEs on evenings, and two FTEs on nights, for a total of about four hours of staff time per resident per day. Although the overall care provision seems appropriate for the level of residents observed, night staffing may be low, and activity staffing—currently 0.25 FTE for all 24 residents—is considerably below best practices.

OBJECTIVE: Utilize cook-chill food preparation to realize the benefits of centralized preparation with small-scale care delivery.

FIELD OBSERVATIONS: Quality food service is central to a successful senior living program. Trondheim's cook-chill

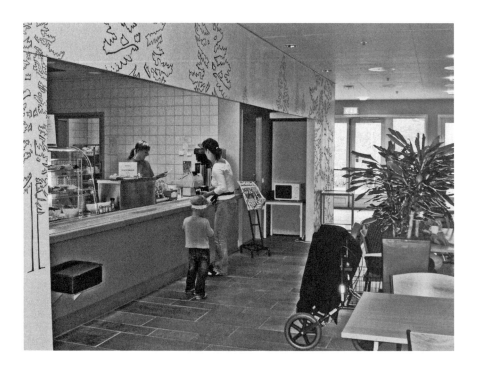

FIG. 22-8 The surrounding community is always welcome in the café; however, the public entrance is difficult to locate   *Photo provided by members of the SAGE POE team*

system is fundamental to the success of a neighborhood-based care model. Consistent preparation, meeting high standards for nutrition, freshness, and cleanliness, plus maintaining proper food temperatures all depend on the cook-chill system working properly.

Each floor of the memory support unit has a dedicated refrigerated pantry and prep area. Meals are reheated in the convection oven and then served family style by frontline staff. Through translators, family members stated that "the quantity of the food is adequate and the taste is good," which suggested room for improvement in both areas. Memory support residents sometimes need snacks and eat at odd hours. Tempe's ability to respond to such à la carte requests was still in development.

OBJECTIVE: Integrate the new health and welfare center into neighborhood life through location, innovative programming, and amenities open to all.

FIELD OBSERVATIONS: Families and staff feel that Tempe still has some distance to go to become fully integrated into neighborhood life, including overcoming some limitations of the physical environment. Tempe's site, at the edge of a neighborhood rather than at its heart, may limit that connection. The closed, solid nature of Tempe's neighborhood face and the partially hidden entrance are not welcoming to outsiders. The inward orientation of the health center does not advertise its services; the café and multipurpose room are shielded from the street.

Physical limitations may yet be counterbalanced by people and programs. The community center amenities can appeal to a wide range of neighborhood residents as interest groups develop. The Kommune recognizes the opportunities, and is encouraging staff to offer more. The adjacent child care center and artist studio are two candidates for expanded roles.

Field Observations: Themes and Hypotheses

Creating Community

The Tempe prototype was designed to foster two types of community: at the small scale, among residents of the assisted memory support program; and, at a larger scale, between Tempe residents and their surrounding neighbors.

In comparison to the larger, more institutional nursing homes being replaced, Tempe's assisted memory support program succeeds in creating a stronger sense of

attachment between residents and Tempe. Family members agreed that their loved ones were happier and more at home in the smaller-scale environment.

At the neighborhood scale, both the Kommune and family members acknowledge that there is much still to be accomplished. The Kommune recognizes that programming is more essential to creating cohesion than they first thought. Expanded activities will include linkages to child care and music programs of general interest. The café is an underutilized resource, capable of a larger role if meals programs for apartment residents are sited there. The café would benefit from signage or more glazing to improve its visibility from the neighborhood, making it less insular and more inviting.

Making a Home

The apartments average 57 square meters each, with eat-in kitchens and wheelchair-accessible bathrooms. Each of the rooms is large enough for the resident's own furniture. The entry hall opens directly into the eat-in kitchen, where a large window with shelf provides a view into the hallway. Most residents kept the café curtains on this window closed, but many used the shelf to display personal items. The living room and bedroom are of almost equal size; sliding doors at either end of the dividing wall give residents a choice of access points. The bathroom, which can be entered from either the bedroom or the entry hall, includes a toilet, a European shower with curtain, a sink, and a washing machine, typical for family housing in Norway.

Residents seem to enjoy their apartments and had space for both prized possessions and favorite furnishings. The large rooms and open layout facilitate care assistance, although the shower and toilet could have more separation. Sliding doors between rooms add to mobility and save space; the sole swing door between the entry and the bathroom is intrusive by contrast. Balconies, about 1.75 by 4 meters, are large enough for furniture and plants. If priced competitively, these apartments would be popular on the general housing market.

Regional/Cultural Design

Tempe's exterior design adheres to a modernist palette, with no attempt to cloak its size in traditional forms. The masonry and wood materials are consistent with local preferences, although even the Kommune admits the design could have been more residential. (See Figure 21 in the color insert.) Inside, the modernist palette is more successful, with railings, light fixtures, and floor finishes combining to create a warm, bright atmosphere.

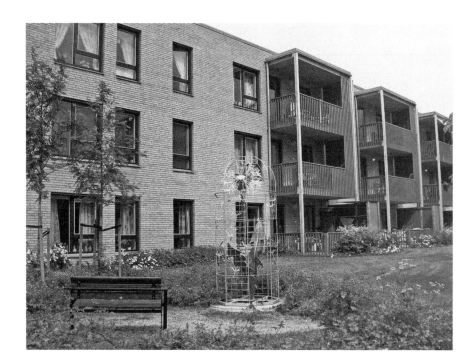

FIG. 22-9 The contemporary exterior is consistent with local vernacular, and artwork from local artists adds an interesting touch
Photo provided by members of the SAGE POE team

Floor finishes were hard surface throughout, which seems in keeping with local preference. In the assisted memory support unit, the hard finishes result in glare that is detrimental to resident mobility. Some apartment residents have throw rugs, and assisted memory support residents are free to use them in their rooms, but this increases the risk of tripping.

Environmental Therapy

With only 18 months of operation at the time of the POE, it was hard for residents, family, or staff to claim evidence-based positive outcomes from the Tempe prototype. However, families do agree that the new environment is better for their loved ones than the previous institutional settings.

Staff's shift from operating two six-resident memory support units to a single 12-resident household, to lessen personality conflicts, reflects ongoing effort to improve the outcomes of the therapeutic environment. Staff look forward to increasing activity programming to further enhance the environment's contribution to resident well-being.

Outdoor Environment

Tempe's wide range of outdoor space is woven throughout the complex, and helps break down the scale of development. Spaces include a large, brick-paved plaza between the community center, memory support unit, and one of the apartment blocks; a linear garden with brook and planting leading toward the river; a private memory support garden bounded by a "living fence"; and sculpture-accented lawn areas bordered by public walking paths between the congregate housing wings.

Most congregate apartments have covered terraces looking onto the lawn areas, and residents appear to use them. Ground-level passages between the congregate housing and community center open exterior spaces to the neighborhood, with activities focused on the brick-paved plaza for neighborhood events. Because of its placement away from the major path from neighborhood to river, the plaza is not as central as it could be. Memory support residents can access their garden or a second south-facing floor balcony that overlooks it.

Quality of Workplace and the Physical Plant

Staff are currently concentrated in the memory support wing, where office areas and break rooms are provided on each floor. A major challenge at all levels of health care in Norway is absenteeism, which tends to reduce Tempe's ability to provide primary caregiver assignments or promote strong identification between residents and caregivers. This was noted by families, who remarked that staff inconsistency caused their loved ones some distress. The Tempe staff are hoping that the new prototype, with its households, smaller size, and noninstitutional feel, will reduce absenteeism and improve staff's sense of responsibility for residents.

Operator Perspectives

The Trondheim Kommune staff who directed Tempe's design and oversee daily operations see the community as a work in progress. They recognize Tempe's difficulties in semi-institutional design, specific problems with glare and underperforming finishes, the lack of connection between on-site residents, and the need to integrate more strongly with the neighborhood.

At the same time, the Kommune sees the cook-chill food service and the 24-bed memory support unit as complementary parts of a successful strategy to decentralize the care of older adults. Engaging these residents through activities is seen as the next step.

The Kommune believes that the congregate apartments are successful as independent living, but knows that these residents may benefit from more communal services, including meals, as they age in place. The Kommune is in the process of discussing when, how, by what means, and under what economic model they can introduce communal services. These issues naturally lead to the future of the community center and its dual role as potential common space for on-site residents as well as a neighborhood center for children, young adults, or families.

The Kommune is applying lessons learned at Tempe to the design of the second- and third-generation projects. As the real-estate component of the new older adult service plan, the Kommune believes Tempe will improve as the "software" side of programming strengthens to match the "hardware" of the built environment.

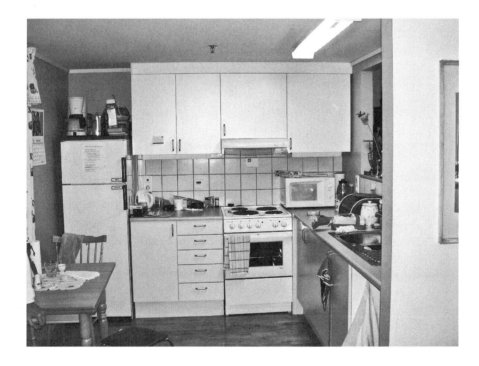

FIG. 22-10 The apartments, complete with kitchens, are intended for independent living. However, it is understood that residents will benefit from the communal services that are offered *Photo provided by members of the SAGE POE team*

General Project Information

PROJECT ADDRESS
Tempe Health and Welfare Centre
Valoyveien 12
Trondheim, Norway

PROJECT STATUS
Completion date: 2003

OCCUPANCY LEVELS
At facility opening date: 95%
At time of evaluation: 95%

RESIDENT AGE (YRS)
At time of evaluation: 84

PROJECT AREAS

SHELTERED HOUSING

AUTHOR'S NOTE: *Although there is no licensure for assisted living in Norway, this care program is comparable to that licensure level in the United States.*

Project Element	New Construction No. Units	New Construction Typical Size
One-bedroom units	61	612–910 GSF
Total (all units)	61	37,819 GSF
Residents' social areas (lounges, dining, and recreation spaces):		1,469 GSF
Medical, health care, therapy, and activities spaces:		0 GSF
Administrative, public, and ancillary support services:		0 GSF
Service, maintenance, and mechanical areas:		13,124 GSF
Total gross area:		54,625 GSF
Total net usable area (per space program):		41,501 NSF
Overall gross/net factor (ratio of gross area/net usable area):		1.32

ASSISTED LIVING

AUTHOR'S NOTE: *Although there is no licensure for skilled nursing in Norway, this care program is comparable to that licensure level in the United States.*

Project Element	New Construction No. Units	New Construction Typical Size
Studio units	24	306 GSF
Total (all units)	24	6,840 GSF
Residents' social areas (lounges, dining, and recreation spaces):		2,164 GSF
Medical, health care, therapy, and activities spaces:		542 GSF
Administrative, public, and ancillary support services:		222 GSF
Service, maintenance, and mechanical areas:		5,380 GSF
Total gross area:		16,500 GSF
Total net usable area (per space program):		11,120 NSF
Overall gross/net factor (ratio of gross area/net usable area):		1.48

OTHER FACILITIES: COMMUNITY CENTER

Social areas (lounges, dining, and
    recreation spaces):   14,629 GSF
Medical, health care, therapy, and activities
    spaces: 463 GSF
Administrative, public, and ancillary support
    services: 1,215 GSF
Service, maintenance, and mechanical areas: 6,957 GSF
Total gross area: 25,693 GSF
Total net usable area (per space program):   18,736 NSF
Overall gross/net factor (ratio of gross area/
    net usable area):   1.37

TOTAL, ALL BUILDINGS

Residence: 44,659 GSF
Social areas (lounges, dining, and recreation
    spaces):   18,262 GSF

Medical, health care, therapy, and activities
    spaces: 1,005 GSF
Administrative, public, and ancillary support
    services: 1,437 GSF
Service, maintenance, and mechanical areas: 25,461 GSF
Total gross area: 96,818 GSF
Total net usable area (per space program):   71,357 NSF
Overall gross/net factor (ratio of gross area/
    net usable area):   1.36

SITE LOCATION

Urban

FINANCING SOURCES

Construction funded by government as part of an oil revenues
    fund
Operations funded by ongoing government taxes and revenues

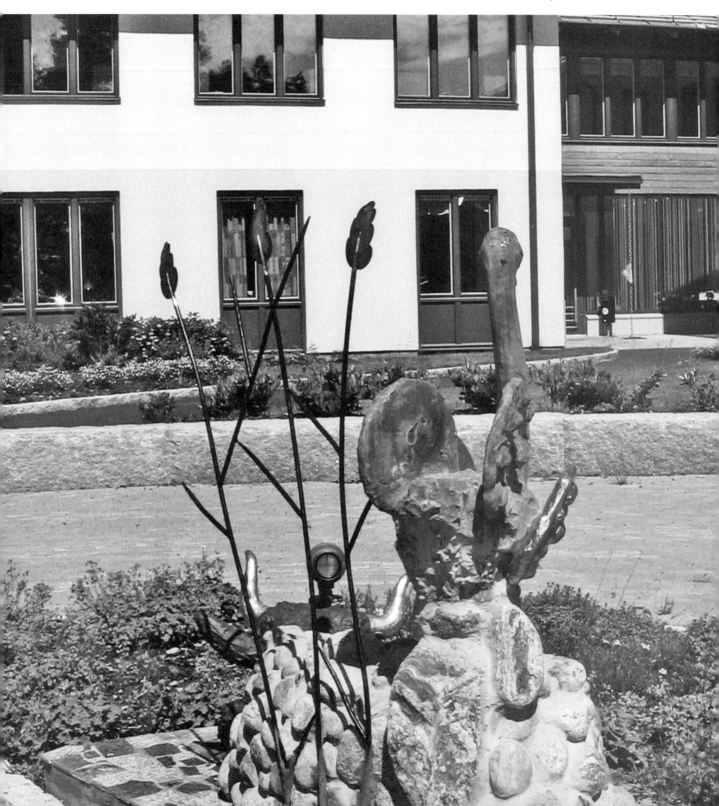

"*The more faithfully you listen to the voices within you, the better you will hear what is sounding outside.*"

DAG HAMMARSKJOLD, 1905–1961

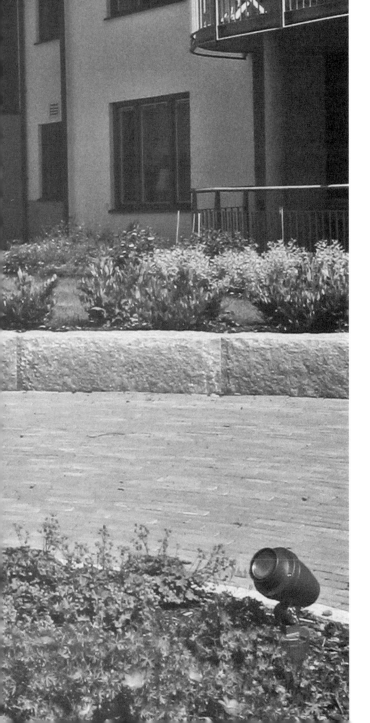

Chapter 23

Swedish Elderly Homes

Long-Term Health Care in Sweden

To fully understand the Swedish approach to long-term elder care, one must first recognize that such care falls under the auspices of the country's national health system and is funded by income taxes and a national insurance system supported by employer contributions. Residents of elderly facilities are required to provide some amount of copayment for housing and services, based on assets, until they have depleted those funds. Between 4 and 5% of the total costs of long-term care are financed through fees charged to residents. Even at this point, residents may maintain a portion of their pension for spending at their discretion.

Elder care facilities are not stratified by licensure, but the majority fall into what would be considered nursing care, although there has recently been a marked increase in assisted-living-level facilities. Since 1992, it has been the responsibility of the Kommun, or state, to provide a health program for the elderly. Both national and local governments have focused upon the ability to allow the elderly to remain within their communities and own residences as long as possible. Because case management is handled by a Kommun nurse, both for home health and facility health care, there is consistency of care for the individual as well as consistency of understanding by the care provider.

This emphasis on home care, coupled with a national policy to maintain the elderly in their homes as long as possible, creates a smaller pool of elderly facility beds than one might expect. Also, as older facilities are decommissioned, the beds are not necessarily replaced. Thus, existing facilities have residents with a lower level of acuity, increased incidence of dementia, shorter resident length of stay, and almost universally full census.

Some Kommuns are beginning to experiment with private care providers that contract to fulfill the Kom-

FIG. 23-1 Local artists provide site artwork for residents to enjoy at Riddarstensgården *Photograph by Jeffrey Anderzhon*

mun's care responsibility. In these cases, as with a newer facility in Lerum Kommun called Riddarstensgården, the government constructs and owns the real estate; the provider leases the property, provides care services and materials necessary for residents, and presumably realizes a profit, while providing the Kommun with less expensive per-person health care.

As in the United States, professional staff are increasingly difficult to recruit in Sweden. Some 10 to 12% of care staff come from outside the country, and it is estimated that by 2010 there will be a 70% turnover of staff due to employees retiring or leaving the professions. Staff-to-resident ratios have historically been set by the facility itself, although in recent years, in the face of significant governmental budget cuts, Kommun governing agencies have begun to take over this responsibility.

Sweden is one of the "oldest" countries, with the world's highest proportion of its population over the age of 65 (about 17.5 percent). Faced with an increasing percentage of the gross domestic product spent on care for the elderly, Sweden will undoubtedly lead the world in finding innovative ways to economically care for its aging population. It is thus important to understand how Swedes deal with this issue, so we all can benefit from their approaches.

Case Study: Klockåreängen

COMMUNITY TYPE: Swedish Elderly Facility

REGION: Western Sweden, rural

OWNER: Ale Kommun, Sweden

ARCHITECT: Unknown

DATA POINTS: Resident Room: 251–434 sf (23.3–40.3 sm)

Residents	48 nursing
Total Area:	692.8 gsf (64.4 gsm)/resident
Total Project Area:	33,255 gsf (3,089 gsm)
Total Project Cost:	Unknown
Investment/resident:	Unknown
Staffing:	4.5 care hours/resident/day
Occupancy:	100% as of June, 2005
Average Length of Stay:	2.5 years

EVALUATION TEAM: Jeffrey Anderzhon, AIA; Uno Claesson; Linda Anderzhon

PROJECT COMPLETED: 1965–1998

DATE OF EVALUATION: June 2005

Introduction

Built in 1965, Klockåreängen would visually fit into any community in the United States and would be immediately recognizable as a structure for the frail elderly. It is not unlike the hundreds of nursing homes built in the United States during the initial years of Medicare. While Medicare was being derided by conservative American politicians as the first step down the slippery slope of socialized long-term care in the late 1960s, Klockåreängen was delivering truly socialized long-term care just north of Göteborg, Sweden.

As have its counterparts in the United States, Klockåreängen has undergone several transformations and endured a 1995 addition and remodeling in search of the ideal environment for the care of an aging population that was itself searching for the ideal provision of care. With these changes came a transformation from a medical-model environment to a household model with small, decentralized, and resident-oriented services. Today the facility takes the form of six households of about eight residents each, all in private studio-style apartment rooms of ample sizes to accommodate a variety of personal furniture. Each household has a kitchen, dining, and living room area, as well as its own staff who become well acquainted with the residents. Of the six households, two are specifically for individuals with dementia.

The shape of this one-story building, which is set in a rural Swedish bedroom community of about 26,000

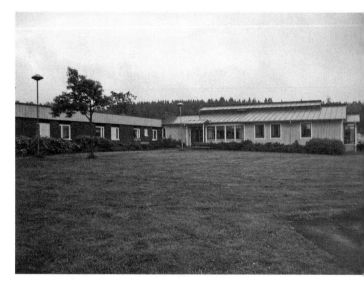

FIG. 23-2 Klockåreängen: Built in the 1960s, this facility for the elderly has had many additions over the years
Photograph by Jeffrey Anderzhon

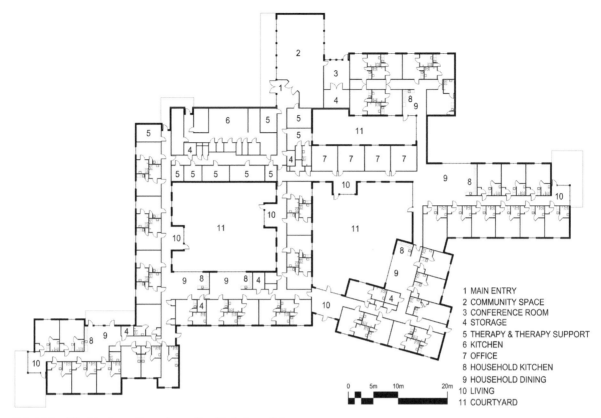

FIG. 23-3 Klockåreängen floor plan *Graphic by Jason Reis*

1 MAIN ENTRY
2 COMMUNITY SPACE
3 CONFERENCE ROOM
4 STORAGE
5 THERAPY & THERAPY SUPPORT
6 KITCHEN
7 OFFICE
8 HOUSEHOLD KITCHEN
9 HOUSEHOLD DINING
10 LIVING
11 COURTYARD

0   5m   10m   20m

residents for urban Göteborg, creates two courtyards fully secured by the surrounding structure. The additions and remodeling have created light-filled passageways for staff and residents to circulate between households to the larger community spaces near the building's main entry. With short summer seasons, exterior space is not only a pleasure but almost a Swedish requirement. The courtyards have both hard and soft surfaces for resident enjoyment, fountains and plants to attract birds and butterflies, and a variety of passive activities for residents to entertain themselves.

Field Observations: Themes and Hypotheses

Creating Community

Set in the middle of a small rural community that is aging in place, this facility has become the center of the community both socially and physically. In one of the several community rooms, dementia support groups or the local Red Cross meet in the evenings. In fact, within

the facility, there are permanent offices for civic organizations, so they can be near the clients they serve. The variously sized rooms allow residents to congregate for holiday meals and parties and even host local family reunions.

The facility, despite its age, is an integral part of the community fabric; residents are not considered to have left the community when they move into the facility, but only to have changed their residence. The benefit of 40 years spent integrating into the community fabric has helped Klockåreängen to maintain strong ties.

Within the confines of the building, there is a true sense of community. The residents recognize their households as their homes, with each resident having an apartment rather than a simple room. The staff is caring and truly concerned about the "family" they care for within the household. When staff members are ill or have a day off, residents ask about them and truly miss them. It is significant to the creation of this community that the staff is consistent, that they are modified universal workers, and that they are vetted during the employment process to be certain they are individuals who have a place in their hearts for the elderly.

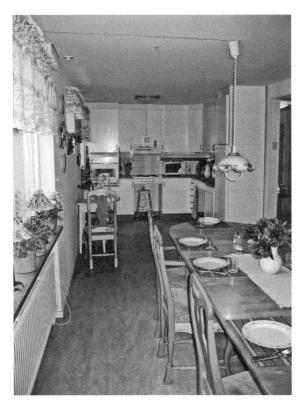

FIG. 23-4 Klockåreängen: A household kitchen where meals are prepared and shared by residents and staff together as a family *Photograph by Jeffrey Anderzhon*

Making a Home

Private apartments, deep connections to the community, and extensive access to the outdoors are important factors that help the facility to be more home-like for its residents. The administration at Klockåreängen takes its commitment to residents seriously and works to make their move from the community relatively easy and beneficial.

Residents' ability to remain connected to the larger community is critical to their feeling at home in this environment. It is commendable that the community outside the facility takes advantage of its social spaces, interacts with the residents, and has installed offices for civic organizations within the facility. This level of interaction not only promotes intergenerational contact, but also reinforces the value and importance residents still have to the larger community; it is an invaluable component of feeling at home in the environment.

Regional/Cultural Design

Klockåreängen is really a design that is somewhat universal in long-term care. The building could fit as easily in the United States as in Sweden. Thus, there is really nothing about the design that specifically relates to the culture of the location or to the region in which it was constructed. This is not to say that it is not a pleasant design, simply that it is a nondescript one. Aside from the operator-generated design of the courtyards, nothing speaks to the visitor as being particularly Scandinavian, although it is clear that the environment is for the elderly. It is not off-putting, neither is it demonstrative of the culture with which it is associated.

Environmental Therapy

Because all competition is controlled through the Kommun, it is difficult to compare environmental therapies to one another. However, Klockåreängen's environment is conducive to a home-like atmosphere and to the therapy of the residents. There really is no question that when the time comes for a member of the community to move to Klockåreängen, the move will be relatively painless and certainly without an overwhelming feeling that he or she has been disconnected from the community.

With the facility divided into smaller households, the therapy provided by the environment is resident oriented and in large part resident directed, in collaboration with the Kommun health authorities. Despite the age of the environment, the facility has been well maintained and updated periodically to meet the needs of residents.

Outdoor Environment

Exterior environments are very important to northern Europeans. The appreciation of these areas is enhanced by the fact that there are only a few months in the year when the outdoors can be enjoyed comfortably. The exterior spaces at Klockåreängen are primarily formed by the construction of the building itself and, as a result, are secure from elopement and extremely accessible to residents, staff, and family members. This accessibility is both physical and visual, with single-loaded corridors providing full visual access throughout the year.

The courtyards provide a variety of plantings, exterior furniture, attractions, and activities. The senses are stimulated by water features, flowering plants, and the birds and butterflies attracted to them.

Quality of Workplace and the Physical Plant

When compared to newer facilities in the western Sweden area, Klockåreängen is feeling its age. Even with this in mind, however, the facility is providing a quality of care that would be the envy of many communities in the

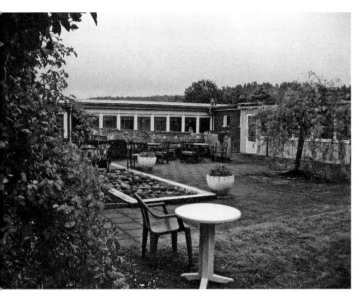

FIG. 23-5 Klockåreängen: In good weather, the outdoors is relished by residents *Photograph by Jeffrey Anderzhon*

United States. The staff may see the environment for what it is, but understand that their work is critically important regardless of the workplace. In many ways they mold the workplace to their idea of a quality environment simply by their love for the elderly.

There are higher-quality long-term care environments in Sweden, largely because of their newer physical plants, but few have been transformed by their staff to the quality of Klockåreängen.

Operator Perspectives

The administrator of Klockåreängen expressed concern about the age of the facility and the costs involved in keeping it functional. The building has undergone a number of both minor and major transformations over the years including the additions of at least two households, the addition of porches or decks to the households lacking access to the courtyards, and upgrades to and modernization of the interiors.

The length of the corridors and distances from the centralized services to some of the households was another concern the administrator expressed. Despite the benefits of single-loaded designs, visual access to the

exterior, and furniture residents have brought from their own homes, the corridors remain a concern to the operator in terms of staff efficiency and fire safety.

During the interviews, the administration was very interested in the trends of nursing environmental design in the United States. This interest was combined with a belief that the Klockåreängen environment was significantly lagging in its approach to long-term elderly care and that the households were deficient in both staff efficiency and resident efficacy when compared to average facilities in the United States. Despite this, it was apparent that the operator and staff have deep empathy for their residents and provide a high level of care for the residents within the constraints of Kommun oversight and the aging physical environment. They creatively integrated a dynamic environment with a dynamic care program to the benefit of both residents and staff.

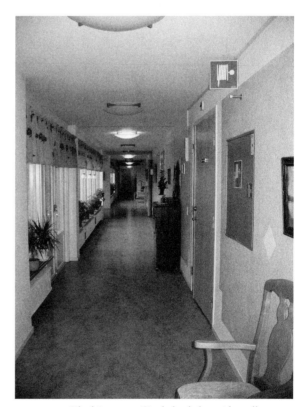

FIG. 23-6 Klockåreängen: Single-loaded corridors allow natural light to flow into the households and provide residents with an outdoor orientation *Photograph by Jeffrey Anderzhon*

General Project Information

PROJECT ADDRESS
Klockåreängen
Odalvägen 2
Skepplanda
Sweden

PROJECT STATUS
Completed in 1998

OCCUPANCY LEVELS
At date of evaluation: 100%

RESIDENT AGE (YRS)
At time of evaluation: 83

PROJECT AREAS

SKILLED NURSING

AUTHOR'S NOTE: *Although there is no licensure for skilled nursing in Sweden, the care program is comparable to that licensure level in the United States.*

| | New Construction | |
Project Element	No. Units	Typical Size
Resident room (average area)	48	300.5 GSF
Total (all units)	48	13,855 GSF
Residents' social areas (lounges, dining, and recreation spaces):		4,741 GSF
Medical, health care, therapy, and activities spaces:		1,528 GSF
Administrative, public, and ancillary support services:		2,785 GSF
Service maintenance, and mechanical areas:		7,148 GSF
Total gross area:		33,255 GSF
Total net usable area:		22,909 NSF
Overall gross/net factor (ratio of gross area/net usable area)		1.45

Case Study: Hedegården

COMMUNITY TYPE: Swedish Elderly Facility

REGION: Western Sweden, suburban

OWNER: Lerum Kommun, Sweden

ARCHITECT: Nils Andréasson Arkitektkontor AB

DATA POINTS: Resident Room: 370–445 sf (34.4–41.4 sm)

Residents	56 nursing
Total Area:	937 gsf (87.1 gsm)/resident
Total Project Area:	52,474 gsf (4,880.1 gsm)
Total Project Cost:	Unknown
Investment/resident:	Unknown

Staffing
(nondementia):	3.64 care hours/resident/day
(dementia):	4.68 care hours/resident/day
Occupancy:	100% as of June, 2005
Average Length of Stay:	1.5 years

EVALUATION TEAM: Jeffrey Anderzhon, AIA; Uno Claesson; Fredrik Zeybrandt; Linda Anderzhon

PROJECT COMPLETED: 1998

DATE OF EVALUATION: June 2005

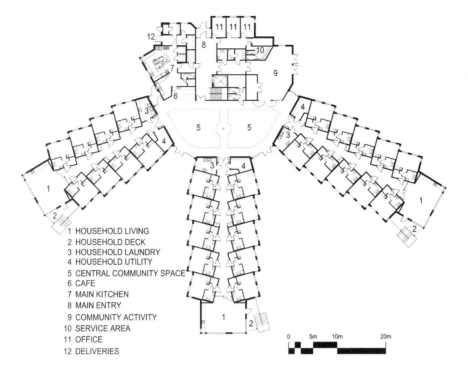

1 HOUSEHOLD LIVING
2 HOUSEHOLD DECK
3 HOUSEHOLD LAUNDRY
4 HOUSEHOLD UTILITY
5 CENTRAL COMMUNITY SPACE
6 CAFE
7 MAIN KITCHEN
8 MAIN ENTRY
9 COMMUNITY ACTIVITY
10 SERVICE AREA
11 OFFICE
12 DELIVERIES

0 5m 10m 20m

FIG. 23-7 Hedegården: first-floor plan *Graphic by Jason Reis*

Introduction

Just outside the city center of Lerum, a suburban community of about 35,000 residents, Hedegården sits on a gently rolling campus of attractive low-rise apartments contemporary with this two-story structure, which was constructed in 1998. As with most elder-care facilities in Sweden, this 56-bed community to the northeast of the city of Göteborg is owned and was built by the Kommun. Organized in a modified-T configuration, the resident wings radiate from a large central community space. The main entry, as well as administrative and support functions, is housed in the structure that encloses the community space, and all are convenient to both residents and staff.

Each floor of two resident wings contains 10 residents, while one two-story wing contains eight residents on a floor. Both floors of the smallest of the three wings are dedicated to dementia units with controlled entry and are programmed for diminished resident stimulation. Aside from the number of residents, each wing is identical, with resident rooms situated along a double-loaded corridor, a resident laundry and staff support space nearest the community center, and a resident gathering room at the termination of the wing.

The resident rooms are organized slightly askew from the corridor plane, which allows the corridor to take on a sort of saw-toothed configuration. This diminishes visual corridor length and has significant additional benefits. The areas created by the configuration in the corridor are utilized for small closets that serve as storage areas for resident supplies, thus decentralizing supply storage and minimizing the use of carts within resident spaces. Residents have also taken ownership of these

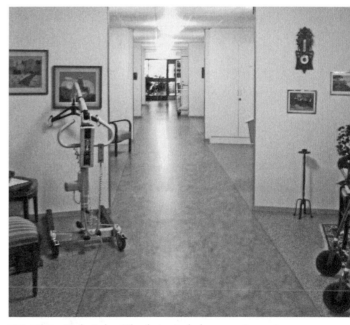

FIG. 23-8 Hedegården: The design includes spaces in corridors that become part of the resident's home *Photograph by Jeffrey Anderzhon*

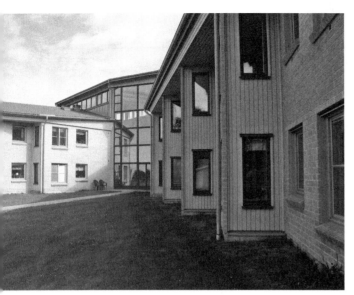

FIG. 23-9 Hedegården: The design provides resident rooms with varying views and a large, centrally located community room *Photograph by Jeffrey Anderzhon*

nooks in the corridor, placing personal items and furniture from their homes in them and thereby creating a welcoming and transitional feeling that delineates public and private spaces.

An added benefit of the offset organization is that each resident room receives a small window within the wall perpendicular to the main exterior wall. This small detail provides additional views, additional natural light, and an opportunity for natural cross-ventilation for the room. The effect is significant and creates options for the resident in furniture placement and environmental comfort that would not be available in a more traditional room organization.

The gathering room creates a natural household on each floor of each wing. Within this nicely proportioned space are a resident kitchen, dining area, and seating area. Aside from the kitchen location, residents are free to organize the large room into divisions that suit each household best. The room has full windows on one wall, as well as a large expanse of glass along a perpendicular wall that also leads to a small patio available to residents.

Field Observations: Themes and Hypotheses

Creating Community

The environmental and programmatic organization of Hedegården contribute to the sense of community within this facility. The large, two-story community space where the three resident wings conjoin provides a multipurpose community gathering space that is well used. Natural light flows generously into the space from full-height windows and clerestories, making it inviting, visually stimulating, and distinctly different from the resident wings. The contrast creates a sense of leaving one's home and joining the larger community on Main Street.

This space is versatile, serving large numbers of residents and visitors for community dining, activities and group celebrations. It is also intimate enough to provide small seating areas for conversation, the resident/staff lunch buffet line, and a bistro dining area. An adjacent two-story area houses the main building entry, administration offices, staff break room, staff exercise area, and a smaller resident activity room. The spaces flow well together for use by the entire community, and the larger community room provides dramatic volumes as the second level of the building traverses this area by means of glass-railed balconies.

Hedegården enjoys a seamless connection to the community of Lerum and the surrounding apartments, whose elderly residents maintain friendships with the residents. Displays in the large central community room are maintained by a combination of staff and community volunteers and are changed on a regular basis. Several community organizations take advantage of the facility space for periodic meetings. As with other Kommun-owned elder-care facilities, there is a sort of natural connection to community that comes from the integration of all levels of elder health-care.

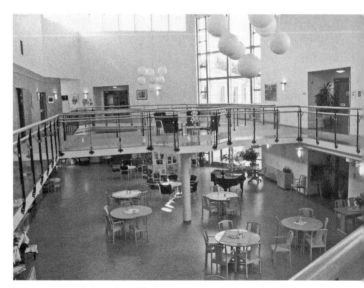

FIG. 23-10 Hedegården: The large community room is flooded with natural light, but the hard surfaces provide acoustical challenges *Photograph by Jeffrey Anderzhon*

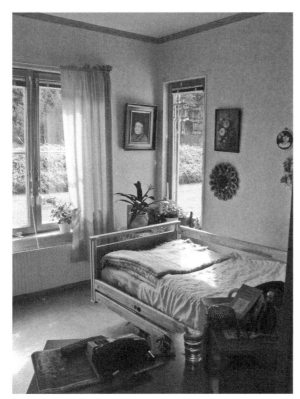

FIG. 23-11 Hedegården: Resident rooms are spacious and airy, with multiple windows *Photograph by Jeffrey Anderzhon*

Making a Home

Just as with Klockåreängen's relationship to the larger community, the connection to Lerum is vital to making residents feel at home in Hedegården. Residents feel valued by the community and connected to the activities and lifestyle they enjoyed before moving to the facility.

The resident rooms, with spacious interiors and private spaces, also help residents to adjust to life in a care facility. The interior windows are an exceptional feature that enhance residents' connection to the spaces outside their rooms, and the ability to customize further familiarizes the space. The ability to customize furniture in the shared spaces extends this familiarization to the semi-public spaces.

Regional/Cultural Design

Hedegården fits well into this relatively new neighborhood of low-rise residential buildings. The exterior design provides interest and begs the viewer to take another look. Certainly the design fits regionally, as it is demonstrably a Northern European structure in its character, complete with faux clay tile and standing-seam metal roofing and eyebrow windows. It is respectful of

established Scandinavian vernacular without being condescending or disingenuous in its execution.

Environmental Therapy

Hedegården's environment provides a light and cheerful ambience and allows resident independence, options, and dignity. Each of the resident rooms is private occupancy and is of a size and proportion that allow wide diversity in furniture arrangement and decoration. Additionally, there is a significant amount of resident opportunity to participate in differing levels of social interaction with other residents, family members, and visitors.

The corridor design allows residents to personalize their spaces and is a convenient area that provides a psychological transition between purely private resident space and that which is shared with others.

Resident and staff traffic flow relatively well in and out of the households, although the placement of the household living area at the end of the wings increases the staff travel distances when that area is used for the care program. The two-story configuration creates some vertical communication issues because there is only one elevator, although staff has quickly learned to utilize the stairs.

The finishes throughout the facility, as is fairly typical of Scandinavian environments, are primarily hard surfaces, with little in the way of flooring or wall coverings to attenuate acoustical problems. This is particularly true in the large central community room, where inti-

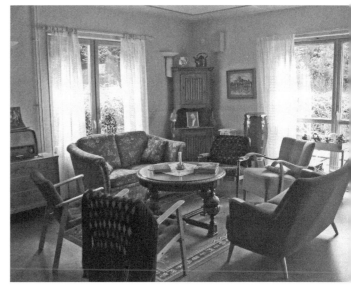

FIG. 23-12 Hedegården: Furnishings for the community activity room are provided by the residents. As a result, many furniture styles are combined, but it looks and feels like home *Photograph by Jeffrey Anderzhon*

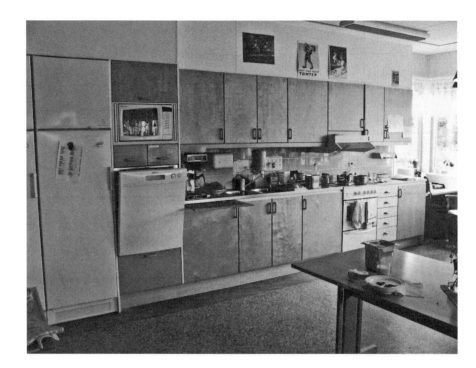

FIG. 23-13 Hedegården: Each household common area has a serving/activity kitchen, dining space, and living space, as well as access to the outdoors
Photograph by Jeffrey Anderzhon

mate conversations are problematic when there are a number of people in the space.

Outdoor Environment

The building shape defines exterior spaces that could be nicely articulated, but have largely been ignored. Aside from one courtyard that is available for dementia residents, there are no secured exterior spaces for resident use without fear of elopement. Each household has a patio or deck that is nicely sized for use by perhaps four residents at one time, but these do not lead to any additionally developed exterior areas. Additionally, the second-level decks require residents to use an exterior stair to access grade-level courtyards.

Perhaps as compensation for the underdeveloped exterior spaces, the central community room does provide lovely natural light and interior areas where residents can appreciate the exterior visually.

Quality of Workplace and the Physical Plant

Hedegården is a well-maintained, pleasant environment for both residents and staff. At the time of construction, there was a concern that staff retention and attraction would be an increasingly difficult issue in a community and nation that is seeing a shrinking professional workforce. A larger amount of facility area has been dedicated here specifically for staff use, including nicely sized locker and break rooms and a staff exercise area.

The vertical communication and, to some degree, the length of the corridors present a counterpoint to the created ambience of the environment. However, care staff primarily remain within their households during their work shifts. This, combined with a modified universal-worker approach to staffing and the decentralized location of supplies, diminishes the need for frequent travel between households.

Operator Perspectives

The operator of Hedegården is Lerum Kommun. Government officials were intimately involved in the planning process for both the environment and the care program for that environment. Having had additional experience with elder care, the Kommun made conscious choices regarding the environment and the use of that environment. It is not surprising, therefore, that they are quite pleased with the environment and its functionality.

They are particularly pleased with the dementia households. Although these differ from the others only in the number of residents in each household, they provide environments in which dementia residents can function well. The one issue that was revealed through an interview with the facility administrator was that the programmatic activities within the dementia courtyard are difficult for residents on the upper-floor level to access.

General Project Information

PROJECT ADDRESS
Hedegården
Ölslanda Gärde 157
443 60 Stenkullen
Sweden

PROJECT STATUS
Completed in 1998

SKILLED NURSING
AUTHOR'S NOTE: *Although there is no licensure for skilled nursing in Sweden, the care program is comparable to that licensure level in the United States.*

OCCUPANCY LEVELS
At date of evaluation: 100%

RESIDENT AGE (YRS)
At date of evaluation: 83

| | New Construction | |
Project Element	No. Units	Typical Size
Resident room (average area)	56	407.5 GSF
Total (all units)	56	23,332 GSF
Residents' social areas (lounges, dining, and recreation spaces):		9,921 GSF
Medical, health care, therapy, and activities spaces:		3,963 GSF
Administrative, public, and ancillary support services:		4,707 GSF
Service, maintenance, and mechanical areas:		8,384 GSF
Total gross area:		52,474 GSF
Total net usable area:		41,923 NSF
Overall gross/net factor (ratio of gross area/net usable area):		1.25

Case Study: Riddarstensgården

COMMUNITY TYPE: Swedish Elderly Facility

REGION: Western Sweden, suburban

OWNER: Lerum Kommun, Sweden

ARCHITECT: Porten Arkitekter

DATA POINTS: Resident Room: 301–334 sf (27.9–31.1 sm)
Residents: 40 nursing
Total Area: 873.2 gsf (81.2 gsm)/resident
Total Project Area: 34,929 gsf (3,248.4 gsm)
Total Project Cost: Unknown
Investment/resident: Unknown
Staffing
  (nondementia): 3.64 care hours/resident/day
  (dementia): 4.68 care hours/resident/day
Occupancy: 100% as of June, 2005
Average Length of Stay: 1.5 years

EVALUATION TEAM: Jeffrey Anderzhon, AIA; Uno Claesson; Fredrik Zeybrandt; Linda Anderzhon

PROJECT COMPLETED: 2002

DATE OF EVALUATION: June 2005

Introduction

An interesting comparison to the Kommun-built and -operated Hedegården, and but a few blocks away, is Riddarstensgården, an elder-care facility that has a rehabilitation clinic component. This facility is also owned by the Kommun, but was constructed to the requirements of a for-profit private care provider that operates the facility on a leased basis. One can immediately see some differences by comparing the data points: for example, the area per resident is less at the newer facility, even though the presented calculation includes the rehabilitation clinic areas.

Riddarstensgården's long-term care residences are housed in two distinct wings that radiate from the main building entry, two stories on one side and three on the other. The rehabilitation clinic is entered opposite the

long-term portion of the building through the same main entry. The entire building is located on a somewhat hilly site that also has a series of mid-rise elder apartment buildings, thus creating a sort of continuing care campus.

The residential wings are designed with a household concept in mind and include eight private-occupancy resident rooms on each household floor, for a total of 40 residents within a total of five households. The household is entered from a small and confining public vestibule. Immediately upon entry, the visitor is thrust into what appears to be a fairly lengthy corridor with resident rooms on either side. Not until the midpoint of this corridor does any visual relief occur. Here is where the household kitchen and dining areas are located. Each household dining area has a patio or deck that is of sufficient size to seat most of the house-

FIG. 23-14 Riddarstens-gården: First-floor plan
Graphic by Jason Reis

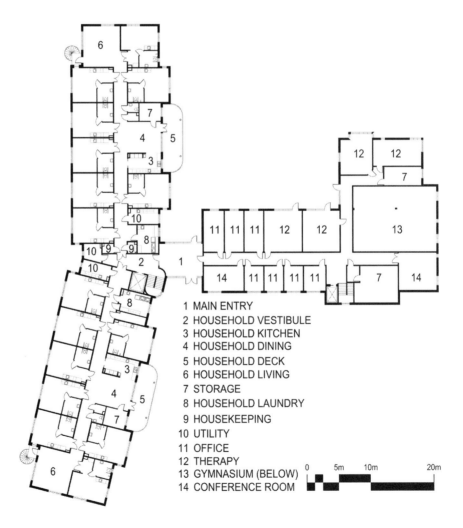

1 MAIN ENTRY
2 HOUSEHOLD VESTIBULE
3 HOUSEHOLD KITCHEN
4 HOUSEHOLD DINING
5 HOUSEHOLD DECK
6 HOUSEHOLD LIVING
7 STORAGE
8 HOUSEHOLD LAUNDRY
9 HOUSEKEEPING
10 UTILITY
11 OFFICE
12 THERAPY
13 GYMNASIUM (BELOW)
14 CONFERENCE ROOM

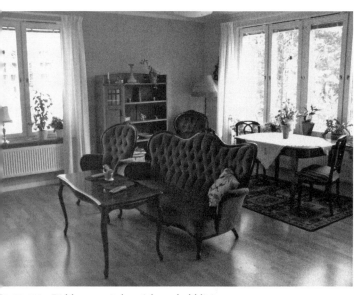

FIG. 23-15   Riddarstensgården: A household living room with resident-provided furniture and accessories   *Photograph Jeffrey Anderzhon*

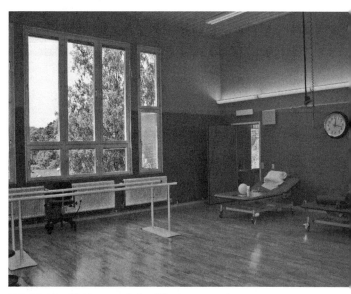

FIG. 23-16   Riddarstensgården: The two-story therapy gym for residents and outpatients is well furnished and well lit with natural sunlight   *Photograph by Jeffrey Anderzhon*

hold residents. The household living room is situated at the terminal end of this corridor and becomes a destination rather than a location for casual resident involvement.

A resident laundry room is located directly adjacent to the household entry. The combination of this household organization is somewhat counterintuitive to a universal residential typology and is also somewhat disconcerting to a visitor. Combined with the restrictive main entry vestibule and entry sequence to each household, the general feeling of the facility is not welcoming.

The rehabilitation wing also houses the administrative offices and a small common social area for the long-term care residents on the second level. A separate entry for rehabilitation patients serves to fully separate these two populations. This clinic is a well-designed, well-organized and well-fitted small rehabilitation clinic, complete with physical, occupational, speech, and audio rehabilitation functions, as well as ample consultation rooms, support offices, and a very nicely equipped two-story gymnasium. This portion of the building is also two levels, with a third level beneath the entry level that takes advantage of a site grade drop. This level also provides a grade-level entry from the space into a small, well-appointed deck and garden area available for rehabilitation patients, as both a resting and a restorative environment.

Field Observations: Themes and Hypotheses

Creating Community

Riddarstensgården is situated within a seemingly tight-knit larger community that tends to respect the elderly and continues to involve them in community activities. Upon this foundation, the facility is situated on a campus that addresses a wider variety of elder-care and retirement options. The adjacent elder apartments have been purposefully situated close to this facility and the two populations play against one another, flowing together visually, aesthetically, and socially.

Ironically, there is a significantly small amount of space for families and visitors to socially interact with residents, or for residents to interact with other residents outside each household. This fact tends to keep residents somewhat isolated, and as a result there does not appear to be an intuitive sense of belonging to a larger community.

The organizational design of Riddarstensgården also tends to work against easy social interaction between households, as well as outside the building. The entry sequence for visitors is restrictive and unwelcoming, as is the area where one moves from one household to another. Once inside a household, the organization strains an easy flow into the social ambience of the

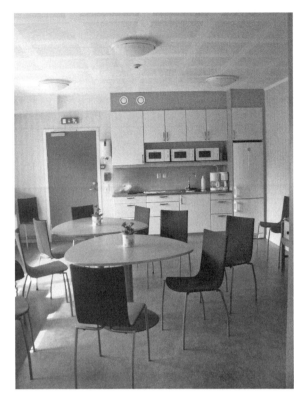

FIG. 23-17 Riddarstensgården: A small community room on the second floor provides space for residents from any household to share time with visitors *Photograph by Jeffrey Anderzhon*

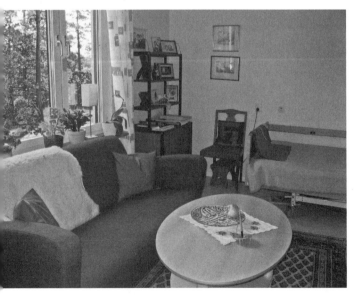

FIG. 23-18 Riddarstensgården: Resident rooms are large enough to accommodate several pieces of the resident's own furniture *Photograph by Jeffrey Anderzhon*

household. Aside from the household living and dining areas, there is really no easily accessible space where residents and visitors can go for a brief out-of-household experience.

Making a Home

The resident rooms are generous, providing residents with ample areas for privacy or for casually entertaining a neighbor. The resident rooms located opposite the dining room are somewhat less desirable, as this area frequently becomes a high-traffic area and somewhat noisy with activity. Nevertheless, the ample space allotted to residents gives them a feeling of independence and dignity.

The furnishings chosen for the household dining rooms are contemporary Scandinavian with bright and cheery fabrics, which helps to make the residents feel more comfortable in their surroundings. The living rooms, however, are furnished with a collection of disparate pieces that appear to have been garnered from residents' homes. This is a refreshing counterpoint to the aesthetic of the building and adds a great deal of character to the living rooms. It also provides a thread of connection for residents and certainly serves to transfigure the household into a home for many.

Regional/Cultural Design

Riddarstensgården was designed with functionality as a primary goal, and in that it succeeds with its compact

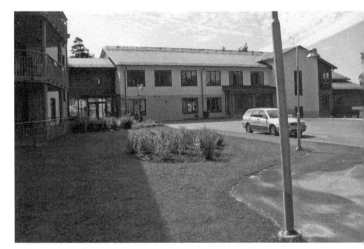

FIG. 23-19 Riddarstensgården: The main entry subtly divides the households from the therapy clinic *Photograph by Jeffrey Anderzhon*

organization and adjacencies. However, the aesthetics of the facility are relatively nondescript and do not relate to a design language of the region. The plain stucco finish, without relief of detail, is somewhat bland; the only visual relief provided on the façade are the balconies where wood siding is utilized, and a seemingly arbitrary change in stucco color on one wing of the building.

Interior finishes are consistent with Scandinavian tastes, being primarily durable and easily maintained. Floors are tile or wood and walls are without wall coverings, with the exception of the bath and toilet rooms, which are finished with ceramic tile.

Environmental Therapy

Resident rooms are generous in size and have very nice natural lighting. This room design allows residents to personalize their rooms with furniture arrangement and decoration, which aids in transforming the rooms into spaces that become their own. The centralized location of the household kitchen and dining is certainly convenient for residents, and as a result this is where most of their time is spent. The attraction of this area is enhanced by access to the only household exterior space—the balcony. Diffused natural light flows into this space and becomes the visual as well as physical center of the residents' living environment. One household has been selected as a dementia-specific household, although no modification was made to the design for this purpose. Additionally, there are residents with earlier stages of dementia throughout the facility, and the design works well for them.

Outdoor Environment

Residents have little direct access to the exterior except at the balconies just off the household dining areas. These are utilized quite extensively by residents simply to sit and enjoy the outdoors. At grade level beyond the main entry connection between the resident wings and the rehabilitation clinic, there is a nicely developed patio area complete with artwork from local artists. However, there is no furniture or shade in this area and it is thus rarely used. This area is also accessible from therapy rooms in the clinic, with the patio surfacing extending to doors from these rooms. Patio furniture, complete with shading umbrellas, is situated here, and it is apparent that clinic patients and staff take advantage of this outdoor environment.

The resident rooms do have very nice visual access to the exterior, and the facility site is surrounded by an

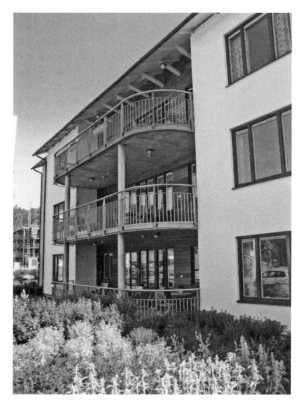

FIG. 23-20   Riddarstensgården: Balconies in each household provide residents with access to the outdoors   *Photograph by Jeffrey Anderzhon*

attractive natural landscape. The thickly insulated exterior building walls provide a deep window sill on which most residents have placed live plants and flowers. This draws the eye to the window and acts as a visual transition from constructed space to the outdoors.

Quality of Workplace and the Physical Plant

The operation of Riddarstensgården was contracted for with Attendo Senior Care, a substantial provider of health care in Europe, and all staff are employees of Attendo. A modified universal-worker approach is utilized for this facility, and a supervising nurse has responsibility for two households during each shift. This becomes somewhat problematic, as one wing has two levels and one has three. However, the separate dementia household on the third level of the larger wing creates a demarcation in the staffing responsibility. Generally, the care providing staff remain within each household. This is possible partly because the supply storage for each household is located within that area.

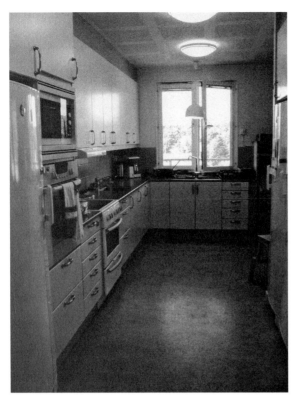

FIG. 23-21 Riddarstensgården: Each household kitchen is fully equipped for meal preparation and food storage
Photograph by Jeffrey Anderzhon

The staff appear to be content in their responsibilities and state that the environment is a pleasing place in which to work. Interestingly, one nursing staff member who was interviewed is a native of the United States, and when asked to compare workplaces between the two countries, she indicated that although there were similarities in care provision, the overall quality of the workplaces in Sweden was far more beneficial to staff and thus to the quality of care provided.

Operator Perspectives

The operator, Attendo Senior Care, was an active participant in the design of this facility and the functionality of the building was obviously of primary concern. There is very little wasted space within the resident households, and some amount of thought was given to understanding the efficiency of caregivers. Within this framework, the operator of the facility is pleased.

From an operational standpoint, the rehabilitation clinic far outshines the long-term care wing. This clinic provides services for the community of Lerum as well as those requiring rehabilitation from the households. Ample space in therapy rooms, convenience of consulting and office space, and intuitive patient wayfinding add to the functionality of this area.

General Project Information

PROJECT ADDRESS
Riddarstensgården
Attendo Senior Care
Riddarstenshöjd 11
443 33 Lerum
Sweden

PROJECT STATUS
Completed in 2002

OCCUPANCY LEVELS
At date of evaluation: 100%

RESIDENT AGE (YRS)
At date of evaluation: 80

PROJECT AREA: SKILLED NURSING

AUTHOR'S NOTE: *Although there is no licensure for skilled nursing in Sweden, the care program is comparable to that licensure level in the United States.*

Project Element	New Construction	
	No. Units	Typical Size
Resident room (average area)	40	317 GSF
Total (all units)	40	12,434 GSF
Residents' social areas (lounges, dining, and recreation spaces):		4,986 GSF
Medical, health care, therapy, and activities spaces:		5,761 GSF
Administrative, public, and ancillary support services:		3,364 GSF
Service, maintenance, and mechanical areas:		8,384 GSF
Total gross area:		34,929 GSF
Total net usable area:		26,545 NSF
Overall gross/net factor (ratio of gross area/net usable area):		1.32

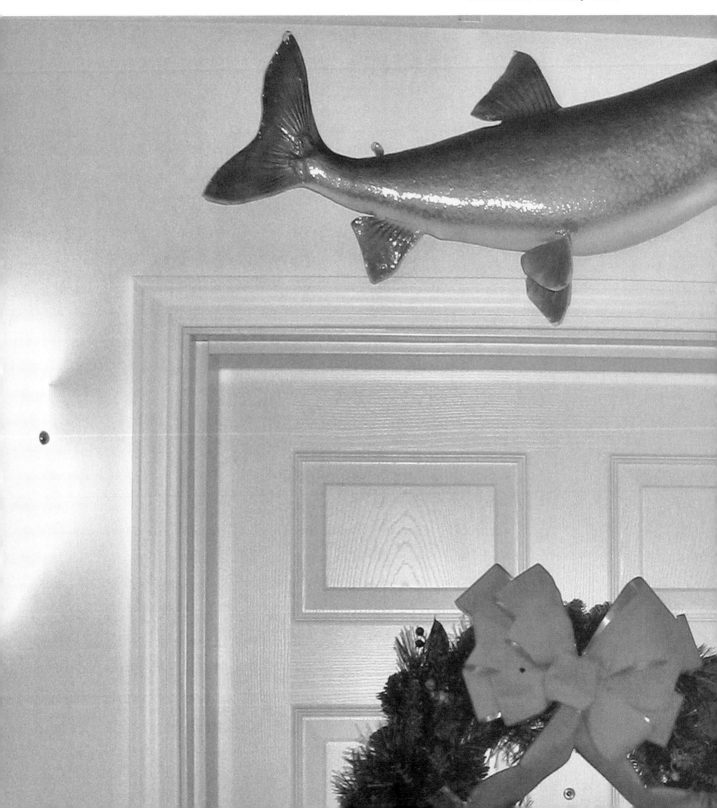

"We've put more effort into helping folks reach old age than into helping them enjoy it."

FRANK A. CLARK, 1911–

Conclusions and Next Steps

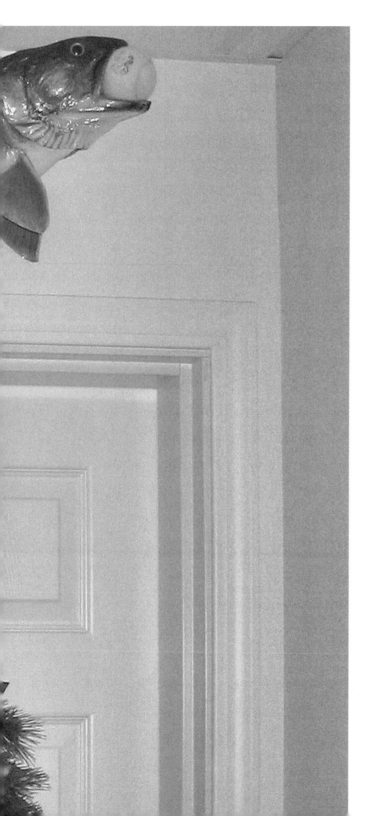

There is difficulty and danger in drawing general conclusions from the evaluations represented in this volume. The danger would be summary judgment of designs without full engagement in the design, construction, and operations processes that produced the communities evaluated.

These evaluations were done on structures that were fully vetted, through rigorous processes, by both owner and architect, and with justifiable reasoning behind decisions and compromises made. It is unfair to make broad generalizations on the basis of these evaluations alone.

However, upon review of all of the evaluations, *general* evidences that were noted in a large number of evaluations can provide some insight as to the success of these projects. In addition, *specific* issues also merit mention, so that they can be avoided, be summarily included, or at least be fully considered when working on future environments for the aging.

Generalized Common Evidences

Successful innovation and successful projects are the result of a committed and consistent board of directors, as well as a strong champion for the project within the organization. A clear mission, vision, and purpose must unite all parties involved.

A certain inner strength is necessary within the champion if an innovative project is to come to fruition and be successful. It is far too easy to fall back on traditional solutions that have served well in the past and to take comfort in the belief that such a solution will continue to serve residents in the future. True advancement in care provision programs and environments is the result of thinking beyond traditional limits and embracing a passion to take something that has been done well and make it even better.

FIG. CONC-1 Allowing residents the freedom and choice to personalize their space will make it their home   *Photograph by Jeffrey Anderzhon*

It should also be noted that the presence of a strong advocate or champion can also quickly lead a project astray, especially if that person is unwilling to fully and systemically understand the ramifications of a wrong-headed decision. This usually coincides with a reluctance to admit that the approach may indeed have been wrong-headed.

CONCLUSION: *Visions of the future are best tested in specific facility situations and, if they pass the test of true and meaningful innovation, become part of a community's unifying mission and purpose. Moreover, sincere dedication to the mission must also demonstrate flexibility to accommodate any "bumps in the road" and to "stay the course."*

Successful innovation in environments for the aging requires considerable time and effort prior to any construction. Time to consider the ramifications of the innovation, time to consider the resource implications of the innovation, and time to refine the innovation are all required steps to success.

Time is money. Without question, quality and innovation take time to envision and bring to reality. In our economically driven world, time translates quickly to resources, and preparation is the passport for this journey. The innovations highlighted in this book were accomplished with a great deal of preparation time in research and in thought about the correct course of action to ensure full value gained from the committed resources.

This is not to say that successful innovation cannot occur on an accelerated schedule, only that the innovative thoughts should be completely researched, fully formed, and well considered. Within a collaborative environment, this can be accomplished expeditiously, and innovations can be tested by all involved and completed in a time frame that incorporates a comfortable and affordable build-out schedule.

CONCLUSION: *Allocate the time to fully form the vision and to collaborate with those who will move that vision into reality. Test the vision, or specific parts of the vision, in an existing environment to discover and address any implementation challenges or unforeseen consequences that arise.*

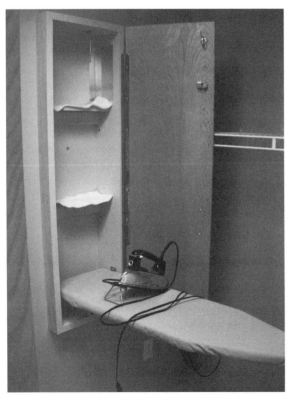

FIG. CONC-2   Residents feel useful and at home when small details that help support routine activities learned from daily living are included in the design   *Photograph courtesy of Jane Rohde, AIA, FIIDA, JSR Associates, Inc.*

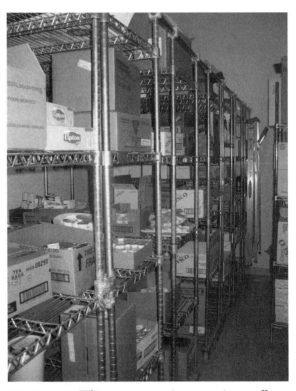

FIG. CONC-3   When storage space is at a premium, staff creativity can help. Stationary food storage shelves are converted to rolling shelves by adding casters on the bottom and track on the top, thereby doubling the storage capacity of a small space   *Photograph by Jeffrey Anderzhon*

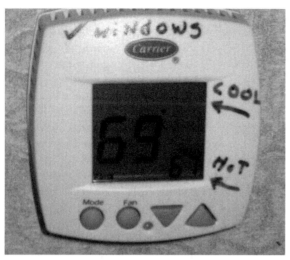

FIG. CONC-4 Modern-day conveniences and improvements in technology can create obstacles for residents. This contemporary thermostat had to be permanently marked to become user-friendly for the assisted living resident. Using common sense, the specification of a simple, inexpensive thermostat would have been a better choice   *Photograph by Jeffrey Anderzhon*

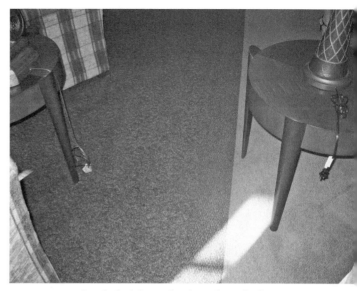

FIG. CONC-5 Overlooked design details can limit the function of a space. When furniture arrangements in the center of the room depend upon table lamps, it is critical to ensure access to electrical outlets   *Photograph by Jeffrey Anderzhon*

Innovations are by definition new methods of doing something that has been done in a certain way in the past. If we are complacent in our routines, innovation will be stifled. Innovative leadership can produce innovative follow-through by our coworkers.

Care innovations are often overlooked. A partially subsidized lunch for staff goes a long way toward improving morale, for example. Implementing "to the table" service provides an opportunity for residents in assisted living to see, smell, and select menu items, thereby increasing resident satisfaction and caloric intake. The presence of a concierge not only provides additional social service but also by strengthening person-to-person relationships, improves the staff's ability to see and sense when something is wrong or someone is ill.

Employee relationships can benefit from a department of "people and culture" rather than human resources, in which increased ethnic diversity, cultural differences, and communication techniques are recognized and utilized rather than ignored.

CONCLUSION: *Innovations do not have to be expensive, only sensible.*

Specific Issues

Evidence of many specific issues can be drawn from each site evaluation; as space allowed, these issues were dis-

cussed within each chapter. A few, however, transcend site specificity and can be recognized, if not as simple common sense, as a product of experience and examination of environment:

- Building and care provision regulations should not be viewed as standards to meet, but as starting points on which to build. Innovation can take the form of creatively working within restrictive regulations to provide environments that improve the lives of residents, staff, and families.
- Simply because it looks good or is expensive to construct does not mean it works well. Putting a derivative façade on an atrium space will not automatically make that space relate to the intended residents. Know the target market and design to it.
- Pay very close attention to details, both aesthetic and functional. They will make the difference between successful innovation and crude experiment.
- Collaborate. Seek out, listen to, and respect the opinions and suggestions of everyone you can. Some suggestions that seem unusual may have amazing results.
- Don't stop refining your ideas. Even when the construction is complete, there can be small, easy-to-implement changes that will have profound results.
- Thoughtful and effective environments empower staff in the fulfillment of their jobs. Empowerment of staff improves the quality of care provided to residents.

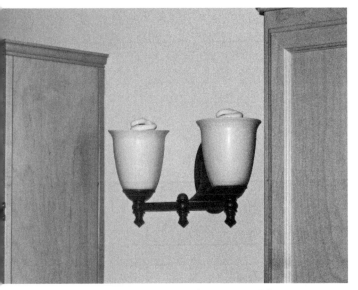

FIG. CONC-6   Selection of furnishings and fixtures requires forethought on the part of both designer and operator. The incandescent light fixture is attractive, but the decision to use low-energy fluorescent bulbs was an afterthought   *Photograph by Jeffrey Anderzhon*

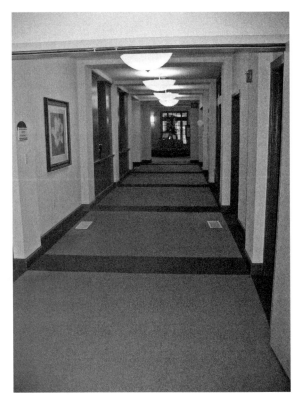

FIG. CONC-7   Collaboration with all parties involved is important to the successful outcome of the design. The HVAC grilles in the floor of this assisted living corridor create a tripping hazard for residents who have difficulty with ambulation   *Photograph by Jeffrey Anderzhon*

- Training is critical to staff understanding of how the environment should function. Orientation within that environment should be ongoing if the desired result is higher-functioning staff who will use the environment as it was intended.
- Meals and food service are paramount to resident happiness. The delivery of the dining experience, from the wait to be seated all the way through to dessert and coffee, will reverberate throughout the building, campus, and community.
- Consider the future and how residents will age in place, what they will want to be doing, and how they will perceive their community.

And most importantly:

- Buildings age along with residents. Successful designs withstand years of changes and challenges. Expect that environments must adapt, adjusting their form and function as needs change. Flexible designs will help keep pace with the physical and mental changes in resident populations and the unique demands of future generations.

Next Steps

Although not a comprehensive research document, this book does provide an important first step in recognizing the importance of studying the interaction of the built environment with older adults, care programs created for them, and the staff which implement those programs. As we continue to increase the quantity of an individual's life, we must also continue to increase the quality of that life. By studying what within our environments contributes to improving quality of life, we can build a foundation on which our society's elders can maintain their dignity as well as their health.

It is hoped that this book of post-occupancy evaluations will encourage increased attention on evidence-based design of environments for the older adults from both the design and care professions. The real next steps are to continue and to refine the process for the greater good, a move that is enthusiastically supported by the American Institute of Architects. For many gathering this knowledge and sharing these lessons learned will undoubtedly lead to improved quality of life and enhanced quality of the workplace.

Appendix 1

PROJECT COST UPDATE AND ESTIMATE

AUTHOR'S NOTE: *This table provides a cost comparison for all evaluation sites updated to December 2006 and equalized for the single geographic location of Baltimore, MD.*

Project Name	Type	City[1]	State	Cost				Estimated		Equalized All in	
				GSF	Date	Total Building Cost[2]	Cost GSF	Cost 12/2006	Cost GSF	Baltimore	December 2006
Parkview at Asbury	ILU	Washington	DC	155,200	10/1/2005	$23,280,743	$150.00	$24,549,543	$158.18	$23,322,066	$150.27
Hallmark	ILU	Chicago	IL	481,180	6/1/1990	$34,747,000	$72.21	$61,335,404	$127.47	$51,521,740	$107.07
Avalon Square	CCRC	Milwaukee	WI	188,810	8/1/2003	$16,084,152	$85.19	$19,783,507	$104.78	$18,398,661	$97.45
Bishop Gadsden	CCRC	Charleston	SC	446,025	4/1/1999	$42,250,000	$94.73	$69,906,850	$156.73	$79,693,809	$178.68
The Jefferson	CCRC	Washington	DC	713,959	6/1/1992	$54,000,000	$75.63	$89,348,400	$125.15	$84,880,980	$118.89
La Vida Real	CCRC	San Diego	CA	353,220	8/1/2003	$40,057,246	$113.41	$49,270,413	$139.49	$42,865,259	$121.36
McKeen Towers	CCRC	W Palm Beach	FL	166,184	1/1/1998	$20,000,000	$120.35	$30,428,000	$183.10	$31,340,840	$188.59
Dominican Center	AL	Grand Rapids	MI	80,190	6/30/2005	$13,556,000	$169.05	$14,847,887	$185.16	$14,996,366	$187.01
Rosewood Estate	AL	Minneapolis	MN	60,663	1/1/1989	$5,000,000	$82.42	$9,027,500	$148.81	$8,124,750	$133.93
Stark Villa	AL	Los Angeles	CA	63,000	10/1/2001	$10,000,000	$158.73	$13,108,000	$208.06	$10,879,640	$172.69
Sunrise of La Jolla	AL	San Diego	CA	39,794	5/1/2003	$8,028,000	$201.74	$9,935,453	$249.67	$8,643,844	$217.21
Cuthbertson Village	AL-Dementia	Charlotte	NC	34,000	5/1/2003	$3,510,660	$103.25	$4,344,793	$127.79	$4,822,720	$141.84
Freedom House	AL-Dementia	San Antonio	TX	45,312	7/1/1998	$6,883,779	$151.92	$10,237,556	$225.93	$11,261,312	$248.53
Forest at Duke	AL-Dementia	Durham	NC	79,346	6/1/2001	$10,579,365	$133.33	$14,006,021	$176.52	$16,387,045	$206.53
Waveny Village	AL-Dementia	Stamford	CT	64,630	9/1/2001	$11,257,838	$174.19	$14,806,309	$229.09	$12,585,362	$194.73
Woodside Place	AL-Dementia	Pittsburgh	PA	23,398	6/1/1991	$2,500,000	$106.85	$4,261,250	$182.12	$4,133,413	$176.66
Abramson Center	NF	Philadelphia	PA	396,850	6/1/2002	$62,115,000	$156.52	$79,587,950	$200.55	$70,037,396	$176.48
The Green Houses™	NF	Tupelo	MS	24,160	8/15/2003	$2,355,313	$97.49	$2,897,035	$119.91	$3,331,590	$137.90
Colo State Veterans Home	NF	Denver	CO	125,000	7/1/2002	$20,459,086	$163.67	$26,130,345	$209.04	$24,823,827	$198.59
Foulkeways	NF	Philadelphia	PA	52,223	8/1/2001	$8,585,429	$164.40	$11,291,556	$216.22	$9,936,569	$190.27
Cody Day Care	Day Care	Denver	CO	49,200	1/1/2004	$5,951,000	$120.96	$7,187,023	$146.08	$6,827,672	$138.77

[1] Costs are provided for nearest major city to project.
[2] Total building costs do not include soft costs.

Appendix 2

Listing of Project Owners and Architects

Independent Living Apartments

Chapter 1—Parkview at Asbury Methodist Village
Owner: Asbury Methodist Village, Inc.
211 Russell Avenue
Gaithersburg, MD 20877
www.asbury.org

Architect: Cochran, Stephenson & Donkervoet, Inc.
The Warehouse at Camden Yards
323 West Camden Street, Suite 700
Baltimore, MD 21201
www.csdarch.com

Chapter 2—The Hallmark
Owner: Brookdale Senior Living, Inc.
330 North Wabash, Suite 1400
Chicago, IL 60611
www.brookdaleliving.com

Architect: John Macsai and Associates (acquired by OWP&P)
111 West Washington Street
Chicago, IL 60602
www.owpp.com

Continuing Care Retirement Communities

Chapter 3—Avalon Square
Owner: Presbyterian Homes of Wisconsin
222 Park Place
Waukesha, WI 53186
www.avalonsquare.com

Architect: KKE Architects, Inc.
300 First Avenue North
Minneapolis, MN 55401
www.kke.com

Chapter 4—Bishop Gadsden Episcopal Retirement Community
Owner: The Episcopal Church Home
1 Bishop Gadsden Way
Charleston, SC 29412
www.bishopgadsden.org

Architect: Cochran, Stephenson & Donkervoet, Inc.
The Warehouse at Camden Yards
323 West Camden Street, Suite 700
Baltimore, MD 21201
www.csdarch.com

Chapter 5—The Jefferson
Owner: Sunrise® Senior Living
7902 Westpark Drive
McLean, VI 22102
http://www.sunriseseniorliving.com

Architect: Cochran, Stephenson & Donkervoet, Inc.
The Warehouse at Camden Yards
323 West Camden Street, Suite 700
Baltimore, MD 21201
www.csdarch.com

Chapter 6—La Vida Real
Owner: Senior Resource Group
500 Stevens Avenue, Suite 100
Solana Beach, CA 92075
www.srgseniorliving.com

Architect: Mithun
Pier 56, 1201 Alaskan Way, Suite 200
Seattle, WA 98101
www.mithun.com

Chapter 7—McKeen Towers
Owner: Carmelite Sisters for the Aged and Infirm
St. Teresa's Motherhouse
600 Woods Road
Germantown, NY 12526
www.carmelitesisters.com
www.noreenmckeenresidence.org

Architect: O'Keefe Architects, Inc.
2424 Curlew Road
Palm Harbor, FL 34683
www.okeefearch.com

Assisted Living

Chapter 8—Dominican Center at Marywood
Owner: Sisters of the Order of St. Dominic of Grand Rapids
2025 East Fulton
Grand Rapids, MI 49503
www.grdominicans.org

Architect: Perkins Eastman Architects, PC
351 West Hubbard Street, Suite 708
Chicago, IL 60610
www.perkinseastman.com

Chapter 9—Rosewood Estate of Roseville
Owner: Care Institute, Inc.
10401 North Meridian Street, Suite 122
Indianapolis, IN 46290
No owner web address
Managed by Sunrise® Senior Living
www.sunriseseniorliving.com

Architect: Arvid Elness Architects, Inc.
No contact information for architect

Chapter 10—The Fran and Ray Stark Villa
Owner: Motion Picture and Television Fund
23388 Mulholland Drive
Woodland Hills, CA 91364
www.mptvfund.org

Architect: SmithGroup
225 Bush Street, 11th Floor
San Francisco, CA 94104
www.smithgroup.com

Chapter 11—Sunrise of La Jolla
Owner: Sunrise® Senior Living
7902 Westpark Drive
McLean, VI 22102
www.sunriseseniorliving.com

Architect: Mithun
Pier 56, 1201 Alaskan Way, Suite 200
Seattle, WA 98101
www.mithun.com

Assisted Living for Those with Dementia

Chapter 12—Cuthbertson Village at Aldersgate
Owner: Aldersgate United Methodist Retirement, Inc.
3800 Shamrock Drive
Charlotte, NC 28215
www.aldersgateccrc.com

Architect: Freeman White, Inc.
8025 Arrowridge Boulevard
Charlotte, NC 28273
www.freemanwhite.com

Chapter 13—Freedom House at Air Force Village
Owner: Air Force Village Alzheimer Care and Research
    Center
Air Force Villages
5100 John D. Ryan Boulevard
San Antonio, TX 78245
www.airforcevillages.com

Architect: Rehler Vaughn & Koone, Inc.
745 East Mulberry, Suite 601
San Antonio, TX 78212
www.rvk-architects.com

Chapter 14—The Forest at Duke
Owner: The Forest at Duke, Inc.
2701 Pickett Road
Durham, NC 27705
www.forestduke.com

Architect: Calloway Johnson Moore & West, P.A.
119 Brookstown Avenue, Suite 100
Winston-Salem, NC 27101
www.cjmw.com

Chapter 15—The Village at Waveny Care Center
Owner: Waveny Care Center Network, Inc.
3 Farm Road
New Canaan, CT 06840
www.waveny.org

Architect: Reese, Lower, Patrick & Scott, Ltd.
1910 Harrington Drive
Lancaster, PA 17601
www.rlps.com

Chapter 16—Woodside Place of Oakmont
Owner: Presbyterian SeniorCare
1215 Hulton Road
Oakmont, PA 15139
www.srcare.org

Architect: Perkins Eastman Architects, PC
115 Fifth Avenue, Third Floor
New York, NY 10003
www.perkinseastman.com

Nursing Care

Chapter 17—Abramson Center for Jewish Life
Owner: Abramson Center for Jewish Life
1425 Horsham Road
Horsham, PA 19044
www.abramsoncenter.org

Architect: EwingCole
Federal Reserve Bank Building
100 North 6th Street
Philadelphia, PA 19106
www.ewingcole.com

Chapter 18—The Green Houses™ at Traceway
Owner: Mississippi Methodist Senior Services, Inc.
109 South Broadway
Post Office Box 1567
Tupelo, MS 38802-1567
www.mississippimethodist.org

Architect: The McCarty Company-Design Group, P.A.
533 West Main Street
Tupelo, MS 38804

Chapter 19—The Colorado State Veterans Home at Fitzsimons
Owner: State of Colorado, Department of Human Services
1575 Sherman Street
Denver, CO 80203
www.cdhs.state.co.us

Architect: Boulder Associates
1426 Pearl Street, Suite 300
Boulder, CO 80302
www.boulderassociates.com

Chapter 20—Foulkeways at Gwynedd
Owner: Foulkeways at Gwynedd, Inc.
1120 Meetinghouse Road
Gwynedd, PA 19436
www.foulkeways.org

Architect: Reese, Lower, Patrick & Scott, Ltd.
1910 Harrington Drive
Lancaster, PA 17601
www.rlps.com

Community-Based Services

Chapter 21—Cody Day Center
Owner: Total Longterm Care, Inc.
200 East 9th Avenue
Denver, CO 80203
www.totallongtermcare.org

Architect: Boulder Associates
1426 Pearl Street, Suite 300
Boulder, CO 80302
www.boulderassociates.com

Scandinavian Comparisons

Chapter 22—Tempe Health and Welfare Centre
Owner: Trondheim Kommune, Norway
N-7004 Trondheim
Norway
www.trondheim.kommune.no

Architect: HRTBAS Arkitekter MNAL
St. Olavs gt. 28, 0166
Oslo, Norway
www.hrtb.no

Chapter 23—Swedish Elderly Homes
Klockåreängen
Owner: Ale Kommun, Sweden
Alafors, Sweden
www.ale.se

Architect: Unknown
Hedegården
Owner: Lerum Kommun, Sweden
443 80 Lerum
Sweden
www.lerum.se

Architect: Nils Andréasson Arkitektkontor AB
Göteborgsvägen 23
443 30 Lerum
Sweden

Riddarstensgården
Owner: Lerum Kommun, Sweden
443 80 Lerum
Sweden
www.lerum.se

Architect: Porten Arkitekter
Gothenburg
Sweden

Index

Abramson Center for Jewish Life, 199–211
Accessibility:
   for aging in place, 14
   Bishop Gadsden, 39, 41
   Cody Day Center, 251, 253, 255, 256
   Colorado Veterans Home, 225, 226, 228, 231
   The Hallmark, 16, 18–19
   Klockåreängen, 276
   Rosewood Estate, 106
Acoustics, 77
Activities of daily living (ADLs), 263
ADLs (activities of daily living), 263
Adult day care:
   Cody Day Center, 249–258
   The Village at Waveny Care Center, 176, 178
   Woodside Place, 188
Advocates, 292
Affinity groups, design for:
   Abramson Center, 199–211
   Colorado Veterans Home, 229
   Dominican Center, 89–90
   Fran and Ray Stark Villa, 115, 117
Aging in place:
   Abramson Center, 202, 204
   Bishop Gadsden, 39, 42–44
   Fran and Ray Stark Villa, 114–116
   The Hallmark, 14, 15, 19
   The Jefferson, 54
   McKeen Towers, 78
   Parkview, 9–10
   Tempe Health and Welfare Centre, 261–271
Aging of buildings, 294
AIA, See American Institute of Architects
Air Force Village Alzheimer Care and Research Center, 147
Aldersgate United Methodist Retirement, Inc., 135
Ale Kommun, Sweden, 274
Alzheimer's care, see Dementia care
American Institute of Architects (AIA), viii, xii, 294
Architects, list of, 297–299
Arvid Elness Architects, Inc., 99
Asbury Methodist Village, Inc., 3, 4
Assisted living, xi–xii
   Abramson Center, 199–211
   Dominican Center, 87–97
   Fran and Ray Stark Villa, 111–121
   Rosewood Estate, 99–109

   Sunrise of La Jolla, 123–132
   Tempe Health and Welfare Centre, 263, 265–266
Assisted living for dementia:
   Cuthbertson Village, 135–145
   The Forest at Duke, 159–171
   Freedom House, 147–157
   The Village at Waveny Care Center, 173–183
   Woodside Place, 185–196
Avalon Square, 25–35

Baby boomers, expectations of, xii
Balconies:
   Abramson Center, 203
   La Vida Real, 66, 68
   McKeen Towers, 80
   Riddarstensgården, 287
   Sunrise of La Jolla, 129, 130
   Tempe Health and Welfare Centre, 267
Bathrooms:
   Abramson Center, 202, 205
   Cody Day Center, 253
   Colorado Veterans Home, 225, 226, 228, 230
   Cuthbertson Village, 138, 140
   Forest at Duke, 166
   Foulkeways at Gwynedd, 243
   Green Houses, 216
   The Hallmark, 16
   La Vida Real, 66
   Parkview, 9
   Tempe Health and Welfare Centre, 266
   The Village at Waveny Care Center, 178, 179
   Woodside Place, 193
Bedrooms:
   Abramson Center, 205
   Colorado Veterans Home, 225–226
   Dominican Center, 90–91, 93–94
   Foulkeways at Gwynedd, 240, 241, 243
   Green Houses, 216
   Hedegården, 279, 281
   private vs. shared, viii
   Riddarstensgården, 287
   Tempe Health and Welfare Centre, 265–266
   The Village at Waveny Care Center, 177–179
Bishop Gadsden Episcopal Retirement Community, 37–47
Boulder Associates, 223, 249

Boundary disputes, 251, 254
Brookdale Living Communities, Inc., 13, 15

Calloway Johnson Moore & West, P.A., 159
Care Institute, Inc., 99
Carmelite Sisters for the Aged and Inform, 73
CCRCs, see Continuing care retirement communities
Champion, 291–292
Child day care:
   Cody Day Center, 251–255
   Freedom House, 149
Circulation:
   Bishop Gadsden, 41
   Cody Day Center, 254
   Dominican Center, 95
   Forest at Duke, 161–164, 167
   Fran and Ray Stark Villa, 115, 117
   Freedom House, 150
   La Vida Real, 63–64
   McKeen Towers, 77, 80–81
   Woodside Place, 188–190
Clock towers, viii
Closets:
   Forest at Duke, 165
   Foulkeways at Gwynedd, 240, 243
Cluster environments:
   Abramson Center, 201–205
   Colorado Veterans Home, 225, 227–228
   Dominican Center, 89, 92–93
   Freedom House, 148–150, 153
   Green Houses, 214
   McKeen Towers, 75
   Riddarstensgården, 284, 285
   Rosewood Estate, 100–106
   Tempe Health and Welfare Centre, 263, 265
   Woodside Place, 188–191
Cochran, Stephenson & Donkervoet, Inc., 3, 37, 49
Cody Day Center, 249–258
Collaboration, 293
The Colorado State Veterans Home at Fitzsimons, 223–235
Common spaces, see Gathering and common spaces
Communication:
   Avalon Square, 32
   barriers to, vii
   Hedegården, 281

Community:
    creating, *see* Creating community
    integration with, 30
Conceptual research, vii
Concierges, 78–79, 81, 293
Connection to outdoor environment:
    Abramson Center, 202–204
    Cody Day Center, 251–255
    Cuthbertson Village, 137, 139
    Dominican Center, 94–95
    Foulkeways at Gwynedd, 239, 242, 244
    Fran and Ray Stark Villa, 114
    The Jefferson, 50, 52
    The Village at Waveny Care Center, 176, 178
    Woodside Place, 188, 190
Construction costs, 296
    Abramson Center, 210
    Avalon Square, 34–35
    Bishop Gadsden, 47
    Cody Day Center, 258
    Colorado Veterans Home, 234
    Cuthbertson Village, 145
    Dominican Center, 97
    Forest at Duke, 171
    Foulkeways at Gwynedd, 246
    Fran and Ray Stark Villa, 121
    Freedom House, 156–157
    Green Houses, 221
    The Hallmark, 22
    The Jefferson, 58
    La Vida Real, 71
    McKeen Towers, 83
    Parkview, 11
    Rosewood Estate, 103, 106, 109
    Sunrise of La Jolla, 132
    The Village at Waveny Care Center, 183
    Woodside Place, 196
Continuing care retirement communities
    (CCRCs):
    Asbury Methodist Village, 4
    Avalon Square, 25–35
    Bishop Gadsden, 37–47
    current trend in, 30
    The Jefferson, 49–58
    La Vida Real, 61–71
    McKeen Towers, 73–83
Corridors:
    Abramson Center, 205
    Bishop Gadsden, 43, 44
    Colorado Veterans Home, 227, 229
    Cuthbertson Village, 139
    Dominican Center, 91
    Foulkeways at Gwynedd, 239–240
    Hedegården, 279, 280
    Klockåreängen, 277
    La Vida Real, 64, 67
    McKeen Towers, 76
    Parkview, 9
    Riddarstensgården, 284
    Rosewood Estate, 103, 104
    Tempe Health and Welfare Centre, 265
    Woodside Place, 191
Cost control:
    Colorado Veterans Home, 225, 227

Green Houses, 215, 217
La Vida Real, 65
Woodside Place, 194
Cost of care, 103, 106
Cost of construction, *see* Construction costs
Courtyards:
    Abramson Center, 203, 206
    Bishop Gadsden, 40–42, 44
    Colorado Veterans Home, 231–232
    Cuthbertson Village, 137, 139
    Forest at Duke, 167
    Freedom House, 154
    Green Houses, 219
    Klockåreängen, 276
    La Vida Real, 63–65, 68
    Sunrise of La Jolla, 129
    The Village at Waveny Care Center, 177, 180
Creating community:
    Abramson Center, 205
    Avalon Square, 30–31
    Bishop Gadsden, 42–43
    Cody Day Center, 255–256
    Colorado Veterans Home, 229–230
    Cuthbertson Village, 140
    Dominican Center, 93
    Forest at Duke, 165
    Foulkeways at Gwynedd, 239, 242
    Fran and Ray Stark Villa, 114–117
    Freedom House, 153
    Green Houses, 216, 217
    The Hallmark, 17–18
    Hedegården, 280
    The Jefferson, 52–53
    Klockåreängen, 275
    La Vida Real, 65–66
    McKeen Towers, 78
    Riddarstensgården, 285–286
    Rosewood Estate, 106–107
    Sunrise of La Jolla, 126–127
    Tempe Health and Welfare Centre, 267
    The Village at Waveny Care Center, 178
    Woodside Place, 192–193
Cues:
    Abramson Center, 205, 206
    Freedom House, 154
    The Village at Waveny Care Center, 177
    Woodside Place, 189, 192
Cultural design, *see* Regional and cultural
    design
Culture:
    institutional, xi
    The Jefferson, 54
    Sunrise of La Jolla, 128
Culture change, xi–xii
    documenting, xii
    Foulkeways at Gwynedd, 242
    Woodside Place, 195
Cuthbertson Village at Aldersgate, 135–145

Decentralization:
    Colorado Veterans Home, 225, 227–228
    Dominican Center, 95
    Foulkeways at Gwynedd, 239–241, 243
    Fran and Ray Stark Villa, 114–115

Green Houses, 214
Rosewood Estate, 100
Tempe Health and Welfare Centre, 263–265
Decision making:
    allowing time for, 292
    knowledge base for, vii
Defined areas, 175–177
Dementia care. *See also* Assisted living for dementia
    Colorado Veterans Home, 226–227
    Fran and Ray Stark Villa, 118
    Green Houses, 213–221
    Riddarstensgården, 287
    Sunrise of La Jolla, 129, 130
Design:
    evidence-based, vii, 294
    research and, vii
    for sensory and mobility loss, 76, 77
    success factors in, 291–294
Design for Aging Knowledge Community (AIA), xii
Design for Aging Review (AIA), viii, xii, xiii
Details, 293
Dining, 294. *See also* Food preparation and service
Dominican Center at Marywood, 87–97
Doors, 94
Drainage, 251, 254
Dutch doors, 192

Eden Alternative, 136–137, 139
Elevators:
    The Hallmark, 14, 15, 20
    McKeen Towers, 77
    and needs for aging in place, 14, 15
    Parkview, 9
    The Village at Waveny Care Center, 177
Employee relationships, 293. *See also* Workplace quality
Engaged wandering, 188–190
Entries:
    Avalon Square, 29
    Cody Day Center, 250
    Colorado Veterans Home, 224, 225
    Cuthbertson Village, 137–138
    Freedom House, 151, 152
    The Hallmark, 16–17
    The Jefferson, 52
    La Vida Real, 63, 64
    McKeen Towers, 78, 79
    Parkview, 6
    Rosewood Estate, 100, 104
    Sunrise of La Jolla, 126, 127
    The Village at Waveny Care Center, 174, 176–177
    Woodside Place, 191, 193–194
Environment:
    home-like, *see* Home-like environment
    integrating programs and, 188
    outdoor, *see* Outdoor environment
Environmental therapy:
    Abramson Center, 206
    Avalon Square, 31
    Bishop Gadsden, 43–44

Colorado Veterans Home, 230–231
Cuthbertson Village, 141, 143
Dominican Center, 94–95
Forest at Duke, 167
Foulkeways at Gwynedd, 241, 244
Fran and Ray Stark Villa, 118
Freedom House, 154
Green Houses, 218
The Hallmark, 19
Hedegården, 281–282
The Jefferson, 54
Klockåreängen, 276
La Vida Real, 67
McKeen Towers, 79
Riddarstensgården, 287
Rosewood Estate, 107
Sunrise of La Jolla, 128–129
Tempe Health and Welfare Centre, 268
The Village at Waveny Care Center,
    179–180
Woodside Place, 193–194
European showers, 179, 239, 240, 243
Evidence-based design, vii, 291–292, 294
EwingCole, 199
Exterior-interior design relationship:
    Cody Day Center, 251
    Dominican Center, 91
    Sunrise of La Jolla, 125, 126
    The Village at Waveny Care Center, 176

Fireplaces, 166
Flexible designs, 294
    Abramson Center, 202, 204, 205
    Foulkeways at Gwynedd, 240–242
    Woodside Place, 190
Food preparation and service:
    Abramson Center, 202, 204, 205
    Avalon Square, 32
    Bishop Gadsden, 42
    Colorado Veterans Home, 225, 228–230
    Cuthbertson Village, 143
    Forest at Duke, 162–165
    Foulkeways at Gwynedd, 239, 241
    Fran and Ray Stark Villa, 114, 118, 119
    Freedom House, 150
    Green Houses, 215, 218, 219
    The Jefferson, 53
    Klockåreängen, 276
    La Vida Real, 66, 69
    McKeen Towers, 81
    Parkview, 7–8
    resident happiness and, 294
    Sunrise of La Jolla, 127
    Tempe Health and Welfare Centre, 264,
        266–267
    Woodside Place, 190, 191, 193
The Forest at Duke, 159–171
Foulkeways at Gwynedd, 237–246
The Fran and Ray Stark Villa, 111–121
Freedom House at Air Force Village, 147–157
Freeman White, Inc., 135
Furniture and furnishings:
    Colorado Veterans Home, 226
    Dominican Center, 92
    Forest at Duke, 166

Freedom House, 150
Hedegården, 280
Riddarstensgården, 285, 287
Rosewood Estate, 104
Tempe Health and Welfare Centre, 266
Future marketability, 89–91

Gardens, see Outdoor environment
Gathering and common spaces, viii. See also
    Creating community
    Abramson Center, 201, 202, 204
    artificial feeling of, viii
    Avalon Square, 31
    Bishop Gadsden, 38, 40, 42–43
    Colorado Veterans Home, 227–230
    Cuthbertson Village, 136–143
    Dominican Center, 90, 91, 93
    Forest at Duke, 165, 166
    Foulkeways at Gwynedd, 239
    Fran and Ray Stark Villa, 114
    Freedom House, 150, 152, 153
    Green Houses, 216
    The Hallmark, 18
    Hedegården, 280, 282
    The Jefferson, 52
    La Vida Real, 66
    Main Street, 139, 141, 143, 165–167,
        174–176, 178–181
    McKeen Towers, 76, 80
    Parkview, 6–7
    Rosewood Estate, 100, 101, 104, 106
    Sunrise of La Jolla, 127–129
    Tempe Health and Welfare Centre, 264
    Town Square/town center, 26, 27, 63, 64,
        137–139, 160, 201, 203, 205, 206
    The Village at Waveny Care Center,
        176–178, 180
    Woodside Place, 188–193
Green building practices, 89, 92
The Green Houses(tm) at Traceway,
    213–221

The Hallmark, 13–22
Hallways, see Corridors
Health and well-being, see Quality of life
Hearth, 215
Hedegården, 278–283
Historic sites, 27, 28
Holistic living environments:
    Cuthbertson Village, 136, 137, 139
    Forest at Duke, 160
Home-like environment:
    Abramson Center, 205–206
    Avalon Square, 31
    Bishop Gadsden, 43
    Colorado Veterans Home, 230
    Cuthbertson Village, 140–142
    Dominican Center, 93–94
    Forest at Duke, 165–167
    Foulkeways at Gwynedd, 242–243
    Fran and Ray Stark Villa, 114, 116–118
    Freedom House, 149, 150, 153–154
    Green Houses, 215–218
    The Hallmark, 18–19
    Hedegården, 281

The Jefferson, 52
Klockåreängen, 276
La Vida Real, 66
McKeen Towers, 78–79
Riddarstensgården, 286
Rosewood Estate, 102–105, 107
Sunrise of La Jolla, 125–128
Tempe Health and Welfare Centre,
    263–265, 267
The Village at Waveny Care Center,
    176–179
Woodside Place, 189–191, 193
Hospice:
    Dominican Center, 94
    Tempe Health and Welfare Centre, 263
Hospital Survey and Construction Act of
    1946, xi
Housekeeping services:
    Abramson Center, 204
    Foulkeways at Gwynedd, 241, 243
    McKeen Towers, 81
    Parkview, 8–9
HRTB AS Arkitekter MNAL, 261

Image, regional, see Regional and cultural
    design
Incontinence, 154, 193
Independence:
    Colorado Veterans Home, 225, 227–228
    Fran and Ray Stark Villa, 114–116
    Freedom House, 154
    Rosewood Estate, 102–103, 106
    Woodside Place, 190
Independent living apartments:
    The Hallmark, 13–22
    Parkview, 3–11
Innovative design:
    Dominican Center, 89, 91
    Freedom House, 149
    Green Houses, 219
    successful accomplishment of, 292
Innovative leadership, 293
Instrumental research, vii
Integration of new and existing construction,
    27–29
Interactive communities, 137, 139
Intergenerational programs, 201–202

The Jefferson, 49–58
John Macsai & Associates, 13

Kitchens, see Food preparation and service
KKE Architects, Inc., 25
Klockåreängen, 274–278

Landscaping, see Outdoor environment
La Vida Real, 61–71
LEED criteria, 92
Lerum Kommun, Sweden, 278, 283
Life expectancy, xi
Lifestyle(s). See also Quality of life
    Foulkeways at Gwynedd, 238–239
    historic changes in, xi
    The Jefferson, 53, 55
    McKeen Towers, 77–79

Light and lighting:
  Abramson Center, 203, 204
  Cody Day Center, 251, 254–255
  Cuthbertson Village, 140
  Dominican Center, 90, 94–95
  Forest at Duke, 163, 164, 166, 167
  Fran and Ray Stark Villa, 119
  Green Houses, 216
  Hedegården, 280
  McKeen Towers, 77
  Rosewood Estate, 104
  Sunrise of La Jolla, 127
  The Village at Waveny Care Center, 175
  Woodside Place, 188, 190, 194
Lobbies:
  McKeen Towers, 77
  Parkview, 6

The McCarty Company-Design Group, P.A., 213
McKeen Towers, 73–83
Main Street:
  Cuthbertson Village, 139, 141, 143
  Forest at Duke, 165–167
  The Village at Waveny Care Center, 174–176, 178–181
Management philosophy, traditional, xi
Marketability, future, 89–91
Materials use:
  Cody Day Center, 253
  Dominican Center, 90, 91
  Forest at Duke, 166
  Foulkeways at Gwynedd, 239–240
  Hedegården, 281, 282
  The Jefferson, 50
  Rosewood Estate, 104
  Sunrise of La Jolla, 125
  Tempe Health and Welfare Centre, 267, 268
  The Village at Waveny Care Center, 176, 180
  Woodside Place, 194
Maximizing limited sites:
  at The Hallmark, 16–17
  The Jefferson, 50–52
  Sunrise of La Jolla, 124
Medicaid, cost of private vs. shared rooms under, viii
Medical model of service, xi
Medical model units, viii
Medicare, growth of nursing home industry and, xi
Memory boxes, 151–152
Memory care, see Dementia care
Mississippi Methodist Senior Services, Inc., 213
Mithun, 61, 123
Mixed-use development:
  Avalon Square, 26–28
  The Jefferson, 52
  Sunrise of La Jolla, 125–126
Mobility:
  Bishop Gadsden, 42
  Freedom House, 150–152
  McKeen Towers, 76, 77

Motion Picture and Television Fund, 111
Multilevel adult day care, 252, 255

Neighborhood(s):
  Abramson Center, 203
  Cuthbertson Village, 139
  Forest at Duke, 160, 162–166
  integration of facility and, 89–90, 100
  setting tone for, 50, 52
  Tempe Health and Welfare Centre, 264
  transitions from, 125, 126
Neighborhood-based services, 263–267
Nils Andréasson Arkitektkontor AB, 278
Norway, Tempe Health and Welfare Centre, 261–271
Nurses' stations, 203
Nursing home industry, xi

O'Keefe Architects, Inc., 73
Operation of facilities:
  Abramson Center, 207–208
  Avalon Square, 32
  Bishop Gadsden, 39, 42, 44
  Cody Day Center, 256
  Colorado Veterans Home, 232
  Cuthbertson Village, 143
  Dominican Center, 93, 95
  Forest at Duke, 168
  Foulkeways at Gwynedd, 244
  Fran and Ray Stark Villa, 119–120
  Freedom House, 155
  Green Houses, 219
  The Hallmark, 20–21
  Hedegården, 282
  The Jefferson, 55
  Klockåreängen, 277
  La Vida Real, 69
  McKeen Towers, 81
  Parkview, 10
  Riddarstensgården, 288
  Rosewood Estate, 108
  Sunrise of La Jolla, 130–131
  Tempe Health and Welfare Centre, 269
  The Village at Waveny Care Center, 181
  Woodside Place, 194–195
Orientation. See also Wayfinding
  Abramson Center, 206
  Forest at Duke, 167
  Fran and Ray Stark Villa, 119
  La Vida Real, 63, 64
  McKeen Towers, 77
  Rosewood Estate, 100
Outdoor environment. See also Environmental therapy
  Abramson Center, 206–207
  Avalon Square, 32
  Bishop Gadsden, 44
  Cody Day Center, 256
  Colorado Veterans Home, 231–232
  connection to, see Connection to outdoor environment
  Cuthbertson Village, 143
  Forest at Duke, 167
  Foulkeways at Gwynedd, 244
  Fran and Ray Stark Villa, 119

Freedom House, 151, 154
Green Houses, 216–217, 219
The Hallmark, 19–20
Hedegården, 282
The Jefferson, 54
Klockåreängen, 275, 276
La Vida Real, 63, 65, 66, 68
McKeen Towers, 76, 79–80
Riddarstensgården, 287
Rosewood Estate, 100, 107
Sunrise of La Jolla, 129–130
Tempe Health and Welfare Centre, 268
The Village at Waveny Care Center, 180
Woodside Place, 192–194
Owners, list of, 297–299

Parking:
  Abramson Center, 210
  Avalon Square, 34
  Bishop Gadsden, 43, 46
  Cody Day Center, 254, 257
  Colorado Veterans Home, 234
  Cuthbertson Village, 144
  Dominican Center, 97
  Forest at Duke, 171
  Foulkeways at Gwynedd, 245
  Fran and Ray Stark Villa, 121
  Freedom House, 156
  Green Houses, 220
  The Hallmark, 22
  The Jefferson, 51, 52, 58
  La Vida Real, 69, 71
  McKeen Towers, 76, 78, 83
  Parkview, 6, 9, 11
  Rosewood Estate, 104, 109
  Sunrise of La Jolla, 130, 132
  The Village at Waveny Care Center, 182
  Woodside Place, 196
Parkview at Asbury Methodist Village, 3–11
Patios:
  Cody Day Center, 253
  La Vida Real, 66, 68
  Sunrise of La Jolla, 129
Perkins Eastman Architects, P.C., 87, 185
Personalization:
  Abramson Center, 205
  Foulkeways at Gwynedd, 243
  Fran and Ray Stark Villa, 116–118
  Freedom House, 151–152
  Woodside Place, 189, 192, 193
Pets, 137
Physical plant:
  Abramson Center, 207
  Avalon Square, 32
  Bishop Gadsden, 44
  Cody Day Center, 256
  Colorado Veterans Home, 232
  Cuthbertson Village, 143
  Dominican Center, 92, 95
  Forest at Duke, 167–168
  Foulkeways at Gwynedd, 244
  Fran and Ray Stark Villa, 119
  Freedom House, 154–155
  Green Houses, 219
  The Hallmark, 20

Hedegården, 282
The Jefferson, 54–55
Klockåreängen, 276–277
La Vida Real, 68–69
McKeen Towers, 80–81
Parkview, 8–9
Riddarstensgården, 287
Rosewood Estate, 107, 108
Sunrise of La Jolla, 130
Tempe Health and Welfare Centre,
    268–269
The Village at Waveny Care Center, 181
Woodside Place, 194
POEs, see Post-occupancy evaluations
Porches:
Bishop Gadsden, 43
Forest at Duke, 163
Freedom House, 154
Porten Arkitekter, 283
Post-occupancy evaluations (POEs), vii–viii,
    xii
evaluation criteria in, xii–xiii
evaluation team for, xiii
site selection for, xii
value of, xiii–xiv
Presbyterian Homes of Wisconsin, 25
Presbyterian SeniorCare, 185
Privacy:
Abramson Center, 205, 206
Colorado Veterans Home, 225–226, 228
Foulkeways at Gwynedd, 240, 241
Freedom House, 153
Green Houses, 215, 216
Sunrise of La Jolla, 128
Private care providers, 15
Private rooms:
cost of shared rooms vs., viii
Cuthbertson Village, 140
Green Houses, 215, 216
Rosewood Estate, 106, 107
Programs:
Abramson Center, 201–202
Cody Day Center, 256
Forest at Duke, 167
Freedom House, 152, 154
Hedegården, 280
integrating environment into, 188, 190
The Jefferson, 53, 54
Tempe Health and Welfare Centre, 267
The Village at Waveny Care Center, 180
Woodside Place, 193
Project areas:
Abramson Center, 209–210
Avalon Square, 33–34
Bishop Gadsden, 45–46
Cody Day Center, 257
Colorado Veterans Home, 233
Cuthbertson Village, 144
Dominican Center, 96
Forest at Duke, 169–170
Foulkeways at Gwynedd, 245
Fran and Ray Stark Villa, 120
Freedom House, 156
Green Houses, 220
The Hallmark, 22

Hedegården, 283
The Jefferson, 56–57
Klockåreängen, 278
La Vida Real, 70–71
McKeen Towers, 82
Parkview, 11
Riddarstensgården, 289
Rosewood Estate, 109
Sunrise of La Jolla, 131–132
Tempe Health and Welfare Centre,
    270–271
The Village at Waveny Care Center, 182
Woodside Place, 195
Public spaces, see Gathering and common
    spaces

Quality of life, 294
Abramson Center, 204
Avalon Square, 31
Forest at Duke, 161, 163–164
Green Houses, 218
McKeen Towers, 76
Rosewood Estate, 107
The Village at Waveny Care Center, 174,
    179, 181
Quality within a budget, 63, 65

Reese, Lower, Patrick & Scott, Ltd., 173,
    237
Refinements, 293
Regional and cultural design:
Abramson Center, 206
Avalon Square, 31
Bishop Gadsden, 38, 40–41, 43
Colorado Veterans Home, 230
Cuthbertson Village, 141
Forest at Duke, 167
Foulkeways at Gwynedd, 243
Fran and Ray Stark Villa, 118
Freedom House, 154
Green Houses, 218
The Hallmark, 19
Hedegården, 281
The Jefferson, 52–54
Klockåreängen, 276
La Vida Real, 63–64, 67
McKeen Towers, 76, 77, 79
Riddarstensgården, 286–287
Rosewood Estate, 107
Sunrise of La Jolla, 128
Tempe Health and Welfare Centre,
    267–268
The Village at Waveny Care Center, 179
Regulations:
Cody Day Center, 251, 254
exemption from, 88, 89
Green Houses, 215, 217
surpassing, 293
Rehler Vaughn & Koone, Inc., 147
Research, vii, viii, 150, 152
Resident-centered care, xii
Residential environment, see Home-like
    environment
Retail spaces:
Avalon Square, 27, 30

The Hallmark, 18
The Jefferson, 52
Riddarstensgården, 283–289
Roof garden, 16, 20, 32
Rooftop patios, 54
Rosewood Estate of Roseville, 99–109
Rural facility, Klockåreängen, 274–278

Safety and security:
McKeen Towers, 79, 80
Woodside Place, 194
Seidel, Andrew, vii
Semi-private rooms:
Colorado Veterans Home, 225–226,
    228
privacy issues with, viii, 153
Senior Resource Group, 61
Sensory loss, 76, 77
Separating levels of care areas:
Avalon Square, 27, 28, 30–31
Bishop Gadsden, 39, 41
Forest at Duke, 161–163
The Jefferson, 50, 52
La Vida Real, 65–66
McKeen Towers, 76, 77
Sheltered housing, 263, 265
Showers:
Abramson Center, 204–205
Cody Day Center, 253
European, 179, 239, 240, 243
Woodside Place, 193, 194
Sisters of the Order of St. Dominic of Grand
    Rapids, 87
Site context sensitivity:
Avalon Square, 27, 29
Bishop Gadsden, 39, 42
Dominican Center, 89, 90
Freedom House, 150, 152–153
Green Houses, 215–217
McKeen Towers, 76, 77
Skilled nursing facilities:
Abramson Center, 199–211
Colorado Veterans Home, 223–235
Foulkeways at Gwynedd, 237–246
Green Houses at Traceway, 213–221
Hedegården, 278–283
Klockåreängen, 274–278
Riddarstensgården, 283–289
Small sites, see Maximizing limited sites
Small town facilities:
Cuthbertson Village, 135–145
Green Houses at Traceway, 213–221
The Village at Waveny Care Center,
    173–183
SmithGroup, 111
Snoezelen, 129
Social interaction. See also Gathering and
    common spaces
Abramson Center, 202, 203
Bishop Gadsden, 43
Cuthbertson Village, 140
Dominican Center, 93
Fran and Ray Stark Villa, 114–117
Freedom House, 150, 152
Green Houses, 217

Social interaction (cont'd)
  Hedegården, 281
  La Vida Real, 66
  Riddarstensgården, 285
  Rosewood Estate, 102, 105–106
  The Village at Waveny Care Center, 175, 176, 179
Social Security Act of 1935, xi
Spas:
  Cuthbertson Village, 140, 141
  Forest at Duke, 166
  Foulkeways at Gwynedd, 243
Space sharing, Cody Day Center, 252, 255
Special care needs. See also Environmental therapy
  Bishop Gadsden, 40, 42, 44
  Forest at Duke, 160
  Fran and Ray Stark Villa, 117
  The Jefferson, 53
Staff. See also Workplace quality
  employee relationships, 293
  empowerment of, 293
  honoring, 189–190, 192
  Rosewood Estate, 104
  training for, 294
Staff/resident ratio:
  Colorado Veterans Home, 225, 227
  McKeen Towers, 75, 76
  Tempe Health and Welfare Centre, 266
  Woodside Place, 194
State of Colorado, Department of Human Services, 223
Suburban facilities:
  Abramson Center, 199–211
  Bishop Gadsden, 37–47
  Dominican Center, 87–97
  The Forest at Duke, 159–171
  Foulkeways at Gwynedd, 237–246
  Fran and Ray Stark Villa, 111–121
  Freedom House, 147–157
  Hedegården, 278–283
  La Vida Real, 61–71
  Parkview, 3–11
  Riddarstensgården, 283–289
  Rosewood Estate, 99–109
  Woodside Place, 185–196
Success factors, 291–292
Sundowning, 179
Sunrise of La Jolla, 123–132
Sunrise(r) Senior Living, 49, 123

Swedish elderly homes, 273–274
  Hedegården, 278–283
  Klockåreängen, 274–278
  Riddarstensgården, 283–289

Target market, designing to, 293
Technology, 55
Tempe Health and Welfare Centre, 261–271
Therapeutic activities, see Environmental therapy
Toilets, 193
Total Longterm Care, Inc., 249
Town centers, viii
  Avalon Square, 26, 27
  Forest at Duke, 160
  La Vida Real, 63, 64
Town Square:
  Abramson Center, 201, 203, 205, 206
  Cuthbertson Village, 137–139
Training, 130, 294
Transition between spaces:
  Forest at Duke, 164
  Rosewood Estate, 100, 103, 106
  The Village at Waveny Care Center, 175–177
  Woodside Place, 189, 191
Trondheim Kommune, Norway, 261

Universal design:
  Colorado Veterans Home, 226–229
  Parkview, 9
Universal worker concept (Green Houses), 215–219
Urban facilities:
  Avalon Square, 25–35
  Colorado Veterans Home, 223–235
  The Hallmark, 13–22
  The Jefferson, 49–58
  McKeen Towers, 73–83
  Sunrise of La Jolla, 123–132
  Tempe Health and Welfare Centre, 261–271
Urban revitalization, 27, 28

Views:
  Abramson Center, 203
  Avalon Square, 29
  Foulkeways at Gwynedd, 242
  The Hallmark, 15–17

The Jefferson, 54
McKeen Towers, 75–77
The The Village at Waveny Care Center, 173–183
Vision (for facility), 89, 292

Walkways:
  Colorado Veterans Home, 231
  Freedom House, 154
  McKeen Towers, 80
  Woodside Place, 194
Water closets, 226
Waveny Care Center Network, Inc., 173
Wayfinding. See also Orientation
  Cuthbertson Village, 137–140
  Forest at Duke, 167
  Freedom House, 151
  La Vida Real, 64, 68
  McKeen Towers, 77
  Woodside Place, 189
Welcoming environment, 251, 253
Well-being, see Quality of life
Woodside Place of Oakmont, 185–196
Workplace quality:
  Abramson Center, 207
  Avalon Square, 32
  Bishop Gadsden, 44
  Cody Day Center, 251, 253–256
  Colorado Veterans Home, 232
  Cuthbertson Village, 143
  Dominican Center, 93, 95
  Forest at Duke, 167–168
  Foulkeways at Gwynedd, 244
  Fran and Ray Stark Villa, 119
  Freedom House, 154–155
  Green Houses, 219
  The Hallmark, 20
  Hedegården, 282
  The Jefferson, 54, 55
  Klockåreängen, 275–277
  La Vida Real, 68–69
  McKeen Towers, 80–81
  Riddarstensgården, 287–288
  Rosewood Estate, 107–108
  Sunrise of La Jolla, 130
  Tempe Health and Welfare Centre, 268–269
  The Village at Waveny Care Center, 180–181
  Woodside Place, 189–190, 192, 194